THE CHANGING FACE OF HEALTH CARE

A Horizon in Bioethics Series Book from

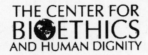

THE CENTER FOR
BIOETHICS
AND HUMAN DIGNITY

The Horizons in Bioethics Series brings together an array of insightful writers to address important bioethical issues from a forward-looking Christian perspective. The introductory volume, *Bioethics and the Future of Medicine*, covers a broad range of topics and foundational matters. Subsequent volumes focus on a particular set of issues, beginning with the end-of-life theme of *Dignity and Dying* and continuing with the genetics focus of *Genetic Ethics*.

The series is a project of The Center for Bioethics and Human Dignity, an international center located just north of Chicago, Illinois, in the United States of America. The Center endeavors to bring Christian perspectives to bear on today's many pressing bioethical challenges. It pursues this task by developing two book series, four audio tape series, four video tape series, numerous conferences in different parts of the world, and a variety of other printed and computer based resources. Through its membership program, the Center networks and provides resources for people interested in bioethical matters all over the world. Members receive the Center's international journal, *Ethics and Medicine*, the Center's newsletter, *Dignity*, the Center's Update Letters, special World Wide Web access, an Internet News Service and Discussion Forum, and discounts on most bioethics resources in print.

For more information on membership in the Center or its various resources, including present or future books in the Horizons in Bioethics Series, contact the Center at:

The Center for Bioethics and Human Dignity
2065 Half Day Road
Bannockburn, IL 60015 USA
Phone: (847) 317-8180
Fax: (847) 317-8153

Information and ordering is also available through the Center's World Wide Web site on the Internet: http://www.bioethix.org

The Changing Face
of
Health Care

A CHRISTIAN APPRAISAL OF
MANAGED CARE,
RESOURCE ALLOCATION,
and
PATIENT-CAREGIVER RELATIONSHIPS

Edited by

John F. Kilner
Robert D. Orr
Judith Allen Shelly

William B. Eerdmans Publishing Company
Grand Rapids, Michigan / Cambridge, U.K.

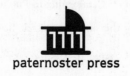

paternoster press

© 1998 The editors and contributors

Published jointly 1998 in the United States of America by
Wm. B. Eerdmans Publishing Co.
255 Jefferson Ave. S.E., Grand Rapids, Michigan 49503 /
P.O. Box 163, Cambridge CB3 9PU U.K.
and in the U.K. by
Paternoster Press
P.O. Box 300, Carlisle, Cumbria CA3 0QS

Printed in the United States of America

03 02 01 00 99 98   7 6 5 4 3 2 1

Library of Congress Cataloging-in-Publication Data

The changing face of health care: a Christian appraisal of managed care,
resource allocation, and patient-caregiver relationships /
edited by John F. Kilner, Robert D. Orr, and Judy Allen Shelly.
p.   cm.   — (Horizons in bioethics series)
ISBN 0-8028-4533-9 (pbk.: alk. paper)
1. Managed care plans (Medical care) — Moral and ethical aspects.
2. Christian ethics.   I. Kilner, John Frederic.
II. Orr, Robert D. (Robert David), 1941-   . II. Shelly, Judy Allen.
IV. Center for Bioethics and Human Dignity.   V. Series.
RA413.C465   1998
362.1'04258 — dc21   98-22481
                                                                    CIP

British Library Cataloguing-in-Publication Data

A catalogue record for this book is available from the British Library.

ISBN 0-85364-864-6

Contents

CONTENTS

ECONOMIC ENCROACHMENT

SELECTED SETTINGS

Contents

Contributors

Mary B. Adam, M.D., Staff Pediatrician, Thomas Davis Medical Center, Tucson, AZ, USA

William K. Atkinson, Ph.D., President and Chief Executive Officer, New Hanover Regional Medical Center, Wilmington, NC, USA

Patricia Benner, R.N., Ph.D., Professor, Department of Physiological Nursing, School of Nursing at the Univ. of California, San Francisco, CA, USA

Harold O. J. Brown, Ph.D., Franklin Forman Chair of Christian Ethics and Theology, Trinity Evangelical Divinity School, Deerfield, IL, USA

Nigel M. de S. Cameron, Ph.D., Distinguished Professor of Theology and Culture, Trinity International University, Deerfield, IL, USA

Scott E. Daniels, Ph.D., Senior Executive, Virginia Department of Health, Richmond, VA, USA

Arthur J. Dyck, Ph.D., Saltonstall Professor of Ethics, Harvard University, Cambridge/Boston, MA, USA

Alieta Eck, M.D., Private Practice Family Medicine Physician, Somerset, NJ, USA

Stephen P. Greggo, Psy.D., Assistant Professor of Counseling Psychology, Trinity International University, Deerfield, IL, USA

J. Stuart Horner, M.D., F.R.C.P., Professor in Medical Ethics at the Centre for Professional Ethics, University of Central Lancashire, Preston, U.K.

CONTRIBUTORS

James M. Hussey, M.B.A., Chief Executive Officer, Physicians Quality Care, Ltd., Chicago, IL, USA

John F. Kilner, M.Div., Ph.D., Director, The Center for Bioethics and Human Dignity, Bannockburn, IL, USA

Janet E. Michael, R.N., J.D., Private Practice Health Care Attorney in Maine, Massachusetts, and New Hampshire, USA

Richard W. Olson, M.A., Vice President of Finance, Covenant Retirement Communities, Chicago, IL, USA

Dónal P. O'Mathúna, Ph.D., Assistant Professor, Chemistry and Medical Ethics, Mount Carmel College of Nursing, Columbus, OH, USA

Robert D. Orr, M.D., Director of Clinical Ethics, Loma Linda University Medical Center, Loma Linda, CA, USA

Edmund D. Pellegrino, M.D., Director, Center for Clinical Bioethics, Georgetown University Medical Center, Washington, DC, USA

Gregory W. Rutecki, M.D., Professor of Medicine, Northeastern Ohio University's College of Medicine, Canton, OH, USA

David L. Schiedermayer, M.D., Clinical Professor, Medical College of Wisconsin, Milwaukee, WI, USA

Judith Allen Shelly, R.N., D.Min., Editor, *Journal of Christian Nursing*, Frederick, PA, USA

Barbara C. Staggers, M.D., M.P.H., Director of the Division of Adolescent Medicine, Children's Hospital Medical Center of Northern California, California, USA

Frank E. Staggers, Sr., M.D., Physician, Alameda County Medical Center, California, USA; and AMA Committee on Minority Physicians

Sondra Ely Wheeler, Ph.D., Martha Ashby Carr Associate Professor of Christian Ethics, Wesley Theological Seminary, Washington, DC, USA

Barbara J. White, R.N., Assistant Professor of Nursing, Regis University, Denver, Colorado, USA

Kenman L. Wong, Ph.D., Professor, School of Business Economics, Seattle Pacific University, Seattle, WA, USA

Preface

The face of health care is changing everywhere. While the particularly rapid change in the United States receives special attention in this book, the lessons being learned there are useful worldwide. The concluding chapter here tells the international story from the vantage point of Great Britain.

Far more than technological advancement is occurring today. The medico-legal climate is changing, the mechanisms of health care delivery are changing, health care financing is changing. Much has been written on these issues in the recent past. Many authors have addressed these changes from a purely economic perspective. Some have looked beyond economics to take a professional approach. In discussing professionalism, many writers have addressed the altruistic nature of health care and the fact that society expects the patient-caregiver relationship to be fiduciary in nature, i.e., a trusting relationship wherein the professional who has more knowledge, skill, and authority is expected to use his or her skills for the benefit of the patient. Relatively few who have addressed these changes have moved beyond mere economics and professionalism to look at these issues from a specifically Christian viewpoint. We have gathered a group of Christian leaders in health care to do just that.

For too long good health care in the United States has been available only to those who could afford to pay their own way, or at least could obtain good health insurance. It did not start out that way. Most American hospitals and nursing homes began as a gift of grace, growing out of the benevolence of the churches. Medical practice included a great deal of charity work, and nursing was a sacred calling from God. Gradually, the churches sold their birthright to the government. As government funding grew, its control expanded and Christian influence eroded. More recently, private industry entered the picture, and the bottom line became a controlling factor, leaving many Christian health care professionals asking, *How can we serve both God and mammon* (cf. Matt. 6:24, Luke 16:13)?

Managed care appeared on the scene as the result of numerous conflicting forces. One element has been the profit drive of business. Too many people, Christians included, merely recognize the danger in this and recoil. We neglect to see that other significant reasons for the advent of managed care include our insufficient concern to conserve health care resources and our unwillingness to share the good gifts that God has given us. We have not been doing our job of caring for the sick, the poor, and the marginalized members of our society. The present turmoil in health care may well be the Lord's way of shaking us out of our complacency to say, "I was hungry and you gave me no food, I was thirsty and you gave me nothing to drink, I was a stranger and you did not welcome me, naked and you did not give me clothing, sick and in prison and you did not visit me. . . . Truly I tell you, just as you did not do it to one of the least of these, you did not do it to me" (Matt. 25:42, 45). The task at hand is not merely to moan about the problems, but to understand and engage them constructively.

It is tempting to be high-minded and assert that altruistic health care professionals should not be concerned about payment for their services, especially if they are practicing their profession as a vocation, a divine calling. This would be both simplistic and unrealistic. In addition to the need to provide financially for oneself and one's family, the rapidly rising cost of education has guaranteed that most young health care professionals can look forward to years of debt repayment. The challenge is to balance the need to serve with the need to survive (by earning a living, in order to serve). While this deduction from biblical principles seems fairly straightforward, the modern industry of health care is very complex. This complexity, combined with our natural tendency to self-interest, has generated new issues and questions.

This book is an honest attempt to grapple with the often-conflicting matters involved in the changing face of health care. We do not have all the answers. In fact, all of the authors do not agree with one another regarding which are the most important problems. But we are trying faithfully to raise the questions and explore some of the potential solutions to the challenges we face. We come from many perspectives, both professionally and theologically, and we have tried to listen carefully to one another and learn from each other. We have organized our effort into six parts.

The book begins by reflecting on the experiences of some of those most intimately involved with the changing face of health care. Physician David Schiedermayer speaks from the perspective of one caught in the middle of patient needs and systemic constraints. Patient Harold Brown shares his personal struggles with a system too cost conscious to treat him well. Nurse Barbara White speaks for many nurses who, with physicians, are wrestling with the tension between economic stewardship and faithfulness to patients. And administrator William Atkinson sees that failing to conserve resources aggressively, where appropriate, means having inadequate resources to meet important health care needs.

With the current situation squarely in view, the next section of the book endeavors to set the stage for further analysis by clarifying essential foundational issues. Nigel Cameron begins with a theological reflection on what the practice of medicine is all about. Judith Shelly extends that reflection to the practice of nursing. Both authors mine the theological and professional traditions for insights to enable health care professionals cope with the profound changes taking place today. Recognizing that much of the contemporary challenge has to do with distributing resources, the other two authors of this section take up the dictates of justice. Sondra Wheeler suggests that justice entails more than many people think, and Arthur Dyck explains why one thing that justice does *not* entail is health care rationing (which he distinguishes from certain forms of health care allocation).

The third section explores the ethical concerns that arise when health care personnel are constrained to pay increasing attention to economic considerations, as opposed simply to pursuing the well-being of their patients. Scott Daniels opens with an overview of the ways that financial incentives are at work in contemporary health care, primarily in managed care. He paves the way for the chapters that follow by introducing competing perspectives on the incentives that are operative today. Proponents of one such perspective are worried about the shift from health care as a profession to health care as a business, with its new economic incentives. Physician Edmund Pellegrino and nurse Patricia Benner raise this concern, buttressed by Gregory Rutecki's examination of the tensions inherent in the physician-as-gatekeeper model. Kenman Wong promotes a very different perspective — one that sees a more community-oriented business ethics as a partner with a more individualistic health care ethics in the task of crafting economic guidelines for the practice of health care. The section concludes with an analysis of professional oath-taking — a telling indicator of the shifts examined in the previous chapters.

Section four provides an opportunity to examine more concretely the changing face of health care in selected settings not explicitly addressed in previous chapters. Stephen Greggo and Richard Olson discuss mental health care and long-term care, respectively. Frank and Barbara Staggers examine what minority communities must contend with as health care delivery changes. The section concludes with Janet Michael's explanation of how the movement toward managed care is creating new legal malpractice issues for health care professionals and organizations.

To this point the book has majored on understanding the nature of the challenge today and assessing it ethically, while minoring on how best to respond constructively to the challenge. In the fifth section the emphasis shifts to a primary focus on constructive engagement. James Hussey begins by highlighting two effective models for meeting the needs of poor persons as the health care system changes. Alieta Eck then looks at some of the creative initiatives that the Church can take. How far should health care professionals themselves go to ensure that changes do not proceed too far in a wrong direction? Mary Adam explores the possibility of physician unions in order to help answer that question. Dónal O'Mathúna completes the section by probing the response of an increasing number of people today to the current predicament: turning to so-called "alternative" or "complementary" forms of health care.

The book closes with a glossary of terms to assist readers with a whole new vocabulary that has developed along with new approaches to health care. But before the glossary, a concluding chapter provides a valuable overview of the international and longer-term significance of this book. Non-U.S. readers will appreciate this explicit bridge from the U.S. scene to other settings. U.S. readers will better understand the importance and impact of changes today by reading this concluding chapter. Change is always occurring to some degree, but not often does it have as intimate an impact on so many people as does today's changing face of health care.

John F. Kilner, Ph.D.
Robert D. Orr, M.D.
Judith Allen Shelly, R.N., D.Min.

INTRODUCTION

A Physician's Experience

David L. Schiedermayer, M.D.

Managed care will succeed if it facilitates communication between patients and their caregivers. Managed care will fail if it cannot improve on the existing communication between doctor and nurse and patient. Because of the additional hassle and bureaucratic parsimony, managed care must be both "high-tech" and "high-touch." A low-tech, low-touch system which interferes with an already tenuous communication link will fail.

I admit that the baseline sitation is already troubled. Communication problems are common in fee-for-service medicine. I remember a Wisconsin farmer who at age 72 was severely bow-legged, had hypertension, and had a detached retina. Eye surgery was scheduled, but the question was whether he should have a scleral buckle, a band around the eye to approximate the retinal edges, or have air bubbles injected to push the retinal edges together.

He didn't have running water in the house. He lived alone and had to make all his own meals. If he had the bubbles injected he'd have to lie face down for several days, an impossibility for this particular patient. A few minutes spent listening to his life situation demonstrated that he needed the buckle. But he told me he hadn't had any guidance on this decision. His eye doctor knew the diagnosis — but not the patient.

Unfortunately, there seems to be a wide variation in the individual physician's ability to listen to patients. Some apparently successful modern physicians would have failed miserably in the past; they don't seem to know how to talk to people. Without their chosen technological procedures they would be therapeutically useless. They lack the common

3

touch; they do not know how to be helpfully present or how to use the power of words.

There is another group of modern physicians, however, who would have been fine doctors years ago, and can now employ their technical skills for the added benefit of the patient. They are talking doctors, even if their specialty involves only a tiny part of the anatomy. They treat their patients like people.

My point is that both kinds of doctors can emerge from our educational system with the means to diagnose illness and intervene in disease. Both kinds can establish practices, perform surgery, and teach students and housestaff. Both kinds can be found in managed care. But only those who are sensitive to the patient's meanings within the discourse of medicine, who try to provide respectful treatment, and who talk to patients, will be successful in their encounters with patients in the sorts of human ways that have always mattered.

If we agree that this kind of treatment has always mattered in the doctor-patient relationship, and moreover that it is the doctor's ethical responsibility to provide this kind of treatment, then we have already accepted the underlying premise that in managed care, the ways physicians use language and communicate really matters. According to Bill Clements,[1] good communication could save $210 for each unneeded emergency visit avoided, $85-115 for each unneeded specialty referral, and $20 for each unneeded office visit. Moreover, only a third of patients fill the prescriptions their doctors give them, and only half of those actually take the medication properly. Good communication will get patients to take their medications, get better faster, sue less often, and recommend the doctor to their friends. Good communication will make managed care or any health care system work better. Perhaps what we need is managed communication, or facilitated communication, rather than managed care.

Whether managed care works is important to all of us, because medicine is actually such an important part of our overall culture:

- Only a stubborn 3 percent of American adults resist going to the allopathic doctor in their lifetimes
- More than 80 percent of the population sees the doctor in a given year
- Patients make more than a billion visits to physicians' offices each

---

1. B. Clements, *American Medical News*, January 22, 29, 1997, p. 18.

4

year, and doctors make still another 400 million visits to patients in hospitals and other facilities

- 20 percent of patients with acute conditions get their medical advice through telephone calls to the doctor; pediatricians average 20 office calls per day and 20 phone calls per day
- In America alone there are more than 527,900 medical practitioners, 1,152,000 nurses, 144,000 pharmacists, 126,000 dentists, 47,300 social workers, 22,000 optometrists, 15,000 physical therapists, 12,000 dieticians, 8,700 podiatrists, 4,200 lay midwives, 5,000 physicians' assistants, 10,000 nurse practitioners, and 18,000 chiropractors
- Medicine is a trillion dollar a year business
- The size of clinic rooms has diminished from 16 feet by 20 feet in 1850 to 8 by 10 feet today, and in big clinics multiple doctors use the same office, decreasing the sense of personalness (diplomas, family pictures, special books, trophies, and knickknacks)
- Photographs of pediatric patients are common, photographs of adult patients exceedingly rare
- The position of desk, chairs, and table may have importance in communication; the doctor's chair is usually an executive swivel and the patient's a straight-backed, fixed chair
- The mean wait in the doctor's office is 27.9 minutes, and a reduction in waiting time signals a more egalitarian relationship or even a shift in relative status (as when the doctor "waits on" a celebrity patient, in the ancient attending-court tradition).[2]

Now how does the discourse of medicine actually work? According to Eliot Mischler,[3] in routine practice, a structural unit of discourse is a sequence of three utterances: physician question — patient response — physician assessment/next question. There are a number of nonlexical utterances, false starts, and repetitions of normal speech. For example:

Doctor: Does drinking make it worse?
Patient: . . . Ho ho uh ooh Yes. . . . Especially the carbonation and the alcohol.
Doctor: . . . Hm hm. . . . How much do you drink?

2. W. Stoeckle, ed., *Encounters Between Patients and Doctors: An Anthology* (Cambridge, Mass.: MIT Press, 1987).

3. E. Mischler, *The Discourse of Medicine: Dialectics of Medical Interviews* (Norwood, N.J.: Ablex Press, 1984).

Through an in-depth analysis of several interviews, Mischler has shown that physicians control the organization and content of interviews. Patient concerns ("the voice of the lifeworld") tend to disrupt the fluent flow of an interview and to be relatively ignored by the doctor. Not only does the physician ask almost all the questions, but these questions are almost always in the "voice of medicine" (quantifying, objectifying) and therefore serve to move the discourse consistently away from topics of the lifeworld.

The author concludes that the discourse of medical interviews is a "dialectic between the voices of the lifeworld and of medicine; it involves conflict and struggle between two different domains of meaning. . . . It is as if a poem in one language that uses qualities of the weather, such as its dampness or coldness, as a metaphor for the feeling state of the narrator were to be translated literally into another language as a description of the weather."

How will managed care respond to this dialectic? I think it is a fascinating question. For example, let us consider the concept of gatekeeping. Gatekeeping limits a patient's unlimited access to specialists or procedures. The gatekeeper's responsibility is

- to be a responsible steward of medical resources
- to use the fewest resources possible
- to authorize only medically necessary diagnostic workups, referrals, medical services, and hospitalizations.

So now the physician's challenge is to use the poetry of the patient, the metaphors of the patient, and translate them both into another language (the doctor's language of the diagnosis) and then to go one step further — to see how this diagnosis fits into the business concepts of authorizations, utilizations, and resource constraints. This is the challenge of managed care; there is a new level of translation, a third language, being superimposed on the process.

Patient's metaphor:

my chest hurts,
maybe it is my heart,
it hurts all day.

Doctor's translation:

this chest pain is atypical,

atypical chest pain is not cardiac,
it is either musculoskeletal or GI pain.

Managed care language:

this patient's symptoms
do not warrant expensive cardiac testing,
only symptomatic measures are authorized.

Eric Cassell argues that "the spoken language is the most important tool in medicine."[4] He encourages students of doctor-patient communication to develop the ability to remember precisely what the patient said and how they said it. I always encourage my residents to repeat exactly what the patient said, and I find it fascinating to hear that they don't repeat it exactly right much of the time. "It is no more complex than the ability to listen with the stethoscope to first one then the other heart sound, or one part of the cardiac cycle at a time," Cassell notes. Careful listening involves listening for paralanguage, word choice, conversational logic, and word meaning in conversation and life context. Careful listening involves listening for the spiritual content in patients' lives as well. How are we to know if we should pray with and for a patient, unless we listen to the patient's story?

Doctors can change the reality of a patient's situation by words, Cassell argues, since language conveys the conception of that reality. For instance, doctors can use pronouns as patients do, to distance the disease and keep the patient in control. I would adapt this to make sure the patient knows that God is in control. Cassell gives this example from his own practice:

> Patient: I want to know exactly where do I stand with this? When can I be up and walking around and go home —
> Doctor: That depends on what happens now. You're — you're obviously, now, gettin' better, gettin' stronger.
> Patient: I see.
> Doctor: Um, a lot of it depends on how you feel about it. A little stronger, then good, fine. 'Cause while I cannot make that liver better, here or at home, I can keep you in control of your situation, so . . .
> Patient: Can you control the liver by medication?

4. E. Cassell, *Talking with Patients*, 2 vols. (Cambridge, Mass.: MIT Press, 1985).

Doctor: Yeah, no — just listen to me. Listen to me carefully. Alright, I cannot make that liver get better, I can't keep it from getting worse. I can only keep YOU on top of things, for as long as that liver holds out for you.

Cassell notes that he did for this patient what language allows a person to do for herself: take the diseased liver and "put it over there" apart from her: "that liver," "it," "the," as distinct from "keep *you* in control," "*you're* getting better," "keep *you* on top of things." "Given an ominous reality," he says, "we can still work in the world of language, in the world of subjectivity, and we can be remarkably effective even after our technical intervention fails." The Christian can go even one step further — pointing out that God is in ultimate control.

Cassell points out that the basic principles of listening and talking can be used in understanding the chief complaint (the story of the illness), the review of systems (asking questions about the body), the history of the present illness (personal history and meaning), and in diagnosis and prognosis (information as a therapeutic tool).

As Marc Lipp writes: "So much of improved function depends upon treasured trifles which cannot all be anticipated or placed on a protocol, e.g., the extra quarter inch on a stump prosthesis that eliminates pelvic tilt, reduces low back pain, and makes ambulation tolerable, or the smuggled aspirin at the hospitalized patient's bedside for self-medication when the overworked nurses can't bring analgesics punctually. Some of the details patients can learn from us, some from other patients, some they can only discover by themselves. What is important is that we help establish an atmosphere in which such exchange of information and such discoveries are facilitated. How do we accomplish that? No one can do it alone, but an empathetic understanding of what it is really like for one human being to suffer from a certain type of affliction is a reasonable point from which to proceed."[5]

Managed care requires another level of translation, because managed care does risk viewing the patient as a commodity. Since people are not foolish, they can tell they are being treated like a piece of meat rather than a person. As William Hurt's character says in the movie *The Doctor*, as he fires his rude radiation therapist, "Someday you will be a patient too. We all get to be patients sometime. When I was a doctor like you I

---

5. M. Lipp, *Respectful Treatment: A Practical Handbook of Patient Care*, 2nd ed. (New York: Elsevier, 1986).

hated patients like me too." Interestingly, Hurt chooses a religious doctor — a devout Jew — to be his surgeon, because he knows he can trust this person. Trust counts, because today, managed care plans are increasingly structured as for-profit rather than not-for-profit corporate entities, and they are developing in an unregulated marketplace. The marketplace rewards efficiency. For example, in California, one nurse recounted the following case: "After complex cardiac surgery, the patients used to be allowed to awaken from anaesthesia naturally. Now they are given a drug used to immediately reverse the effects of anaesthesia right after the surgery so that they spend 8 hours instead of 36 hours in the ICU. . . . We used to keep patients very sedated for a day or so, and in our experience this led to better outcomes . . . they simply get less pain meds now. It is cheaper. And the patients don't even know what is happening, they just think that surgery hurts a whole lot. But we know the difference, how the bottom line has dramatically affected the most basic aspects of care we provide."[6]

In light of all these changes, physicians and nurses need to recognize their personal vulnerability and their individual and clinical limitations, and they need to maintain a sense of high morale. In short, they need to respect themselves as well as the patient. What I personally fear most about managed care is that it will diminish the sense of professionalism and morale of medicine and surgery and nursing. Then we will be unable to hear even our own language above the language of strict business. I really don't think that is what our patients want.

Solutions? We need to preserve the language of medicine during this time of change. It is the essence of our work. I hope managed care does a proper self-assessment too. I suspect that if it doesn't, it will go the way of previous health care initiatives, and be subsumed by the government or by insurance companies. I don't call it a fad, but I really believe it is a phase. The passing of this phase will be even more certain if managed care takes itself too seriously and doesn't take the patient seriously enough; if it fails to remember that managed care executives will be patients too.

---

6. L. Zoloth-Dorfman, "Just Managing: Ethical Obligations in the Managed Health Care Marketplace," in J. C. McCloskey and H. K. Grace, eds., *Current Issues in Nursing*, 5th ed. (St. Louis: Mosby, 1997), pp. 679-85.

A Patient's Experience

Harold O. J. Brown, Ph.D.

As the son of a medical specialist and the grandson of a country doctor, I have always had a kind of filial respect for the medical profession, and a willingness to obey "doctor's orders." I also developed a dislike for hypochondriacs and malingerers. Among my father's many excellent diagnostic skills there was one rather disturbing feature: When it came to diagnosing members of his own family, he inevitably tended to suspect the worst. For example, once when I bloodied the nail on a big toe with running shoes that were too tight, he looked at the blackened nail and suggested that I consult the staff oncologist at the hospital where he worked to be sure that there was no malignancy under the nail. During my childhood, these apprehensions proved universally unfounded. Although my father regularly predicted his own early death, saying that he would not live to see me graduate from college, he lived to be almost 83, by which time I had been out for 25 years.

As a result of this experience, when I had troublesome but not particularly painful symptoms, I tended *not* to suspect the worst, and was ready to listen to soothing statements from medical experts. The expression, "You're getting older," played a role in what happened to me between 1993 and the present.

The Introduction of Managed Care

In 1987, following my return to the United States from service in an Evangelical-Reformed parish in Switzerland, I moved to rural McHenry County in Illinois, and there enjoyed the care of a local general practi-

10

tioner. However, a few years later, in 1992, Trinity Evangelical Divinity School decided to change from its old-fashioned employee medical insurance system to a more modern HMO type of program. The new insurers offered three different levels of service, and for a variety of reasons my wife and I chose the fullest and most expensive level. As a result of this change in insurers, we were forced to designate a primary care physician. Since our general practitioner in McHenry was not part of the program, we elected to return to the family physician who had been our family doctor before we went to Switzerland, who was and is in the HMO plan.

For the first time I was in a program that covered full-scale, regular annual check-ups and began to take advantage of that. It is bizarre that the difficulties arose only after I began to get intensive check-ups. One small incident sticks in my mind. Noticing some small keratoses on my skin, I asked my primary care physician to refer me to a dermatologist — indeed to the one who had removed such blemishes in previous years. He demurred, stating that the care would be cosmetic rather than medically necessary, and that the insurers would object to his referring patients for such a banality. This seemed reasonable, but it should have alerted me to the fact that my doctor was reluctant to use up too much of his credit with the insurance companies.

In 1993 I experienced some persistent sinus congestion and, upon complaining, was finally referred early in 1994 to a local in-network hospital for a CAT scan. The results of the scan were reported back to my doctor, who told me that I probably had sinusitis and prescribed an antibiotic and from time to time antihistamines. The sinus condition was never very painful, but persisted. It would frequently wake me up at night with the sensation of being unable to breathe through the nostrils. I also complained of some strange facial sensations, such as the feeling that my nose was running, although it was not, and a wandering, intermittent sensation of anesthesia on the left side of my face. None of these symptoms was severe, but they were puzzling. Remembering a bit of anatomy, I asked if it were possible that the trigeminal nerve was damaged, perhaps by a dental procedure. The physician demurred. Facial neuralgia, he said, would be quite painful, and this was not. He suggested the possibility of a temporary obstruction of one of the carotid arteries, but since the symptoms were mild and intermittent, he did not order further testing.

On one occasion in May of 1995, having had sinus symptoms for two years, I experienced double vision, but it quickly disappeared. It recurred again — I remember the day well, for it was our wedding anni-

11

versary — but the double vision lasted for only an hour or two. In August, driving together with two students to Wyoming for a climbing expedition, I noticed a tendency in my left eye to be distracted by lights in the side mirror. Again double vision occurred. Two days later, while climbing to Disappointment Peak in the Tetons, I had considerable vision difficulties in the left eye, and in fact could see only lights and blurred shapes.

Because it was hot and I had been sweating profusely and was plagued by insects, I thought that perhaps a bug had flown into the eye. I do remember praying, as I lay down in my tent, that I might not be going blind. The next day we prepared for an ascent up Mt. Owen. I covered the troublesome eye with a sweatband and attempted to carry on with one eye functioning. I did not realize how disorienting this was. At least we were doing nothing very daring or dangerous. We climbed a snowy slope on Disappointment Peak, and after a time decided to descend to our campsite at Amphitheater Lake and try again the next day. Four of my fellow-climbers preceded me in a sitting glissade down the icy slope. To start the glissade, we had to jump a gap of about two feet over a crevasse about ten feet deep — no problem for an experienced mountaineer. But for some reason I felt extremely unsure of myself and refused to jump, instead walking around the end of the crevasse.

My own attempt to perform the glissade ended in a disaster. For no evident reason I suddenly veered off to the right, tipped over, lost my ice-axe in a failed attempt at a self arrest, and slid 300 feet down the steep, icy slope, striking numerous rocks with my left side and left shoulder before my trusted teaching assistant caught me. We rolled a few more feet entangled together, and then I wound up on my back on the snow. It was apparent that I was seriously injured. My companions summoned help, and I was transported by a rescue helicopter to St. John's Hospital in Jackson. My injuries were said not to be life threatening, but this was an incomplete diagnosis, for I had a punctured lung with hemothorax. By the time the nurses identified this and put me in intensive care, I had lost a liter and a half of blood. After that, my recovery was slow but unexceptional. When it came time to discharge me from the hospital, I was unable to secure air transportation, because President Clinton with his entire entourage was vacationing in the area and all flights were fully booked by press and hangers-on. The attending physician, a Christian and former army doctor, then took me into his home for four days until I could get a flight. This was an unusual experience of personal, Hippocratic care!

Back in Illinois, I consulted my primary care physician, who found no special problems; I did ask him about the facial anesthesia, which continued to puzzle him. When I was sufficiently recovered, I went to my local ophthalmologist — an eye surgeon of some repute — to see about the now frequent double vision. He diagnosed a palsied sixth cranial nerve and prescribed prismatic eyeglasses, which indeed cleared my vision. However, now in addition to the double vision, I noticed some blurred vision in the left eye and consulted him by telephone. He said that this could result from diabetes. Yet, when I consulted the primary care physician — or rather his younger associate — I was told that my recent complete physical excluded diabetes. So the ophthalmologist told me that if the double vision persisted, I could see an associate of his who specialized in double vision. Not one of the several physicians warned me that the palsied nerve could be a sign of a severe problem.

I continued to visit my primary care physician, now seeing only his associate. He diagnosed moderately high blood pressure — in the range of 145-160 over 85-95 — and wanted me to take an anti-hypertensive drug. However, he agreed to let me try exercise and diet for a time instead. A cardiologist who was a student in one of my bioethics courses provided me with some extensive literature on moderate hypertension and suggested that I wait a while before attempting medication. I continued to complain to my primary care physician about the eye, which was becoming ever more troublesome. He referred me to an ophthalmologist in the insurance plan. At this time, the end of 1995, my left eye was still seeing clearly, but was now consistently swinging out to the left, causing double vision. The second ophthalmologist also suggested the problem was a palsied cranial nerve. When I asked him the reason for it, he suggested that I had had it for some time, but as I became older, I was less able to compensate for it. In other words, "You're getting older, after all." He also told me, "You don't need one of those thousand-dollar workups."

As the spring wore on, I had ongoing problems with my vision, and told the primary care doctor, whose attention was fixated on my blood pressure, that I wanted to see an eye specialist. He advised me that I could do so on my own, and suggested that the facial symptoms and the new symptom that felt like water in the left ear could be caused by what he called high blood pressure. For a time, I did receive a prescription for hypertension. Two days before my departure to teach in France during July, I finally consulted my ophthalmologist in McHenry. He became concerned, diagnosed optic neuritis, and referred me to a neurological ophthalmologist and ordered an MRI. He told me that if I could not do both, I should see the specialist. The specialist told me that I did not have optic neuritis, that I had some hemorrhaging in the region of the optic nerve, but that the condition was unlikely to deteriorate rapidly and that I could go to France. This man kept me waiting so long in his office in Skokie that I missed my MRI appointment, which was postponed until my return from France.

On my return from France, I consulted my primary care physician, telling him that I had been advised to get an MRI. He had his receptionist tell me that he would not refer me for anything. Under the circumstances I decided not to plead with him and finally changed primary care physicians.

The True Picture Emerges

A new general practitioner referred me for the MRI, which revealed a "large necrotic mass spread through most of the left sinuses." The Skokie ophthalmologist, on reading the report, said, "This should not be happening." He was under the impression that the tumor had entered the brain, which subsequently proved not to be the case. At this time I saw my medical records for the first time, and saw that the original CAT scan had reported "opefaction in the ethmoid sinus," and "opaque mass in the ethmoid sinus." If I had seen this report early in 1994, when it was fresh, I would certainly have asked for further clarification and would never have let myself be put off with the statement, "You're getting older." I was inclined to trust my physicians, and inasmuch as I had never gotten older before, I could not say that the explanation made no sense.

When I told some of my medical friends about the diagnosis of an extensive tumor, likely to be malignant, they were aghast at the reports and at the situation in which I found myself. They put me in touch with a Christian otolaryngologist in Evanston, who in turn recommended a famous surgeon at Rush-Presbyterian-St. Luke's Medical Center. I consulted Dr. William Panje, who ordered a biopsy. The diagnosis was cancer — adenoid cystic carcinoma, to be specific. Dr. Panje recommended a course of chemotherapy before surgery. During the months of September, October, and November, 1996, I experienced some of the consequences of a heavy course of that strong medicine. In December Dr. Panje performed a nine-hour operation and removed the tumor mass; in the process he was forced to remove the left eye, which by now was sightless.

While in the hospital I was troubled by a racking cough, which prevented me from sleeping, and found it almost impossible to get the resident to prescribe an antitussive. I received some seeding with radioactive cobalt before being discharged.

When I arrived home, I was extremely weak and had a rather troublesome loss of a considerable amount of clear fluid from my right nostril, virtually soaking a towel. I had to be virtually carried up the stairs to my bedroom, although I was able to walk on the level. The post-operative course began well enough, and I seemed to get stronger every day. However, when after twelve days I went back to Rush to have the stitches removed, complications developed. I had been finding it difficult to eat and drink and more or less refused to take nourishment. In addition, I continued to lose a lot of clear fluid through my nostrils and was losing the ability to talk coherently. In the meantime Dr. Panje had gone on vacation, so I frequently called his surgical fellow at Rush for advice. So did my wife, on several occasions, as she felt that I was not describing my situation adequately to the doctor. He told us that this was a normal post-operative phenomenon, and that I should be urged to drink much fluid and to walk and to come in after New Year's Day for an office visit.

By the day after Christmas I had become much weaker and unsteadier. I ate Christmas dinner in my room. More than once my wife found me on the floor, where I had fallen in an attempt to get to the toilet. Two M.D. friends who came to see me found my condition threatening, and called the resident, telling him that they thought that I might have had a stroke. The resident continued to trivialize the problem, telling my wife to wait until January 2 and then to bring me into his office. Finally, he did agree to send a nurse to evaluate me. This was on December 31, but the nurse was never called, because neighbors who came to see me told my wife that my situation was desperate; she must call 911 and get me to a hospital, which she did in mid-morning of December 31.

I was totally incoherent mentally by this time and unaware of what was happening. I was sent to the local medical center, where the emergency room physician took my vital signs, pronounced me all right and wanted to send me home. My wife absolutely refused. If it had not been for her stubbornness and I had gone home, I probably would not have been alive for the office visit January 2. She called our former McHenry general practitioner, who ordered me admitted to the local hospital, the Northern Illinois Medical Center, for 24 hours of observation. He came by himself later in the day, found me rather irrational, and demanded an immediate CAT scan, which revealed an absence of cerebrospinal fluid, air on the brain, and some swelling. Needless to say, he found this situation alarming. He told my wife that she should give some thought

15

to the question of whether to utilize heroic measures if my condition continued to deteriorate.

Northern Illinois considered my condition to be beyond their capacity to treat. Dr. O'Rourke finally succeeded in persuading Rush-Presbyterian to readmit me. I was supposed to be flown in by helicopter, but when the machine arrived, the crew found the fog too heavy to continue, and instead accompanied me in an ambulance to Rush. I was oblivious to all of this and remember only a brief impression of Dr. O'Rourke examining me in my room. I was admitted to intensive care at Rush, where I stayed for a few days and was then transferred to the neurosurgical floor. There I received considerable attention from several neurologists, including Dr. James D'Angelo, who had participated in the December 11 surgery.

One rather amusing thing happened. A young Iranian resident called me one morning and asked, "Do you know Dr. C. Everett Koop?" I told her that we had worked together for some years. She replied, "That's a relief. A man called me, said he was Dr. Koop, and asked about you. I told him everything. Then I was afraid that I had violated medical confidentiality." After that, I received regular visits from several staff physicians, including Dr. Panje's surgical fellow who had minimized the complications and had not wanted me readmitted. I was grateful for the attention, but wondered whether a call from the former U.S. Surgeon General really ought to be necessary for such good care. Finally, 18 days later, I was able to return home, in a much debilitated condition, but clearly on the mend. During late February and March, after I had recovered considerable strength, I received ambulatory radiation therapy, and finally was discharged at the beginning of April.

Since then, apart from the loss of an eye, I seem to be relatively intact. I thank God for my recovery. I am grateful for the brilliant surgical work of Dr. Panje, as well as to Dr. Stephen Yeh, the otolaryngologist who recommended him. However, as I think of the many missed opportunities to diagnose the tumor long before its spread had caused such damage, I certainly find fault with the system that encouraged my physicians to keep the expenses down at the cost of their patient's chances for recovery.

A Nurse's Experience

Barbara J. White, R.N., M.S.

Last Tuesday morning I was talking with my friend and colleague, Sue. After 18 years of critical care experience, Sue recently left her position as nurse manager of critical care services in a large acute care hospital in Denver. "Why did you leave, Sue?" I asked. "You are one of the best nurse managers I know. Your expertise in critical care is outstanding. You're a leader in the field. Your staff respected you."

"I left because I could no longer sleep at night. I had always prided myself in providing the best care possible for patients. And when I became a manager, my goal was to provide my staff with the environment in which they could provide the best care for their patients. But we were forced to drop patient care hours significantly over the last year. Unit secretarial support was no longer present. I couldn't get administration to listen or respond. I had never asked staff to take a patient assignment that I myself couldn't handle. Suddenly, I was asking the nursing staff to do what I knew was unsafe. Ethically, I could no longer do the job, so I had to resign."

Change within the health care industry is placing growing pressure on the more than two million registered nurses in the United States. From staff mix changes, to nursing staff being supplemented with unlicensed aides, to overall restructuring and downsizing in health care, job security and job stability are a thing of the past for working nurses. Health care reform is changing health care financing, care delivery, resource allocation, and patient-caregiver relationships. The focus of reform inevitably addresses the three broad issues of cost, access, and quality. These seemingly simple concepts become complicated when they are intertwined in the complex array of financing arrangements, delivery mechanisms, market forces, professional interests, government structures, and political realities. Transition is difficult. And no one is more acutely aware of the real issues than the nurses themselves. In an attempt to hear their voice and relate their stories, I recently surveyed more than fifty registered nurses, practicing in a variety of settings. I asked them just one question: How have the changes in health care impacted your nursing practice? The nurses' experiences in the changing health care environment speak to high standards, deeply held convictions, realistic frustrations, and intense emotions.

Nurses are struggling to balance care with limited time and resources. Staffing issues are intense. Patient safety issues are the primary concern. Diane, an expert ICU nurse, states: "Last weekend, we were short-staffed and were not able to get pool nurses. The unit was full and the charge nurse requested that we divert any other patients to other facilities. But administration refused and sent us three more patients. One of my patients coded [stopped breathing] and didn't make it. The family is very angry and will probably sue. I will probably lose my job. I feel just terrible. What should I have done?"

Another expert ICU nurse reports: "Our staffing grid is the standard used to staff the unit no matter what the acuity level of patients. It is supposed to keep us within budget. This is fine unless we have open heart surgery patients. The first few hours after surgery, these patients need one-to-one nursing care. Management is strict about using the grid. When we complain about patient safety, we are told, 'It should work. Just triple-up on your other patients.' We staff nurses feel this is very unsafe, especially after 2:00 P.M. when we also have to clean rooms because our environmental service staff has been cut. Patients have extubated themselves, climbed out of bed, and gone into ventricular tachycardia when we nurses are cleaning toilets."

Nurses are concerned about staffing in other settings as well. A psychiatric nurse states: "New graduates don't get the precepting and orientation they need. Recently two new grads were hired on a unit where all the expert nurses had resigned because the company had cut back full time nursing staff to 24 hours per week." Mary, a clinic nurse, reports: "We recently had a physician and two RNs leave. Administration says we cannot replace them." On a general medical-surgical unit, a nurse states: "Sometimes it is truly a night for *survival of the fittest*. As a seasoned nurse, I have learned to prioritize. Now I must prioritize who, literally, gets seen and who is on autopilot. I just can't be there with the patients anymore. This hurts the most."

Nurses today are finding restrictions and limitations on the care they provide. Nursing care frequently ends before patient needs are met. A conflict of values arises when nurses must choose between insufficient care and no care at all. The frustration is expressed by a nurse with 18 years' experience in the psychiatric setting when she states: "In the past few years I have seen resources decrease for psychiatric patients, greatly impacting their lives. Funding for services has been severely cut. Patients without insurance have less or no treatments available. Only the most severely ill get admitted. We joke that there must be blood on the floor for some insurance companies to authorize admission for suicidal patients. Many are discharged onto the street or to shelters. Some end up in jails."

A clinic nurse reports she now has only 15 minutes to see each patient. To make matters worse, she is now being timed and given 3-5 minutes per phone call to handle patient concerns. Another nurse is concerned about a stroke patient not getting rehab because of lack of insurance coverage. And a nurse in home care states: "As a nurse specializing in non-surgical management of urinary incontinence, I have had outstanding results with a bladder training program. In 4-6 visits, I have been able to instruct people and enable them to incorporate new behavior and skills into their lifestyle. Eight out of ten clients have great outcomes and new hope. Now with managed care, I'm getting referrals for only two visits. I have written many letters and made many phone calls to the people who are making the decisions, trying to give them rationale and telling them that it will save money and avoid unnecessary surgery in the long run. There are so many hoops I must go through that by the time I am blessed with visit #3 and maybe #4, the patient has forgotten everything and I must start again."

Nurses are dealing with situations which generate feelings of discouragement, fear, abandonment, and anger. One nurse states: "I have not had management accessible to me to gain more wisdom or clinical judgment. They are so busy in meetings that I rarely have supervision at all."

An operating room nurse reports: "I have had to stand alone many times to ensure patient safety. Just last week our unit had an emergency surgery on a high-risk baby at 5:30 P.M. There was no back-up help. The RN asked for me to stand by. I stayed, with much resistance given by management. I know money was the decision-maker. But when a coworker feels there is a need for me to stay, I will be there."

An intensive care nurse, working with aides and technicians instead of RNs, expressed anger as she gave examples of aides filling in for RNs, passing medications, and carrying out physicians' orders. And Vicki, a competent and compassionate rehabilitation nurse, states: "I find that the changes in health care have impacted the personalization of nursing. There is decreased time to spend with patients' emotional needs. It takes time to listen to the patient who is over 80 years old. They don't speak fast and they take longer to form their ideas. It is so very rude to rush through care. I find it very difficult to know the whole patient and what impacts them. Sometimes all the patient needs is someone to listen and skip the narcotics. Could their pain be taken care of in diversional ways? A young patient with multiple trauma lies in bed and 'runs the tapes' of his life and can't cope, and the nurse has no clue of the real issues. I find that the decreased time spent with patients impacts my desire to treat the human spirit."

Trends Impacting Nursing

Several trends are influencing the delivery of care and the roles nurses play in today's health care arena.

- *Health Care Restructuring.* Nursing has traditionally been a service-oriented profession with attention to patient care rather than the bottom line. Changes in hospital structures and the business of health care are greatly impacting nurses. Hospitals have restructured, consolidated, merged and/or diversified. As a result, nurses once employed by small, private hospitals find themselves working for national chains or regional multisystem corporations. Many hospitals now contract with outside services to provide entire management teams, educational inservices, or clinical services. Other hospitals have entered into arrangements in which two or more organizations share staff, services, and facilities. No matter what the arrangement, the objective has been the same — reduce cost and increase productivity and profit.
- *Workplace Redesign.* Nurses who have been functioning under total-patient-care models of delivery are now being forced to return to a partnership model in which RNs are required to delegate tasks to nurses' aides. Safe delegation of nursing tasks has become a critical issue. In some instances, however, unlicensed assistive personnel are being used to replace rather than augment nursing care. Nurses

are being required to work in multiple specialty areas with minimal training and experience. Patient acuity and earlier discharge characterize the "sicker and quicker" reality of patient care. Nurse workloads have increased, computer documentation has expanded, and nurses are being required to perform duties of other departments in addition to nursing care measures, thus detracting from the time available to meet patients' needs.

- *Career Retraining.* In the early 1990s, over two-thirds of RNs were employed by hospitals. It is anticipated that by the year 2000, less than half the RNs will be employed in acute care settings.[1] With fewer hospital admissions and shorter hospital stays for patients, more health care is being provided in outpatient settings such as homes, ambulatory care centers, and extended care facilities. Greater emphasis is being placed on health promotion and disease prevention. Nurses are finding increased job availability and career enhancement opportunities in home care and community-based settings, but are also needing to retrain and retool their areas of expertise to function competently in these settings.

In today's health care environment, novice and experienced nurses alike are having to cultivate unique workplace skills in addition to clinical expertise. Parameters of managed care, capitation, and fiscal benchmarks are forcing nurses to do more with less. According to Leah Curtin,[2] the clinician's ethical focus has changed from that of patient advocate to responsible steward of society's (and the institution's) resources. One nurse describes it this way: "we are moving in nursing from patient advocacy — giving the patient every service needed — to figuring out what the patient really needs . . . then providing it at the right time in the right setting at the lowest possible cost."[3] Clearly, the challenge is to become more business-minded professionals, more effective leaders in the workplace, and more discerning employees.

1. American Nurses Association, *The Acute Care Nurse in Transition* (Washington, D.C.: American Nurses Publishing, 1996).

2. See her three-part article: "The Ethics of Managed Care — Part 1: Proposing a New Ethos?" *Nursing Management* 27 (8) (1996): 18-19; "The Ethics of Managed Care — Part 2: Diagnosis: The World as It Is . . . ," *Nursing Management* 27 (9) (1996): 53-55; "The Ethics of Managed Care — Part 3: Toward a Common Vision," *Nursing Management* 27 (10) (1996): 71-74.

3. American Nurses Association, 1996.

Nursing's Response

Nursing's responses to the changes in health care are varied. Some nurses, too timid to speak out about unsafe conditions and convinced that their jobs are on the line every day, choose to respond by quiet compliance. Others, who see no way that they alone can penetrate management's wall of denial, are turning to unions to protect themselves and their patients. Some suggest that nurses should respond politically through the collective action of professional organizations; others suggest that the educational imperative is the solution. Some nurses rationalize, such as the manager who stated: "What good does it do if I resign? Administration will just bring in someone else who will get the job done. And it will probably be a business person rather than a nurse." Others compromise their values for the sake of their patients, like one nurse who states: "According to my value structure, telling a lie, as I need to tell it, is bothering my conscience. Many times I have to stretch the truth to get an appropriate stay for a mom and baby or a 78-year-old gynecological surgery patient without family support. Almost daily, I have to lie to insurance companies to get what the patient needs." Still other nurses choose to stand firm and not compromise their value system. Sally, an experienced RN, states: "While I was employed as a medical case manager for insurance carriers, I was instructed to 'shut down' treatment when it was not felt necessary by the adjusters. The adjusters had limited medical knowledge and were basing their directives on reports from disgruntled employers or the projected cost of treatments. I found it against my own personal ethics to be a part of a system that denied treatment to injured individuals. I could not compromise my standards and had to find employment elsewhere."

The response of nurses to the changing health care environment must incorporate the value of nursing's unique contribution to the care of patients. A recent study published by the American Nurses Association[4] confirmed the positive link between adequate nursing care and patient outcomes. RN staffing was significantly related to shorter lengths of stay and morbidity indicators for preventable conditions. Over a decade of research shows that when there are more RNs, patients experience fewer complications, hospitals show lower readmission rates, and there are fewer deaths. In the long run, this means overall lower health care costs.

4. American Nurses Association, *Implementing Nursing's Report Card: A Study of RN Staffing, Length of Stay and Patient Outcomes* (Washington, D.C.: American Nurses Publishing, 1997).

The response of nurses must also include collaboration. Through dialogue, nurses, physicians, and other health care providers must recommit to the common values we share and collaborate for the good of our patients. Nursing needs to join with others to provide the leadership in health care reform.

Indeed, the system must change. The old ways were, at times, extravagant. All of us were at fault to greater and lesser degrees. Nevertheless, health care reform does not justify abandoning patients. Health policy is too important to be left to businesspeople and politicians. Health services are too vital to be left to contracts and protocols. People need to know that they can find help when in need, and that the health care they receive will be competent, compassionate, available, and affordable.[5]

Opportunities for Christian Nurses

God's purpose for the ministry of Christian nurses in health care is quite different from the world's agenda. In these chaotic times, God is calling us to maturity in Christ. Ephesians 4:11-16, addressing the spiritual gifts given by Christ to prepare God's people for works of service, commands us to become mature and to speak the truth in love. We are called to present the living and true God to a suffering and lost world. The changes in health care exert external pressures on nurses, creating internal feelings of fear, anger, compromise, and discouragement. But as Christian leaders we must help other nurses develop a truly Christlike ethical system, a framework that will allow them to live fearlessly, to redeem their time, to hold fast to their values, to overcome discouragement, and to advance the cause of Christ in our current health care environment. Today, God is calling us all to commitment:

- commitment to Christian ethical values and to a clear understanding of how we can apply them to the real world of practice
- commitment fervently to practice the disciplines of the faith — prayer, study of Scripture, and fellowship
- commitment to encourage and counsel one another in the ways that Christ would respond to our daily circumstances
- commitment to spiritual growth and maturity, remembering that in

5. Curtin, see note 2.

Christ, we are more than conquerors through him who loved us (Romans 8:37).

In Acts 17, Paul's approach to the chaos of his day illustrates how we are to be well informed on the issues, to be persuasive and compelling in our speech, and to be spiritually sensitive to our environment. God, through the indwelling power of the Holy Spirit, assures us that he is involved in the very details of our lives. He knows the problems and issues in health care. He is at work in the world and invites us to join in his work.[6] God is calling us to moral leadership in these changing times. Today, more than ever, we need discernment, boldness, and faith. Christ told us in John 16:33 that in this world we will have trouble. But we are to take heart — to be encouraged. He has overcome the world. "And who knows but that you have come to royal position for such a time as this?" (Esther 4:14). Let us rejoice in the challenge.

6. H. T. Blackaby and C. V. King, *Experiencing God: How to Live the Full Adventure of Knowing and Doing the Will of God* (Nashville, Tenn.: Broadman & Holman Publishers, 1994).

An Administrator's Experience

William K. Atkinson, Ph.D.

The world is undergoing a time of tremendous change. In the military, banking, engineering, science, and education, phenomenal changes are being experienced as we move toward a global economy. The major advances in civilization are processes that all but wreck the societies in which they occur. Although persons in the health care field often feel like major changes are happening only to them, they need to be reminded that the world at large is indeed undergoing transformation. Many of the current presentations and materials on health care convey the feeling that the world is coming down around us. This process of rapid, immense change certainly is affecting major medical environments, be they private practices, specialty practices, or institutions involved in health care.

We have seen phenomenal changes in the way things happen in American health care, and will continue to see more. These changes have had and will have major effects on those who are involved in the actual hands-on delivery of care and the clinical application of the arts and sciences of medicine, nursing, and other fields. We must consider what impact we can have on this dynamic health care system — or non-system, depending on our perspective.

Much of the upheaval is being felt even outside of the major cities where managed care now prevails. In the workplace, people encounter massive changes ranging from technologies, mergers, acquisitions, and right-sizing (or perhaps wrong-sizing), to reorganization, new policies and procedures, and constantly shifting duties and responsibilities. As a result of such instability, people may receive mixed messages about where values, ethics, belief in God, and health care fit into the overall process of change. Some people may conclude that certain factors do not fit with the changing system at all, while others may believe that they do. Compounding the disorientation is the speed with which this change is occurring and the resultant ups and downs of health care that we all experience.

For many, it feels like a roller coaster ride, even if it's only a small roller coaster at a local fair. For others, though, even for those not yet directly affected by the changing system but merely contemplating its future effects, the changing health care system is more like the *ultimate* roller coaster — a scary and nauseating experience.

Proactive Involvement

Many of us may sense that religious and other values we hold dear may be less and less respected. Yet we must remember that the way we experience what happens in the health care system is not beyond our control. Many people have the attitude that changes in the health care system are going to affect them negatively and that there is nothing they can do to prevent it. However, we can choose to let things happen to us or we can recognize that systems cannot run our lives. They can influence how we do things, but we do not have to let them ruin our day.

Being from the South, I am a bluegrass fan. As one particular bluegrass group puts it, in a popular song: "It doesn't matter what I want, it doesn't matter what I need, it doesn't matter if I cry, it don't matter if I bleed. You been on a road, don't know where it goes or where it leads." These lyrics could be describing what it feels like these days to be a nurse, physician, or patient. It is not a good feeling. However, as we look at the question of pursuing change we can take as a starting point this kind of doom-and-gloom attitude and use it as an opportunity to alter fundamentally the way we view ourselves, the health care system, and where we fit into this system. We need to sit down with people of diverse views and hear what is happening in health care around the country and around the world. We may then focus or refocus on the important issues. Our Christian faith and ethics at this point must be central.

One way that people commonly react to a sense of danger is to take steps backward and to shut down their systems. People facing danger often shut down their ability to interact with the changes that threaten them. In terms of health care, this means the negative aspects of these changes tend to harm those who fail to confront them.

A more productive response would be to see near, to see far, and to

26

see further. Of course, we must also not forget where we have been. History is extremely important. It reminds us how health care began and some of the values that must be carried forward with us. Yet, more is needed. First, we must see near. People must be aware of the things that are happening every day. They must attend to the things they have to deal with each day because, practically, if people do not deal with daily issues arising in their practice sites, hospitals, clinics, and teaching activities, there will be no tomorrow. This is one of the urgencies people in the health care professions now face.

Second, people need to see far. They need to think about what's going to happen in health care in the next year or the next couple of years. In my current work environment, we commonly focus on a very short time period: the next operating quarter. This focus is pragmatic in terms of survival, at least in the short run, but not a strong position to operate from.

People also need to see further. They must learn how to see beyond the horizon, beyond what the average individual would normally think about in terms of the future. While many people follow the beaten path — and the beaten path is easy to pick out — there may be signs in our lives that tell us to go another way. We need to consider those signs, whether they are rooted in the Word of God, in experience, or in intuition.

For example, seeing the coming danger of economics eclipsing ethics, I have not allowed finances to drive my decisions. We discuss policies and initiatives on their non-economic merits first. We have to analyze our ideas at some point on the basis of whether they may potentially threaten the continuing existence of the institution, but that is not the first way we look at things. Many people consider this a very foreign concept in the delivery of health care, but I have a strong conviction that bad medicine is bad business. Bad health care is extremely bad business. Both the medical care and the business aspects of a health care system ultimately have to be carried out adequately and ethically.

Changes in Health Care

From my perspective, the changes in health care may be characterized as follows. In the 1970s, medical facilities were committed to offering as many services as possible. Every hospital seemed to offer every service — they all wanted to have women's centers and other centers which offered specialized care, and they each wanted to be the first with new technologies. Then, in the 1980s, we saw the niches and carve-outs begin to appear. These were the freestanding psychiatric hospitals, the freestanding rehabilitation hospitals, and the birthing centers, all of them operating separately from the major hospitals.

In the 1990s, we began to see the development of significant networks. Networks are interesting entities because generally they represent all the verbiage of coordination, yet are free of the realities and the heartaches of coordination. This is because hospitals and other groups such as physician groups come together under the premise of working together, but no integrated leadership is established. As a result, each organization still has an equal vote, and no significant change really occurs in many of the networks that formed in the 1990s. In fact, the formation of such networks actually generates additional cost because an additional tier of operational administration is added without the benefit of being offset by any significant changes. Many communities have lived through this network development, which in most cases has been ineffective.

In the late 1990s, we have begun seeing some comprehensive, fully integrated networks, and the changes are likely to continue. Certain basics are always involved in clinical care, but the organizational structures have changed and will probably continue to change forever. I predict that we will return to niches and carve-outs around the year 2005 because big will not be so glorious then. People are going to want independent services again, and I expect to see a new cycle begin.

Health care today has become big business, whether we like the term "business" associated with health care or not. Health care involves billions of dollars: even if there were no corporations involved in hospital ownership, it would still involve billions of dollars. Fundamental to health care are hundreds of millions of customers; millions of jobs; thousands of schools with their entire economy built around teaching, training, and educating; thousands of vendors; ties to all segments of the economy; and involvement with every single government agency and military service that exists. Health care also has ties to many political, cultural, and spiritual organizations. This was true 25 years ago, it was true 40 years ago, and it will be true 100 years from now. Health care is big business simply in the sense that it involves economics on a huge scale, regardless of who is in charge of the organizations. That does not change.

Even though "national health care" did not pass in the United States during the 1990s, it is my opinion that we now have such a health care system, for better or worse. National health care is typically characterized

28

by the domination of large systems. In our current system, the larger insurance companies prevail, the larger medical groups succeed, and the larger hospitals are doing fairly well within systems. We see a lot of subcontracting, especially military styles of subcontracting for delivery of care. A national data and records system is growing at a rapid pace. Such systems are typical of national health care as well.

We are also witnessing the rapid growth of large health care companies. Columbia HCA, one such company, in less than ten years became one of the largest companies in America and the largest health care provider in the world. In the state of Florida, Columbia facilities are very concentrated. From an operational perspective, South Florida has 15 hospitals (with close to 4,000 beds), psychiatric services, and a wide range of other services concentrated in three counties.

The effects of such concentration can be positive, though they are not necessarily so. One advantage is that when health care institutions are brought into a real system — be it Columbia, an Adventist system, a Catholic system, or another system — clinical issues like the need for trauma centers can be realistically assessed. Where needed, such centers can then be created. Neonatal intensive care issues may be realistically assessed in a manner that bypasses political issues. Efficient transport systems can be built to support large systems and to make sure that patients are treated in a way that is economical and also clinically sound. Similarly, putting a patient under the care of a qualified medical and nursing team makes good economic sense. Even if there is more initial cost in doing so, long-term cost may be less than the cost of opting for lower-quality care.

Health care continues to change in other ways as well. We are witnessing the emergence of trends such as home health service, outpatient diagnostics, outpatient emergency services, specialty centers, rural health centers, and subcontracting for skilled nursing. Technology, communications, health care consolidations, and global economy are all change factors in health care. With changes in demographics and population mobility and recent advances in science such as laser technology and minimal-access surgery, the face of health care has also begun to change in major medical centers. This trend will certainly continue. Minimal-access heart surgery, which shortens the length of a patient's stay to one day — or provides it on an outpatient basis entirely — is changing the nature of tertiary health care.

The microprocessing world's technological ability to make so many things mobile allows an increasing number of services and procedures that have commonly been done in the hospital to be moved to other settings. We have seen this happen to a great extent in home health care. Home health care today in the U.S. is about a $25-billion business. Ten thousand public and private agencies are now involved in the delivery of home health, which is increasingly being supported by public policy and by technology. Nevertheless, the roots of home health care are in our history, not in our current economic conditions. Home health care is the foundation of medicine; it is where medicine started before hospitals arose.

Federally-funded home health visits in the United States have increased at a dramatically rapid pace. I believe that, ultimately, people are entering the home health business primarily because they understand the economics of being in home health today. Home health care is, for all practical purposes, unregulated from a reimbursement standpoint, but it will probably become regulated in the very near future. Because governmental regulation is soon to occur, it is probably not a good time to begin investing in home health if one is not already involved with it.

Managed Care, Economy, and Quality

What is the future of managed care? I believe that managed care is here to stay, whether we like it or not. This does not mean that we must accept the form it is currently in, but simply that the concept of managed care is much more acceptable to the average person than the concept of unmanaged, overly expensive care. Managed care companies are looking at price first and they are seeking to identify services, not offered by other companies, that they can obtain for their patients at no additional cost. Eventually, they are going to be concerned with quality. In my eleven years in Denver, however, only one managed care company has asked for quality outcome data as part of a bid for a managed care contract — only one — and that company went out of business. Managed care is not primarily concerned with quality; it views the meter as running when the patient walks through the door. That is not a good way to think about health care, but it is the way that managed care operates.

Where should quality fit in the managed care system? The first challenge is to define quality, especially in changing economic times. Quality is very difficult to define, and there is really no national definition of quality that is generally accepted, even among caregivers. If caregivers cannot get together to define quality, someone else is going to define it for them. Determining an acceptable standard for quality of health care is one of the biggest challenges society faces. This is most appropriately a clinical task. People who are delivering the care need to define its quality standards.

In the meantime, quality of health care is going to be defined by many organizations, it is going to be tracked by more and more interested parties, and it is ultimately going to emerge as the main managed care focus after the initial price wars are over. Prices in many parts of the country are about as low as they can go with managed care. Therefore, after the cost of health care ceases to be the dominant issue, companies will probably shift their focus more to quality issues. Good medical practice is good business also, even for managed care companies. It does not make sense for these companies to offer compromised health care and as a result find themselves involved in the types of lawsuits that are occurring today. That is not good business. A $25-million settlement does serious economic damage to a company.

True Leadership

One of the most important things health care providers can do is to intertwine their spiritual and moral commitments with what they do. It is important that they have some core of understanding of why they are doing what they are, and why they are involved in health care. They need to have a moral compass built inside, a basis for evaluating those things they are asked and told to do. If they do not believe in what they are being asked to do, they need to have the moral courage to say no. They need to be willing to accept the short-term economic ramifications of their decision.

Many people will claim that there is only one way to go in health care. However, pioneers are the ones who go in other directions, who go to places where no one has ever been. People who are willing to accept this role can say no to managed care. They can suggest and demonstrate a better way for the delivery of health care. This is something each of us is in a position to do, though it requires passion. A visible passion for what we do often inspires others. If we believe in something and we believe that it is spiritually based, or clinically based, or hopefully both, we must use our internal passion to convince others that it is right or to bring them the information that will allow them to make appropriate decisions.

Christians understand the importance of at least one Carpenter in their lives. The standard rule of carpentry — measure twice, not once — should be applied to the building of a health care system. As we create the health care system, we must measure it twice before we make decisions, because managed care companies and other groups have a large saw. The key is for Christian health care professionals to be involved in the measurement of what they do in health care in order to make sure that the dimensions are right before they allow someone to cut away.

In fact, all members of the Christian community, with their various areas of expertise, need to work together on this. And all must pray about the challenges they face and the decisions they must make. On my very first day at the hospital I direct, I sat outside before I went in and prayed, "Lord, show me how to make this work. Please guide my hands and guide what little bit of leadership I am going to be able to exercise." Every morning I repeat the same ritual when I arrive, because health care is complex. Of course it is not too complex for God; nor is it for us if we are willing to place what little we have to offer at God's disposal.

SETTING THE STAGE

A Theological Mandate
for Medicine

Nigel M. de S. Cameron, Ph.D.

The task of elaborating a Christian perspective on contemporary questions in bioethics is a complicated one. The very novelty of *bioethics,* symbolized in the coinage of this special term a generation ago, suggests that the context of contemporary discussion is to be separated from all previous reflection on the questions under consideration. This is ironic, since there lies a long history behind them, all the way back to the Greek philosophers for whom issues like abortion and euthanasia were talking-points as they are for us. The advance of technology, in medicine as elsewhere, imparts a fresh context and raises some wholly new matters. Yet just as political philosophy boasts fundamental continuity in a world of modern media and election funding, so one would have anticipated that such a continuity would have been admitted in the case of the ethics of medicine, science, and the human person.

One component in the claimed discontinuity is to be found in the pluralistic nature of current discussion.[1] Until the 1950s and 1960s there prevailed a widespread consensus in the Western tradition going back at least to the first centuries A.D. and the cultural currency of the Judeo-Christian worldview. The sudden shift from consensus to debate was signaled in Jospeh Fletcher's book *Morals and Medicine,*[2] one of the first

1. See Nigel Cameron, "Bioethics: The Twilight of Christian Hippocratism," in D. A. Carson and John D. Woodbridge, eds., *God and Culture* (Grand Rapids: Eerdmans, 1993), pp. 321-40.
2. Joseph Fletcher, *Morals and Medicine* (Boston: Beacon Press, 1954; and London: Gollancz, 1955).

contributions to the modern discussion of bioethics which suggests across a range of questions that the tradition has been wrong. Fletcher writes in the 1950s, well before the term *bioethics* was coined. But in his preface, he declares that "medical ethics" must be discussed in terms of Christian theology and ethics, and proceeds, chapter by chapter, so to do, even though this is often a rather challenging exercise! This dramatic shift in discussion is also well illustrated by the work of Paul Ramsey.[3] In the 1960s and early 1970s Ramsey was the major figure in this nascent field and brought to it a conservative and candid understanding of the Christian context of the conversation.

This analysis does not suggest that the development of an understanding of bioethics which is rooted in the profession[4] and set within the context of Christian faith[5] will either answer all our current problems or readily commend itself to the secularists who largely adorn the bioethics academy. But it will achieve two vital results. First, it will enable those many physicians, nurses, administrators, and ethicists who work self-consciously within the context of their Christian faith to be freed from the notion that they must do secular bioethics. Although they will still need to engage in the wider secular discussion within their professional contexts, their own position can be informed by the commitments of Christian faith before they seek to translate it into terms that resonate with the secular marketplace of ideas. They do not need to *begin* with secular starting-points. Secondly, and partly as a result, the development of a thriving Christian bioethics will itself challenge the raw secularity of the field, since only by the exclusion of Christian sensitivities has bioethics been able to ignore its own long tradition, and its grounding in the identity of medicine. Yet evangelical Christians have been slow to articulate their understanding of medicine in theological terms aside from its offering a context for Christian service and mission.[6]

---

3. See, for example, Paul Ramsey, *The Patient As Person* (New Haven and London: Yale University Press, 1970).

4. For an example of the potential significance of this kind of approach, see Edmund Pellegrino and David Thomasma, *The Virtues in Medical Practice* (New York and Oxford: Oxford University Press, 1993).

5. For example, see Edmund Pellegrino et al., *The Christian Virtues in Medical Practice* (Washington, D.C.: Georgetown University Press, 1996).

6. See Appendix to Nigel Cameron, *The New Medicine: Life and Death After Hippocrates* (Wheaton, Ill.: Crossway Books, 1992), pp. 171-82; and "Soundings in a Theology of Medicine, *Trinity Journal* 14, n.s. (1993): 123-41.

The Need for a Dissident Community

Some assessment of the strategic situation at this point would be helpful. As we survey the current ethical debates around medicine, with health care restructuring and allocation issues now high on the agenda, we should note that they are proceeding in a context in which the moral consensus upon which Western medicine has long been founded is facing collapse. That consensus stemmed from the blend of Christian Hippocratism that was still remarkably intact a little more than a generation ago, though in bioethics discussion it is now ignored or, when noted, generally reviled.[7] In its place, as the basis for the moral structure and integrity of medicine, we see the rise of a post-Hippocratic tradition which has been enshrined in the mainstream bioethics of the last 25 years. As it is post-Hippocratic, it is also post-professional in character. The marriage of skills and values that characterized Hippocratism and laid the foundations of professional identity has crumbled. It is no surprise that these changes have gone hand in hand with a growing reduction of the medical "profession" to essentially a consumerist-corporatist exercise in the delivery of saleable skills to the market.[8]

How then should Christian physicians — and those who would support them — position ourselves? We would do well, above all, to cultivate and even endeavor to regenerate that dying tradition of professional Western medicine (albeit refined in light of Christian understanding). It is hard to overstate the significance of this endeavor for our culture. Indeed, the professional medical tradition is a jewel in the crown of the Western tradition. How shall we proceed? First, it is plain that we must seek to maintain a presence within the medical culture of our day. But it must be a presence characterized by dissidence. As in the culture at large, so here, there is no virtue in withdrawal. By the same token, there is not much more in simply conforming to the image of the new medicine and being absorbed. We must be present, but present as dissidents. And that conception is of special importance in this discussion. The pattern of dissidence set in the latter years of the Soviet empire is a possible model for us — if we would seek a way of understanding the kind of role we can play in the post-Christian West and, in particular, in the post-Hippocratic Western medical culture.

7. See Nigel Cameron, 1992.

8. Needless to say, many individual physicians do not agree with but are being swept up in these trends.

It is salutary to note what the Soviet dissidents did and did not do. They did not withdraw (for example, by emigration, or by withdrawing into communities hidden from view); they did not keep silent. They stayed, and they spoke. Finally, their testimony to the truth, and to the corruption of the Soviet system, helped bring it down. But if that is our model, we must nurture an alternative community, a community which is radically countercultural in its values and its testimony. It will be a community bound together by the ties of faith and theological understanding, and by the ties of commitment to an alternative professional model. It will be marked by an eager interest in the past, that other territory which has been almost entirely excluded from consideration in contemporary bioethical discussion. If we would do that, we must educate ourselves in order to sustain, nurture, and cultivate the alternative community. For we must be able not simply to survive as physicians, nurses, patients, and clergy; we must challenge the culture, throw down the gauntlet of a yet more excellent way to care for the sick. And in so doing we may hope to rekindle and encourage the original Hippocratic vision of a guild of professionals committed above all else to helping the sick. If we forget that medicine is about helping the sick, we have forgotten what it is about.

In order to prepare ourselves to engage in that kind of task, the dissident task, we must turn first of all to a theological understanding of medicine, which in turn derives from a distinctive perspective on the nature of human beings. The Christian worldview is founded deep in a theological understanding of who we are. We are made in the image of God, and find our being in our redemption in Jesus Christ, and in his resurrection, ascension, and final return, as well as in the resurrection of the dead. That is the matrix of Christian understanding in which we make sense of ourselves in the world in which we live.

As we debate the intricacies of health care restructuring, of costs and consent and the growing corporatization of American medicine, we above all need to gain a fundamental perspective on the crisis through which our medical tradition is passing. If we are to engage effectively in the debate and help chart the wisest course for this increasingly and depressingly post-professional medical enterprise, nothing can be more important than to gain our theological bearings to understand what medicine truly means — to peer over the wall, as it were, and see how medicine looks in the eyes of God. That is to say, our point of departure will lie in our Christian conception of what it means to be human in the face of life, sickness, and, finally, death.

In other words, those who would engage in these many discussions as Christians must first attain at least the rudiments of what we should properly call the theology of medicine. This is a task that has been little attempted. Indeed, the general failure of Christians to think about medicine as a theological question is extraordinary. An example of this lies in the manner in which our theological seminaries have shown scant interest in this whole area, such that the development at Trinity International University (Deerfield, Illinois) of graduate-degree programs in bioethics remains unparalleled. While bioethics raises many technical questions that may seem to be of only highly specialized interest, basic issues of life and death, such as abortion and euthanasia, are among the most controversial in the world. At the same time, pastors regularly encounter such issues in the course of pastoral care.

Moreover, throughout the Christian centuries the story of the church has been interwoven at every point with the story of medicine. The story of the original hospices, which were monastery hospitals, the story of physicians, the story of nurses, the story of various imperatives of the care of the sick — these have been largely Christian stories. And the reason for this is not hard to find: the Bible itself is replete with sickness and healing, with the fragility of life and the inevitability of death, with the imperative of care, and with the hope of something far better than merely the temporary restoration of bodily health.

Sickness and Healing in Theological Perspective

Consider more carefully, first of all, the question of sickness.[9] Sickness is the shadow of death. That was much more evident in earlier times, of course, than it is now. Today we are more likely to see sickness as the shadow perhaps of medical treatment, or the shadow of insurance, or the shadow of medical malpractice. But not so long ago — before anesthesia, antisepsis, and antibiotics — sickness was other than that. When the armamentarium of the physician was drastically limited, the sick bed and the grave lay side by side. If they do not for us it is partly because technology

9. See two of my other essays for a discussion of the centrality of the meaning of death and suffering in this debate: "Theological Perspectives on Euthanasia," in Nigel Cameron, ed., *Death without Dignity* (Edinburgh: Rutherford House Books, 1990); and "Autonomy and the Right to Die," in John F. Kilner et al., eds., *Dignity and Dying: A Christian Appraisal* (Grand Rapids: Eerdmans; and Carlisle, Cumbria, U.K.: Paternoster Press, 1996).

has come a long way, and can now do so very much more for us when we are sick. But it is also partly because we have become a less candid people and a less far-sighted people. We have developed a new conception of sickness that has little connection with our understanding of mortality.

Yet it is surely true today, as it ever was, that sickness precedes death, the final sickness. And this is where we enter what we may call the mystery of medicine. We find our fragility exposed, our hearty neglect of our mortality on trial, and our desperate will to live forever in an entropic universe exposed as a tragic lie. We confront what George Bernard Shaw called "the ultimate statistic, that one out of one dies" (which is almost true, despite a few biblical counterexamples). While actuarial tables have been steadily rewritten, and the exponential curve of medical success has risen upward, we know too well that death will still get us in the end. And we may note in passing that much of the social significance of HIV and AIDS lies precisely in the fact that we inhabit a culture seemingly convinced that death will not succeed. We see paraded before us the tragedy of a large class of persons, most of them young, seemingly condemned to a young death, and we are thus forcibly reminded in our most unwilling culture of our final mortality.

Of course, if we compare the present situation with that of a century ago or earlier, the process of dying takes longer and is therefore delayed; and it will surely cost more. Our "passing," that old word, will likely be through cancer, or coronary heart disease, in place of the vicious infections that used to carry us off as children; but pass we shall. And we must ask the question: when did the pastor last preach a sermon about death? The problem here does not simply lie outside the church, among the unbelievers; not simply in "the culture" out there, but in the culture of which we also partake. Moving death from the sickroom and the nursery to the nursing home and the hospital has helped obscure it from view. Yet its incidence remains as sure as Shaw's ultimate statistic suggests.

The key point here is that we have lengthened the connection between sickness and death. Every year it is lengthened further. This truly represents extraordinary progress. We have been given dominion over this world. It is not just a world of rain forests and rare species. It is a world of the microchip and of nanoseconds. It is a world that extends to cosmic time and space. Woe to us if we seek to exclude God from that world by denying that we have been commanded to possess it, thereby aiding the grim process of its secularization. We have lengthened the move from the sickbed to the grave, but the connection has not been severed. The connection remains, and if we seek in death the meaning of sickness we

40

find it of course in that terrifying monosyllable, sin. The wages of sin is death. The sin/death causality runs through the biblical-theological understanding of the nature of reality, and offers one of the foundation-stones of the Judeo-Christian worldview.

The most fundamental Christian perception of death is that it is profoundly unnatural — which in turn explains our deep-seated ambivalence toward our mortality. Hear Tennyson, the massive romantic intellect of the Victorian crisis of faith, in his remarkable, sustained encounter with grief and mortality entitled "In Memoriam":[10]

> Thou wilt not leave us in the dust,
> Thou madest man — he knows not why,
> He thinks he was not made to die,
> And thou hast made him: thou art just.

"He thinks he was not made to die." And as Holy Scripture confirms, he is right. It is not that we each die for our own sins. As they said to Jesus, "Who sinned? This man or his parents?" (John 9:2). It is rather that humankind is subjected to mortality because "all have sinned." The sinful race, contrary to its original creation, is a mortal race. This is the reason why we find death so hard; the reason why we intuitively cry out with Tennyson as he mourns over the death of his old friend; the reason why we shield death from our everyday life; the reason why our pastors do not preach about it; the reason why our own feelings about it, even as Christian believers, are so profoundly ambivalent. If we think we were not made to die, we are right.

This sin/death causality lies at the heart of Christian understanding of what it means to be human. It is part of the key to our interpretation of the fulfillment and the dismay of the inexorable longing and its final extinction which are the subjective measure of the human condition. In other words, as we seek to understand the predicament of our mortality, we find that our ground for hope lies in the radically unnatural character of death. If the cause of death is not natural, if it is both moral and supernatural, if it is sin and the divine judgment upon the sin, then we also believe in a final great reversal in which, after weeping has lasted for a night, joy comes in the morning. Sickness, the shadow of death and its foretaste — indeed every sickness — brings with it evidence of our final mortality.

10. Alfred Tennyson, *Poems* (Boston: J. E. Tilton and Company, 1866), p. 303.

Next, let us examine the conception of healing. If sickness is the shadow of death, healing is the foretaste of the resurrection of the body. Now if this is true, it is a matter of some moment. Because the gospel record on page after page is that Jesus Christ of all things went about healing the sick. They brought him all the sick and he healed them. And that line seems to recur like a chorus in a hymn. As theological scholar Benjamin Warfield has observed, to say that Jesus abolished sickness and death from Palestine for the three years of his ministry would be an exaggeration, but a pardonable exaggeration.[11]

Jesus Christ, whom Christians worship, was a healer, a miracle worker, whose encounter with disease and even death itself proved one-sided, such that the blind saw and the deaf heard and the lame walked and even the dead were raised. We do not know how many of the dead were raised. We have several specific accounts, such as the widow of Nain's son, and the daughter of the centurion. The most detailed, and plainly the most remarkable, is that of the raising of Lazarus in John 11:17ff. We ask the question, why? Why the constant reiteration of a healing ministry coming to a final climax in this extraordinary account of the resuscitation of a decaying corpse, that of the man Lazarus who had been Jesus' friend? And yet we know the answer. Here Jesus challenges the curse which brought death into the world. He takes on the moral and supernatural forces which have made his friend die. He challenges death as he has for three years, in confronting its precursor, sickness. And he does so within days of his own personal engagement of death on the cross, which gives place to his final victory over it in resurrection.

The gospel record of Jesus is one in which he has gone around bringing balm — palliation is our term — to the suffering people to whom he ministered in anticipation of the final resurrection of the dead. Supremely in the resurrection of Lazarus, but in principle in every act of healing, we have a sampling of the resurrection of the body and the life of the world to come. We have a foretaste of the day when the dead will be raised incorruptible. We have anticipation of one of the most interesting phrases in the whole New Testament, in Romans 8:23, "the redemption of our bodies." These vile bodies will finally gain their restoration and renewal. We shall be restored in body, mind, soul, and spirit. "Thou wilt not leave us in the dust," cried Tennyson. Just as every sickness brings a foretaste of the final sickness of death, so every healing brings a

11. Benjamin Warfield, *Counterfeit Miracles*. Reprinted in 1996 by Banner of Truth.

foretaste of the resurrection. And so in 1 Corinthians 15:51ff. we find the words of the apostle:

> Listen, I tell you a mystery:
> We will not all sleep,
> but we will all be changed. . . .

The Challenge Before Us

What follows from all this? Those who would stand with the sick to restore them or bring balm to their symptoms, the physicians and nurses and others in allied professions, join in a unique vocation, the first and last task of which is to mitigate the sad effects of the curse of sin, the universal fact of death and its life-long anticipation of death in disease. Let us review some particulars.

First, we note the realism with which we can face human mortality. Once this recognition has been grasped, the therapeutic imperative remains an imperative. There is here no short-circuiting of the sanctity of the human life. But there is a therapeutic imperative always conscious of its final limitation. The physician is called to heal, but to heal mortal creatures.

Secondly, we see indeed how great a stress such a model will place upon palliative care, because the final futility of the therapeutic task is built into our understanding. Therapeutic endeavor, we may softly suggest, plays a secondary place in the care of mortal men and women. It must ultimately give place to a preparation for their "passing," for death itself.

Thirdly, we may note the hope that pervades such a vision for medicine. It is not a hope based upon the contingencies of the fragile skills of a human being or even the wonders of medical technologies, or the quest for a perfect health care system; rather, it is rooted in the infinite and enduring goodness of God. God himself determined the mortality of his human beings, and yet extends his hand of hope to those who will go down into the grave, for they will rise again. Every patient is finally lost; but whoever is finally lost to medicine is found to God, and will be found once again by us all in the resurrection of the dead.

Such is the framework for a theological understanding of medicine. Here is a way in which the hallowed task of the physician — and indeed all of health care by implication — finds itself center stage in the divine human theater of sin and redemption, of death and the redemption of the body. Here too is a final ground of hope. The single most significant beneficial development in medicine in our generation has been hospice care, and the rise of palliative medicine as a central specialty. It is no coincidence that this was from the start a Christian project, devised by the remarkable Dr. Cicely Saunders back in the 1960s. Because Christians can face death with a steady eye, we are not like those without hope. We can see beyond the grave, though the grave can have a place on our horizon. We are aware of the fragility of human nature under the curse, and therefore the sheer contingency of the context of the medical exercise that is brought to bear on mortal beings. Yet in this awareness we find either a ground for despair or a ground for turning in hope to this Jesus Christ, who was born, lived, and died; who was raised, glorified, and seated; and who will return — and whose resurrection will be the pattern for ours and all those who are found in him.

Nursing:
Remaining Faithful
in an Era of Change

Judith Allen Shelly, R.N., D.Min.

The nurse-patient relationship, like the physician-patient relationship, is coming under escalating economic and structural pressure. In the rush to trim costs and increase efficiency, the danger is real that the essential role of nursing in the healing process will be overlooked, or at least undervalued. While much of the discussion about the future of health care has revolved around medicine and technology, the heart of caring for the sick (and keeping people well) comes in the uniquely Christian contribution to the health care system — nursing. We must have a clear understanding of what nursing is all about if we are to secure its important role in an era of change.

Christian Roots

Although some forms of health care were provided in ancient cultures,[1] nurse historian Patricia Donahue states, "The history of nursing first becomes continuous with the beginning of Christianity."[2] Nurse historians Dolan, Fitzpatrick, and Herrmann state,

---

1. These health care providers include midwives, shamans, and wise women, but none of these roles meet the criteria for professional nursing as defined in this chapter.
2. Patricia Donahue, *Nursing: The Finest Art — An Illustrated History* (St. Louis: C. V. Mosby, 1985), p. 93.

The teachings and example of *Jesus Christ* had a profound influence on the emergence of gifted nurse leadership as well as on the expansion of the role of nurses. Christ stressed the need to love God and one's neighbor. The first organized group of nurses was established as a direct response to His example and challenge.[3]

This movement began when the first-century Christians began to teach that all believers were ministers and expected to care for the poor, the sick, and the disenfranchised.[4] As the churches grew, church leaders appointed deacons to care for the needy within the church.[5] Eventually, more men and women were added to the roll of deacons and their designated responsibilities grew to include caring for the sick.[6] Phoebe, the deacon mentioned in Romans 16:1-2, is claimed to be the first visiting nurse.[7] By the third century organized groups of deaconesses were caring for the sick, insane, and lepers in the community at large.[8] In the fourth century the church began establishing hospitals. Most of these hospitals did not have a physician; they were staffed by nurses. In fact, there were several periods when the early church did not condone the practice of medicine, which they viewed as a pagan art.[9] Nurse historians Lavinia Dock and Isabel Stewart state:

> The age-old custom of hospitality . . . was practiced with religious fervor by the early Christians. . . . Their houses were opened wide to every afflicted applicant and, not satisfied with receiving needy ones, the deacons, men and women alike, went out to search and bring them in. The private homes of the deacons were turned into hospitals called diakonia, and the name deacon became synonymous with that of a director of hospital relief.[10]

3. Josephine Dolan, M. Louise Fitzpatrick, and Eleanor Krohn Herrmann, *Nursing in Society: A Historical Perspective,* 15th ed. (Philadelphia: W. B. Saunders, 1983), p. 43.

4. Matthew 25:31-46, Hebrews 13:1-3, James 1:27, 1 Peter 2:9.

5. James Monroe Barnett, *The Diaconate: A Full and Equal Order* (Valley Forge, Pa.: Trinity Press International, 1995), pp. 28-42.

6. David Zersen, "Parish Nursing: 20th-Century Fad?" *Journal of Christian Nursing* 11 (2) (Spring 1994): 16-45.

7. Dolan et al., *Nursing in Society,* p. 45.

8. Mary Haazig, "Historical Presence of the Nurse in the Church," in *Oneness in Purpose — Diversity in Practice* (Park Ridge, Ill.: National Parish Nurse Resource Center, 1989), p. 3.

9. Bonnie Bullough and Vern L. Bullough, "Our Roots: What We Should Know about Nursing's Christian Pioneers," *Journal of Christian Nursing* 4 (1) (Winter 1987): 12.

10. Lavinia L. Dock, R.N., and Isabel Maitland Stewart, A.M., R.N., *A Short History of Nursing, From the Earliest Times to the Present Day* (New York, London: G. P. Putnam's Sons, The Knickerbocker Press, 1931), p. 51.

As nursing history demonstrates, something radically different happened in society through the early Christian church. Second-century theologian Tertullian remarked:

> It is our care of the helpless, our practice of loving kindness that brands us in the eyes of many of our opponents. "Only look," they say, "how they love one another! Look how they are prepared to die for one another."[11]

Third-century historian Eusebius of Caesarea recorded during a devastating plague:

> The Christians were the only people who amid such terrible ills, showed their fellow-feelings and humanity by their actions. Day by day some would busy themselves by attending to the dead and burying them; others gathered in one spot all who were afflicted by hunger throughout the whole city and gave them bread.[12]

Nursing grew out of a Christian worldview, in response to Jesus' teaching and example of caring for the sick. What was it about a Christian worldview that motivated the early church to reach out to the poor, the sick, and the marginalized?

While other worldviews of the time focused on gaining control of the physical elements and spiritual powers, the early Christians looked instead to God as one who deserved love and obedience, and inspired loving service to others. That tradition of caring for others in the form of nursing has continued throughout church history (with a few bleak periods). What we believe about God shapes our understanding of human persons and the environment in which we find ourselves. That, in turn, informs our concept of health and directs us to the means by which we nurture one another toward health and healing. Hence, as Christians, we begin with a *theology* of nursing, more than a philosophy. If we truly believe what we say we believe about God, we cannot help but act in obedience to him — which means communicating the good news of salvation, health, and healing through word and deed. A Christian worldview is neither the mechanistic understanding of Western dualism, nor the impersonal energy field of Eastern philosophy, but is characterized by personal relationship with God and other people.

---

11. As quoted in Dolan et al., *Nursing in Society*, p. 44.
12. As quoted in Dolan et al., *Nursing in Society*, p. 44.

A Christian worldview affirms good empirical science and the appropriate use of technology. They are gifts from God to be used for the benefit of creation. The methods of science give us knowledge of the physical aspects of creation. However, science has its limits. The personal, spiritual aspects of creation are veiled, and while manifested in the physical world, cannot be explained by science. The meaning of the personal and spiritual are seen only in the context of a larger worldview.

Christians can also affirm many of the concerns and goals of our postmodern society (as expressed in the rush toward alternative therapies), although our understanding of many concepts may differ. We share the concern for a more personal approach to health care, including the use of touch. We hold a holistic view of the person, and affirm the need to provide comfort in human suffering. A Christian worldview includes the reality of the spiritual and unseen, and the importance of faith and prayer. We recognize that there may be forms of physical energy that we cannot yet measure, and we reject *scientism*, which reduces all reality to physical/material phenomena.

The uniqueness of Christ-inspired nursing lies in its emphasis on caring for the whole person as embodied. It is both a science and an art, but primarily it is a response to God's grace and a reflection of his character.

After a professional nursing conference where several alternative therapies based on the concept of *chi* (spiritual energy) had been presented, a group of Christians gathered to discuss the implications of what they had heard. Several presenters had attributed their new understandings of *energy fields* to Buddhism, Hinduism, and Shamanism. "With increased diversity and the rapid proliferation of other religions in our society, nursing has to become more inclusive," one nurse explained, then continued: "We have to be more open-minded and approach spirituality from a broader perspective." Another nurse added, "It is presumptuous for Christians to think they can know God better than people of other religions do. Although the Christian faith is right for me, I think we have to respect their traditions as well." "All truth is God's truth," interjected another; "if alternative therapies work, we should use them, regardless of the worldview behind them." While all of these nurses were Christians, they were also postmodern in their understanding of spirituality. Their comments echoed the spirit of our age.

One of the unique features of Christianity — the one that grates most on the postmodern conscience — is the *scandal of particularity*. The Bible teaches that God singled out one people (the Hebrews), at a particular time and place in history, and revealed himself to them as the only true God. He drew firm boundaries, requiring absolute faithfulness. Any worship of other gods he labeled *idolatry* or spiritual adultery. He then took on human flesh in the one person of Jesus Christ, who said, "I am the way, and the truth, and the life. No one comes to the Father except through me" (John 14:6). One cannot be much more exclusive. However, Jesus also said:

> I am the bread of life. Whoever comes to me will never be hungry, and whoever believes in me will never be thirsty. . . . This is indeed the will of my Father, that all who see the Son and believe in him may have eternal life; and I will raise them up on the last day. (John 6:35, 40)

God's offer of salvation is, in reality, the most *inclusive* belief system. He calls all of creation into relationship with himself. Salvation is a free gift, but it is on his terms.

When we presume to know a better way than what God has revealed to us in Scripture, we are like children crying, "Everybody else is doing it!" Every wise parent knows that what "everybody else" is doing, is not necessarily right or good. The call to be spiritually inclusive falsely masquerades as virtue, when in truth it is simply rebellion against God. Furthermore, the kind of tolerance advocated by many people in our society borders on indifference, not kindness and compassion.

The Trinitarian nature of God — Father, Son, and Holy Spirit — forms the basic structure of Christian theology. The Scriptures reveal God as the Creator of the universe who established both time and eternity, the Redeemer of the world who entered history in human form, and the Sanctifier of his people who continues to dwell among and within them. We can know God personally, but we cannot become God or force him to do our bidding. Furthermore, we can only know God as he reveals himself to us. We cannot merely shape God into whatever we want him to be. The Bible calls that *idolatry*.[13]

Throughout history, the way people viewed God affected not only their worship and personal salvation, but also shaped their ethics and morality, the way they related to one another, and to their use and abuse of power. We can see these effects in nursing history. With a few exceptions, during times that the church remained faithful to Scripture and orthodox in beliefs, nursing flourished. When the church grew weak and corrupt, nursing suffered and declined.

---

13. See Isaiah 44 for a graphic description of how God views our idolatry.

The Rise of Secular Nursing

We have seen how nursing as a public role first developed in the Christian church; however, by the seventeenth century nursing had degenerated into a sorry state. When Pennsylvania Hospital, the first hospital in America, opened in 1752, nursing care was provided by nurses who were expected to be "trustworthy and experienced" but had no formal training. Their duties, which included preparing food and feeding patients, washing and ironing the linens, and keeping the rooms clean, were shared by the patients as they were able.[14] However, during this period, nursing occurred primarily within the family as an extension of motherhood. Hospital nursing was not considered a respectable vocation for a young woman.

The Crimean War forced Florence Nightingale to reinvent nursing. She defined nursing as having "charge of the personal health of somebody . . . [knowing] how to put the constitution in such a state as it will have no disease, or that it will recover from disease."[15] She believed that every woman was a nurse, and wrote her little book, *Notes on Nursing*, to help them "think how to nurse."[16] The women she took with her to Scutari were not formally educated as nurses. Nightingale taught them after they arrived. Following the war she established the first secular school of nursing.

However, war alone did not define nursing. Catholic monastic orders maintained the role of nursing sisters throughout the history of the church. The nineteenth century also brought a revival of nursing in the Protestant church, especially in northern Europe. The deaconess movement sprang up as a response to the gospel. These early deaconesses lived in community and cared for the sick and poor without charge. They established hospitals and schools of nursing. Florence Nightingale learned what she knew about nursing from these Christian communities.[17]

The nuns and deaconesses were never overly concerned about defining nursing; they just did it. When the nuns first arrived in America in the eighteenth century, they were not educated as nurses, but as teachers. However, they found that the people they had come to teach

---

14. Roberta Mayhew West, R.N., *History of Nursing in Pennsylvania* (Philadelphia: Pennsylvania State Nurses' Association, N.D., circa 1932), p. 6.

15. Florence Nightingale, *Notes on Nursing: What It Is and What It Is Not* (New York: D. Appleton and Company, 1860), p. 3.

16. Florence Nightingale, *Notes on Nursing*, p. 3.

17. Catherine Herzel, *On Call: Deaconesses Across the World* (New York: Holt, Rinehart and Winston, Inc., 1961).

needed health care, so they started a hospital and nursed. Others became social workers, but when health needs surfaced, they too became nurses.[18] The deaconesses demonstrated a similar flexibility. Their primary commitment was not to a professional discipline, but to God and service.[19] This strength may have led to the eventual decline of Christian nursing. The pursuit of a "secular order" by Nightingale and the early public health nurses in America gradually became more energized by the optimistic spirit of the age than by Christian commitment.

In the early part of the twentieth century secular nursing was still not clearly defined, but to a large extent nurses became physicians' assistants — a role that still shapes the public image of nursing. In an attempt to provide nursing with a stronger identity, set standards for nursing education, and work toward greater autonomy, nurses began to organize into state and national associations. A body of thoughtful literature began to develop as a growing number of professional nursing journals began publication. These associations and journals became a forum for discussing the nature of nursing. World War II set the stage for increasing activism and assertiveness among nurses. By 1946 the American Nurses Association had plans for the future that included improved working conditions, educational standards with federal subsidies, and increased professional organization.[20]

In 1955 the American Nurses Association approved a definition of nursing practice that was adopted by most state boards of nursing:

> The practice of professional nursing means the performance for compensation of any act in the observation, care, and counsel of the ill, injured, or infirm, or the maintenance of health or prevention of illness of others, or in the supervision and teaching of other personnel, or the administration of medications and treatment as prescribed by a licensed physician or dentist; requiring substantial specialized judgment and skill and based on knowledge and application of the principles of biological, physical, and social science. The foregoing shall not be deemed to include acts of diagnosis or prescription of therapeutic or corrective measures.[21]

18. Suzy Farren, *A Call to Care: The Women Who Built Catholic Healthcare in America* (St. Louis: The Catholic Health Association of the United States, 1996).

19. Rev. C. Golder, *The History of the Deaconess Movement* (Cincinnati: Jennings and Pye, 1903).

20. "Platform for the ANA," *American Journal of Nursing* 46 (11) (November 1946): 729.

21. "ANA Board Approves a Definition of Nursing Practice," *American Journal of Nursing* 55 (12) (December 1955): 1474.

This definition made a clear break with the tradition of volunteer nursing or Christian communities providing care without charge. Professional nursing required compensation. This focus on compensation would become a rising theme. Another significant contrast to the nursing of nuns and deaconesses also occurred. While the nurse's responsibilities of observing, caring, counseling, supervising, and teaching seemed to be a step toward autonomy, the definition engraved the physicians' assistant role into nurse practice acts. Nurses were not allowed to diagnose or treat. Treatments and medications could only be prescribed by a physician.

While the ANA definition remained the legal definition of nursing, the 1950s and 1960s brought a ferment of thinking about the nature of nursing. New definitions began to emerge. They focused more on nursing's uniqueness and less on its subservience to medicine. Virginia Henderson's classic definition of nursing has been ingrained into nurses since 1960, when it was adopted by the International Council of Nurses:

> The unique function of the nurse is to assist the individual, sick or well, in the performance of those activities contributing to health or its recovery (or to peaceful death) that he would perform unaided if he had the necessary strength, will or knowledge. And to do this in such a way as to help him gain independence as rapidly as possible.[22]

Most nurses feel this definition in their gut. It identifies who they are, what they are concerned about and what they do. It also allows for an increasing sense of self-sufficiency.

All of these early definitions focus on maintaining and restoring health to the individual and assume a positive direction toward health (or peaceful death). However, by 1980 new definitions began to proliferate. Some of them were based on radically different understandings of nursing concepts. The American Nurses Association's 1980 *Nursing: A Social Policy Statement* definition did not even articulate the promotion of human health as the goal of nursing care.[23] The statement defined nursing as the "diagnosis and treatment of human responses to actual and potential health problems."[24] As such, it was an attempt to

---

22. Virginia A. Henderson, *Basic Principles of Nursing Care* (London: International Council of Nurses, 1961), p. 42.

23. Rozella M. Schlotfeldt, R.N., Ph.D., F.A.A.N., "Defining Nursing: A Historic Controversy," *Nursing Research* 36 (1) (January-February 1987): 64-67.

24. American Nurses Association, *Nursing: A Social Policy Statement* (Kansas City: American Nurses Association, 1980). According to Donna Diers, "What Is Nursing?" in

wangle around the prohibitions against diagnosing and treating disease in nurse practice acts.

In response to protests about the lack of focus in the 1980 definition, the 1995 revision of this statement maintains the original wording, but adds that more recent definitions "frequently acknowledge four essential features of contemporary nursing practice:"

- attention to the full range of human experiences and responses to health and illness without restriction to a problem-focused orientation;
- integration of objective data with knowledge gained from an understanding of the patient or group's subjective experience;
- application of scientific knowledge to the processes of diagnosis and treatment; and,
- provision of a caring relationship that facilitates health and healing.[25]

This revision also states that "nurses intervene to promote health, prevent illness, or assist with activities that contribute to recovery from illness or to achieving a peaceful death."[26] Although this definition seems more in line with Florence Nightingale's, nursing is no longer the calling of every woman. It is a "scientific discipline as well as a profession"[27] that requires education (with a baccalaureate degree recommended) and national examination for licensure. Furthermore, this definition takes a bolder step toward the issue of diagnosing and treating. However, its scope of practice remains fuzzy, with a "flexible boundary that is responsive to the changing needs of society and the expanding knowledge base of its theoretical and scientific domains."[28]

Nurse practice acts in most states now permit advanced-practice nurses to make simple diagnoses and prescribe certain classes of drugs,

---

Joanne Comi McCloskey and Helen Kennedy Grace, (eds.), *Current Issues in Nursing* (St. Louis: Mosby, 1997), pp. 6-7, this wording was first adopted by the New York State Nurses Association in 1976 on the recommendation of their counsel that "the diagnostic privilege was the *sine qua non* of independent practice." This, then, set off the nursing diagnosis movement with its attempt to establish a unique taxonomy for nursing. The whole process was essentially a political movement to separate nursing from medicine.

25. American Nurses Association, *Nursing: A Social Policy Statement* (Kansas City: American Nurses Association, 1995), p. 6.

26. *Nursing: A Social Policy Statement* (1995), p. 13.

27. *Nursing: A Social Policy Statement* (1995), p. 7.

28. *Nursing: A Social Policy Statement* (1995), p. 12.

further blurring the line between nursing and medicine.[29] Nurses can practice independently, own and manage extended care facilities, establish their own companies to deliver care and receive compensation from third party payers. Insurance companies now hire nurses as case managers with the authority to grant or deny reimbursements for physician-ordered medications and treatments.

The current upheaval in health care delivery, and nursing's frantic scrambling to redefine itself in order to advance (or even survive), present us with an open opportunity to reassess where nursing has come and to determine where it should go. To do so, we need to back up and look at nursing from a Christian worldview. Reacting from the midst of the whirlwind and jumping on the current trends without thoughtful examination could prove disastrous for nursing. Many of today's trends are contradictory, and lead to fragmentation of the profession. For example, while there is tremendous push for more education (nursing masters and doctorates), most of the bedside care is provided by those with less education (institutional training and associate degrees). Nurses are gaining more of that long-sought autonomy (advanced practice, community health, entrepreneurship), but they are becoming more isolated and alienated from one another in the process. Although parish nursing brings nursing back into the church, the churches increasingly find their funding through health care conglomerates, which then maintain the continuing education and supervision of the nurses.

Defining Christian Nursing

Just what is *Christian* nursing? How do we gain the perspective needed to define it? Many contemporary nursing leaders (and theologians) are saying that we are defined by our stories. To some degree, this is valid. Throughout nursing history we can catch a glimpse of what Patricia Donahue calls the *nursing impulse,* a uniting of "the head, the heart, and the hands" to nurture health and overcome disease.[30] However, there are also low points and digressions in the story of nursing that should not be incorporated into nursing's identity. Rather, nurses need to repent of willfulness and neglect, and turn again to Jesus Christ for a vision of nursing.

29. "More Power to the Nurses," *Chicago Tribune,* Monday, April 14, 1997.
30. M. Patricia Donahue, *Nursing: The Finest Art,* 2d ed. St. Louis: Mosby-Year Book, 1996), pp. 2-7.

Instead of looking primarily to nursing history, or even current practice, to find nursing's true story, we must begin with God's story in the Scriptures, for that is where Christian nursing began. However, consulting a concordance and Bible dictionary, one will not find much about nurses or nursing per se. The term *nurse* in the Bible implied a woman who fed and cared for infants and young children, not today's professional role. However, health care figured prominently in the life and teachings of Jesus. He healed the sick, cared for the poor and oppressed, sought out those that society rejected, and instructed his followers to go and do likewise. After Jesus' death and resurrection, health care — including the physical, psychosocial, and spiritual dimensions — became the concern of the whole church.

Several characteristics of Christian nursing stand out from the Scriptures. First, nursing is a response to God's grace and flows from a dynamic personal relationship with God. Second, it is a ministry of the church and functions in the context of the body of Christ. Third, it recognizes the role of sin in a world created good and seeks to restore justice and righteousness. Fourth, it views the person as created in the image of God. Fifth, it works toward the goal of *shalom* as ultimate health. Sixth, it is demonstrated in compassionate care that is characterized by the fruit of the Spirit. These characteristics, and a theological understanding of the concepts in the nursing paradigm, will help us to both define nursing and shape the future of nursing practice.

Based on these considerations, Christian nursing can be defined as *a ministry of compassionate care for the whole person, in response to God's grace toward a sinful world, which aims to foster optimum health (shalom) and bring comfort in suffering and death for anyone in need.*

A Ministry

Ministry in the New Testament and the early church was understood to be the work of every Christian. The Greek term translated as ministry, *diakonia*, essentially means service. It incorporates everything from preaching the gospel to waiting on tables and delivering relief to the poor. Jesus demonstrated this spirit of service by washing his disciples' feet, then telling them to follow his example (John 13). In fact, the term *diakonos* (servant) is often used synonymously with *doulos* (slave). When Jesus' disciples began to seek power and privilege, he told them: "It is not so among you; but whoever wishes to become great among you must be your servant, and whoever wishes to be first among you must be slave of all" (Mark 10:43-44).

The ministry of nursing is servant work. Sometimes it is dirty work like washing feet and emptying bedpans. It is the visiting nurse who returns on her day off to clean a patient's apartment, or buys dressings for another who cannot afford them. It is the critical care nurse who pulls double shifts to cover for a sick colleague. It is the nurse practitioner who gives up a lucrative position to work in an inner-city clinic that pays him less than he made before his advanced-practice certification. It is the nursing instructor who spends extra hours encouraging and counseling students. It is the nursing leader who pours tremendous time and energy into serving on a professional organization's task force to develop documents that will shape the future of nursing. It is the nurse who gets involved in the political system to work for justice in health delivery.

To a large extent these servant-nurses remain unheralded and invisible.[31] That is not a problem, though, because their fulfillment comes not from who sees them but from whom they ultimately serve. They are servants of the Lord Jesus Christ, who has reminded them, "I do not call you servants any longer, because the servant does not know what the master is doing; but I have called you friends, because I have made known to you everything that I have heard from my Father" (John 15:15).

Today, when nurses are clamoring for autonomy, we have to recognize that Christian nursing is never an autonomous role. The Christian nurse functions as part of the body of Christ and is always accountable to the church (even when in secular employment). Because health care is the concern of the whole church, the boundaries of nursing's ministry will always remain fuzzy.

As we have seen, the history of nursing and compassionate health care has been intricately interwoven with church history until fairly recently. It was when nursing moved away from its association with the church that it degenerated into an independent profit-making scheme practiced by the Sairey Gamps of Charles Dickens's day. We are seeing a

---

31. Journalist Suzanne Gordon presents some interesting suggestions about this problem of invisibility in "What Nurses Stand For," *The Atlantic Monthly* 279 (2), February 1997, p. 88. "Because nurses observe and cushion what the physician and writer Oliver Sacks has called human beings' falling 'radically into sickness,' they are a reminder of the pain, fear, vulnerability, and loss of control that adults find difficult to tolerate and thus to discuss. . . . [Nurses] are our secret sharers. Even though they are our lifeline during illness, when control is restored the residue of our anxiety and mortality clings to them like dust, and we flee the memory."

similar decline today as hospitals and extended care facilities, which were once church owned and operated, have become dependent on federal funds, and then on conglomerate buyouts, simply to survive.

If nursing is a part of the body of Christ that has been particularly gifted with the ability and responsibility to care for the health needs of others, then one of its primary roles must be to awaken the church to its mission of healing. Jesus sent out his followers in Luke 10:8-9, saying: "Whenever you enter a town and its people welcome you . . . cure the sick who are there, and say to them, 'The kingdom of God has come near to you.'" Proclamation is only part of Jesus' commission. Demonstration of the gospel through compassionate health care is the other part.

Compassionate Care

Jesus gave the most comprehensive description of compassionate care when he told the story of the Good Samaritan in Luke 10:30-35:

> A man was going down from Jerusalem to Jericho, and fell into the hands of robbers, who stripped him, beat him, and went away, leaving him half dead. . . . But a Samaritan while traveling came near him; and when he saw him, he was moved with pity. He went to him and bandaged his wounds, having poured oil and wine on them. Then he put him on his own animal, brought him to an inn, and took care of him. The next day he took out two denarii, gave them to the innkeeper, and said, "Take care of him; and when I come back, I will repay you whatever more you spend."

The Samaritan in this story had no legal responsibility to stop and help. Two religious leaders had already passed by the wounded man without getting involved. The man could have been a ruse set up by the robbers in order to claim another victim. Yet the Samaritan pitied the man and risked his own welfare to intervene, using his own limited supplies. Furthermore, he took his patient to an inn and stayed with him as long as he could, then provided for continuity of care after he left.

Christian caring is not just an emotional tug, intellectual concept, or metaphysical event. It is hands-on, patient-centered physical, psychosocial, and spiritual intervention to meet the needs of a patient *regardless of how the nurse feels*. Nurses' skill in caring develops as they receive care from others, and ultimately as they grow in their understanding and acceptance of God's care for them. Caring is an act of faith, for it involves the risk of opening oneself to another who may not want to care or be cared for. But unless nurses take that risk they cannot claim to be truly nursing.

For the Whole Person

Christian nursing is holistic, caring for the person in all the interrelated dimensions — physical, psychosocial, and spiritual. In fact, Christian nurses know that ultimate healing cannot occur unless patients are placed in the hands of Jesus, the Great Physician (Isa. 53:5).

In Response to God's Grace toward a Sinful World

The motivation for Christian nursing comes primarily from a sense of gratitude to God, not merely a reaction to human need or a sense of duty (although they, too, flow naturally from a grateful heart). Nurses can say, with the apostle John, "We love, because he [God] first loved us" (1 John 4:19). The contrast between gratitude and duty results primarily in a difference in attitude and approach. Nurses who care out of a sense of gratitude for what God has done for them can view patients as persons of great value, worthy of respect, interest, and attention. When nurses care out of a sense of duty, patients become objects. Nurses do what they have to do and get out.

Even as Christian nurses care out of a sense of gratitude, there is always a sense that God is still working on them, making them more like Christ (2 Cor. 3:18). They do not always care in the way they would like to care. Sometimes only a sense of duty enables them to press on. They humbly struggle with their own sinfulness, their inability to truly care, and draw their strength from him (Phil. 4:13).

Aims to Foster Optimum Health

Health is being able to live as God created us to be — as an integrated whole, living in loving relationship with God, self, and others (Ps. 16). It is dependent on the cross and resurrection of Jesus Christ (Isa. 53:5, 1 Pet. 2:24). Health is central to the Old Testament concept of *shalom* (Ps. 38:3, Jer. 33:6) and the New Testament understanding of *salvation*

(Luke 18:42). Healing results in praise to God and restoration to the believing community, not mere improvement in physical functioning.

Health cannot be separated into isolated compartments, and neither can nursing care. We deceive ourselves to think that nurses can care only for physical needs while ignoring the emotional, spiritual, and social needs of their patients. If nurses are concerned only for the mechanical functioning of the body, they would do better as pure scientists or car mechanics. On the other hand, nurses cannot fully meet the health needs of anyone while ignoring physical needs. Pastors and counselors focus on the spiritual and emotional components of health, but nurses incorporate all dimensions. They need not duplicate the services of other members of the health care team, but they function as coordinators of care, making referrals, communicating across the disciplines, and keeping the whole person in view.

The presence of sin in the world, and the predilection of each person to sin, impinge on health spiritually, physically, and psychosocially (Exod. 20:5, Ps. 32:3-4, Luke 5:17-25). Physical or psychosocial dysfunction can also cause spiritual distress (Job 16:7-9, Pss. 13, 22). Nurses stand in a unique position to assess the interrelationship between these dimensions. The intimacy required in caring for the body often leads patients to be more open in sharing emotional and spiritual concerns. For example, a woman who feels guilt over a past abortion may feel freer to confess her sense of guilt to the nurse who already knows her medical history, than to a pastor whom she perceives as "too holy" to understand. A man with bleeding ulcers may be able to tell a nurse about his anger toward his son, or his alcohol binges, but hesitate to seek professional counseling.

While God's ultimate plan for us is complete health, a person can be spiritually healthy when physically or psychosocially limited (2 Cor. 11:7-9, 1 Cor. 1:27-29). Consider the wheelchair-bound woman with multiple sclerosis who loves life, continues to care for her children, cook and clean, and teach a Sunday school class of rambunctious five-year-olds each week. Public figures such as author, speaker, and radio personality Joni Eareckson Tada and baseball player Dave Dravecki demonstrate health in the midst of physical limitation. They have turned their serious disabilities into an opportunity for ministry. Another example of health would be the young adult with Down's syndrome who cheerfully serves as a church greeter, handing out worship programs and hugs to people at the door.

Nursing works toward the healing of the whole person in the context of communities. This broad understanding of health — *shalom* — is the goal of nursing. Furthermore, it is the goal of the entire Christian community and a sign of the kingdom of God (Rev. 21:1-7). Within that broader view of health, nursing finds a unique place in keeping people healthy, holistically intervening to restore health, and enabling the body of Christ and the health care system to work together toward healing.

Comfort in Suffering and Death

Optimal health means enabling people to live as fully as possible while they are alive. However, despite increasing lifespans in many countries, we are mortal beings; the human death rate is still 100 percent. We live in a world that has been corrupted by the effects of sin. Not all patients will get well. Some may live with severe physical and mental limitations due to brain damage, loss of limbs, suppressed immune systems, or other conditions. Those with degenerative diseases may experience remissions, but the course of the illness causes their bodies, and often their minds, to deteriorate. If health is the only aim in nursing, nurses can only feel futility and despair in the face of these conditions. Christian nursing means providing comfort, hope, and compassionate presence for those who are suffering and will not recover. As two hospice nurses explain,

> Caring requires a commitment . . . and a willingness to do the unlovely. Neither education nor experience quite prepare you for doing the unlovely. . . . Caring demands listening and observing with your whole person. . . . To care means to be trustworthy. . . . Caring is costly. It takes a great amount of physical, emotional, and spiritual energy.[32]

For Anyone in Need

A willingness to do the unlovely entails a willingness to care for the unlovely, whoever they are. Even the "least of these" (Matt. 25:20) are included in those whom Jesus would have us serve. As long as the dying are living, as long as the suffering are surviving, Christian nursing will endeavor to meet their needs.

How can nurses keep going when they cannot see physical improve-

32. Roberta Lyder Paige and Jane Finkbiner Looney, "Hospice Care for the Advanced Cancer Patient," *American Journal of Nursing* 77 (11) (November 1977): 1813-15.

ment? Many in our society believe that the answer lies in ending the suffering by terminating life, but Christian nurses are not free to participate in active euthanasia. Only God has the authority to determine when a person should die. Nurses can provide those who are suffering with comfort by keeping them clean, controlling their pain, and turning and positioning them. Nurses can advocate for discontinuing futile heroics and unnecessary painful treatments. Nurses can stay with patients, surround them with peace and beauty, facilitate relationships with their loved ones, encourage them spiritually, and walk with them through the valley of the shadow of death — eventually placing their hands into the hands of Jesus for the rest of the journey.

A Work of God

In order to provide that kind of care, nurses need to be walking moment-by-moment with Jesus themselves. He is the only one who can prepare them and sustain them in the face of suffering and death. Otherwise they will be overcome. Death is an enemy with deceptive strategies. It tempts us either to seek it (through suicide or euthanasia) or frantically hold it at bay (through futile heroics or placing hope in miracle cures). Only in Christ can nurses find realistic hope in the face of suffering and death, and the depth of character needed to provide compassionate accompaniment when hope for recovery is gone.

Based on the hope given in Christ Jesus and the presence of the Holy Spirit, Christian nursing should be characterized by love, joy, peace, patience, kindness, goodness, faithfulness, gentleness, and self-control (Gal. 5:22). This "fruit of the Spirit" results from a dynamic, personal relationship with God through Jesus Christ. Nurses cannot work it up on their own. The fruit develops as they put their faith into practice. When they do not feel loving, they act lovingly anyhow. Eventually, the feelings will catch up with their actions. Joy and peace do not come naturally, especially in a chaotic working environment where staff do not trust or respect each other. However, by focusing on Jesus, nurses can begin to see God at work in difficult situations. Joy and peace grow in the light of eternity. Patience, kindness, goodness, faithfulness, gentleness, and self-control sound like characteristics of the ideal nurse. They also come with practice, refined in the furnace of difficult patients, substance-abusing nurse managers, surly nursing assistants, arrogant physicians, and dieticians who cannot seem to get their orders straight.

The common theme in all these aspects of Christian nursing is the glory of God. Nurses, committed to Jesus Christ, holistically caring for the sick, the poor, and the needy, demonstrate the character of God to the world. They bring the light of Christ into dark situations, with humility, love, passion, and power.

When asked to summarize his theology, the eminent theologian Karl Barth is said to have replied, "Jesus loves me this I know, for the Bible tells me so." In the face of a complicated technological society and an uncertain future, Christian nurses might do well to stick with such a basic assertion. God's love, demonstrated in the person of Jesus Christ and recorded in the Bible, certainly provides the heart of a theology of nursing.

Because God's love is active and empowering, nursing must also be practical and dynamic. Knowing God's love impels nurses to care for anyone in need, as it has inspired nurses for the past 2,000 years. Nursing demonstrates God's love in a ministry of compassionate care for the whole person. It aims to foster optimum health and bring comfort in suffering and death. The health toward which nurses strive is part of the greater work of God in his people to bring completeness, soundness, and well-being *(shalom)* to the total person — in relationship to God, self, others, and the environment. Nursing is a work of God's grace. Nurses are privileged to share in that work.[33]

33. An expansion of this discussion will soon be available in Judith Allen Shelly and Arlene Miller, *Called to Care: A Christian Theology of Nursing* (tentative title), forthcoming from InterVarsity Press.

Broadening Our View of Justice in Health Care

Sondra Ely Wheeler, Ph.D.

Medical ethics often sounds like something that was dreamed up very recently. That is because most of us encounter it chiefly through whatever current controversy is making headlines. We read in the paper about the dilemmas of selective reduction by abortion of multiple pregnancies which resulted from the use of drugs to stimulate ovulation. We find articles in popular magazines about genetic testing and genetic therapies, and even about therapeutic interventions on tiny patients still in the womb. We have also heard much about the possibility of human cloning, with all the fears it raises about genetic engineering techniques being applied to humans in ways that evoke Huxley's *Brave New World*[1] and similar nightmares. Then there is the renewed controversy about physician-assisted suicide (which is just a variation on the active euthanasia debate), as the U.S. Supreme Court has refused to allow two lower courts to void state legislation against assisted suicide.[2] Some states such as Oregon have now legalized or are working to legalize assisted suicide. This issue is in turn a spin-off from (and often confused with) the related questions of when and to what end we should use or forgo advanced life support technologies. All these are questions which have arisen, and could have arisen, only in very recent decades.

1. Aldous Huxley, *Brave New World* (San Francisco: Harper and Row, 1960).
2. United States Supreme Court, in re Ninth Circuit Court of Appeals, Compassion in Dying et al. v. State of Washington, and Second Circuit Court of Appeals, Quill et al. v. Vacco et al.

But in truth, medical ethics is as old as medicine, and in fact substantially older than what we would recognize as medicine, if by "medicine" we mean the modern sense of an empirically-based and measurably successful intervention in human disease and dysfunction for the sake of improving health. Long ago when surgeons were still doubling as barbers, and still being paid in chickens (Socrates, on his execution, is reported to have left instructions to pay a rooster to his faithful physician); back when people had a slightly better statistical chance of recovering if they could *not* afford a doctor, there was already extensive instruction and reflection (and substantial debate) about the obligations of doctors and the nature of the relationship between doctor and patient.

A Moral View of Medicine

Perhaps the antiquity of this body of reflection and teaching, some of which is captured in the original Hippocratic Oath and its modern variants, helps to explain the power of a certain moral view of medicine which we as a society continue to honor even as we recognize that it is being pressed out of existence. This is the model which sees the relationship between doctor and patient as a relationship of personal trust and individual loyalty. This is the view presupposed in those discussions which speak of the "covenant" between doctor and patient.[3] According to this conception, adapted from the Old Testament account of God's relation to Israel, the physician stands in a fiduciary relationship with patients, as one entrusted with responsibility for their well-being. According to this model, justice is done when the doctor rightly fulfills her or his responsibility to act as a patient's benefactor, protector, and advocate.

Both for its theological grounding and for its exalted picture of the virtue of human fidelity, this is a very attractive picture, and one that continues to instruct us. But it would be a mistake to imagine that this model of health care, and the delivery system that has embodied it, does not have its own structural problems and characteristic failures. To begin with, health care in this view is highly individualistic, considering the doctor/patient relationship to be essentially dyadic. The physician is left to determine the patient's interests largely on his or her own, although based on broad standards of practice. On the other side, the patient and

3. William F. May, *The Physician's Covenant* (Philadelphia: Westminster Press, 1983).

her or his interests are thought of in isolation from the other people and relationships which make up the context of human life, and provide so much of the content to our experiences of illness and recovery. Such a model can distort or obscure crucial dimensions of what is at stake for both patients and providers in the giving and receiving of care.

With its focus on individual doctors and patients, this understanding of health care may also be characterized as privatized, that is, the physician is seen as a separate actor and the patient as a single recipient of care. The work of the physician is not seen as representative of a broad social ethos, nor is medicine seen as a social enterprise relying on the contributions of all members of the society or directed toward a well-being in which all have a stake. This individual and private construction of caregiving might be unproblematic in some contexts. Indeed, it has the strength of emphasis upon the personal nature of health care and the human particularity of both doctor and patient. But what the model makes invisible is still a reality. Under the fiduciary and covenantal moral model of health care, despite its appeal, there is a rationing of access to care using the blunt instrument of who can afford to see a doctor. Another level of selectivity occurs when doctors simply do not prescribe modes of treatment for which a particular patient lacks the resources.

The edges of this *de facto* rationing have been softened by personal and community connections some of the time, as physicians have provided free care for members of their communities who could not pay for needed treatment. But optimal treatment has not been provided universally under this model any more than under alternative constructs. The poor have been and continue to be under-treated. Similarly, there have always been incentives toward, and instances of, corruptions of this version of the doctor-patient relationship — for example, in the prescribing of unnecessary drugs and procedures and in unjustified paternalism. The weaknesses of this personalized moral model are simply the obverse of its strengths. It depends on the quality of personal, professional relationship as the mediator of justice. And the focus of care is narrowed to the patient at hand in contrast to other actual or potential patients. Nonetheless, both physicians in their training and patients in their understanding of what they do when they seek treatment frequently still operate under this picture of the doctor as a personal caregiver, committed to the individual patient's welfare above and in spite of every other thing.

The Effects of Changes in Health Care Financing

In the decades of the 1930s and 1940s, health care financing in this country moved from almost exclusively private fee-for-service arrangements to include various types of health insurance. The landscape was permanently reshaped by newly created social insurances of Medicare, Medicaid, and Veterans' benefits, and by the proliferation in the 1950s and thereafter of the private health insurance market that was part of the growth and ascendency of corporations. During this historical transition, the ethical model for practice and the moral assumptions that accompanied it did not change very much. But the realities underlying the delivery system, and the constraints operating within it, changed quite a bit. Now we had insurance companies deciding (not without medical advice, but obviously with nonmedical agendas) what was a normal and appropriate "standard of care," and what was "extreme" or "experimental" or "not indicated." The same companies exerted direct pressure on the cost of treatment as well, by determining what could be reimbursed for a particular service in a given region. Even more fundamentally, with the rise of health insurance the basis for assessment of appropriate treatment shifted from individual to group, mediated by actuarial analysis of costs, risks, and distribution of need. This is a crucial shift in the meaning and determinants of justice. But much of this was hidden, and most of it passed without serious public comment or debate, or even public recognition. We still went to our doctors, handed over our Blue Cross cards or whatever, the doctor (usually it was a he) decided what treatment was indicated, and that — as far as we were concerned — was that.

But in fact that wasn't that, as the faster-than-inflation rate of health care cost increases soon made clear. Suddenly, starting about 20 years ago, the cost and terms of health insurance were on the table in employer-employee struggles over contracts and compensation. Complaints began to be heard about what insurance companies would or would not cover, and whom they would or would not accept as a subscriber. At about the same time, universities, large employers, and others responsible for the health care of large groups began to find it cheaper and more efficient to manage their own primary health care professionals and facilities, with out-referencing as necessary for special needs. The pressure of institutions to meet and control the costs of the health care they needed to provide for employees or student populations led to the development of health maintenance organizations and other managed care plans.

These innovations in financing and delivery systems achieved many of their aims. In those initial settings, membership in the sponsoring institution determined coverage, and a covered population of full-time active employees and full-time college students ensured a relatively young and healthy group upon which to practice the principles of health maintenance: preventive medicine and early intervention. Per capita costs went down, and patient satisfaction was generally high. But immediately there was a different kind of rub, as physicians began to chafe at being expected to see more patients per hour, and to account for their time and their prescriptions and the tests they ordered. Already there was a new layer of management accountability where diagnostic and treatment decisions were questioned not by other physicians, but by administrators and financial officers. This, some practitioners felt, was an intrusion into the practice of medicine itself, and it affected not only their professional autonomy but the quality of care.

More fundamentally, it created moral confusion and ambiguity as it placed doctors and other providers of health care in a situation where their loyalties and responsibilities were divided, and their internalized norms regarding the moral practice of medicine could not be applied without revision. On the one hand, they still had the privileged relationship with patients and the duties it entailed; on the other, those patients tended to come and go rather quickly as their relationship with the sponsoring entity was often temporary. For caregivers, their "employer" was no longer the set of patients who constituted their practice; now it was Yale University or Community Health Care Inc., and that employer could place constraints on what care was delivered to whom — demands that doctors and nurses had to meet. When those demands conflicted with what the providers thought of as appropriate care and professional conduct, it created tensions and moral crises for medical staff. Barbara White has vividly delineated how acute and how pressing these can become.[4] The old understanding of justice as the fulfillment of a fiduciary relationship between an individual patient and her or his physician was under assault.

But tempting as it is to regard this straightforwardly as the intrusion of crass financial concerns into the pure moral realm of medical practice, this is not an adequate construal of the problem. Remember that HMOs and managed care operations arose because of a significant degree of failure of the old system. A system of health care in which an ever-shrinking proportion of relatively affluent citizens can afford a dedicated personal

4. See Barbara White's essay earlier in this volume.

physician to protect their interests is not necessarily more just than one in which more people have access to more limited forms of health care. There has always been a mechanism for distribution. Large-scale funding decisions (macro-allocation) have always directly or indirectly affected small-scale possibilities (micro-allocation), such as whether Aunt Lily gets her hip replacement. The rise of managed care and the development of for-profit hospitals have just made more direct and more visible (and thus more open to scrutiny) a set of moral and social problems endemic to the application of finite resources to needs that outstrip them.

In addition, a concern for the economic viability of institutions that provide health care is itself a moral concern. When public hospitals are forced to close because they lack operating funds, poor and vulnerable populations in already under-served areas have that much less recourse for treatment. The bankruptcy of San Francisco General is a moral disaster as well as a fiscal problem. In asserting our ethic of care we cannot wash our hands of questions about what care we can afford to give and how we will pay for it. But as more and more diverse groups of citizens have moved under the umbrella of managed care (a trend that is bound to continue as we experiment with HMOs for Medicare patients), the difficulty and the moral ambiguity of the allocation and access decisions these systems will have to confront have become ever more apparent. The question is not *whether* we as a society will make painful and difficult allocation decisions, including decisions to deny care that might be beneficial in order to provide some other care to someone else. The question is *who* will make them, and *how* will they be made? According to what version of justice will they be made and defended? It is here that Christian convictions and the understanding of justice that they shape have an important and distinctive contribution to make, both to the moral formation of Christian health care professionals and administrators, and to the wider public discussion.[5]

Biblical Justice

The general theological foundations of justice in Christian thought are threefold. First there is the lordship of God over all of creation, and God's

---

5. An excellent and illuminating discussion of this necessity, and Christian theological warrants for addressing it, are found in Hessel Bouma III et al., *Christian Faith, Health and Medical Practice* (Grand Rapids: Eerdmans, 1989), ch. 6.

claim of final ownership of all the material resources over which we exercise stewardship. Thus God's will for the distribution of the means of life is the ultimate ground of justice.[6] Second there is the basic equality and dignity of every human being, founded in their common origin and their shared status as the bearers of God's image and the subjects of God's care.[7] Thus every person as a matter of justice has claims to freedom from attack, to fair treatment, and to an equitable share of the resources which God provides for the well-being of all. Third there is the gospel's demand that our treatment of one another imitate and reflect the graciousness of God toward us, revealed preeminently in the redemptive grace of Jesus Christ. Our understanding of what we owe to one another is decisively shaped by our consciousness of the enormous debt in which we all stand before God.[8] The Christian idea of justice is rooted firmly in the biblical story which forms the church. And that has a marked effect on what versions of justice Christians can embrace.[9]

Whereas individualism and privatism characterized the traditional understandings of justice in medical care, the biblical picture of human life is social at its very heart.[10] The human person comes into being already in relation, and all dimensions of moral life including the individual's relationship with God are seen in terms of their impact upon a community. Justice as described in the Old Testament is thus a feature of interpersonal relationships, and includes such obligations as truthfulness, fair-dealing, and the avoidance of harm, as well as positive duties like loyalty and gratitude. Justice is also, however, a feature of much broader social relationships and of the structures that mediate and regu-

6. For a rhetorically fierce account of the implications of God's ownership for human obligations regarding the distribution of goods, see John Wesley's 1781 sermon, "The Danger of Increasing Riches," in *John Wesley's Sermons: An Anthology*, ed. Outler and Heitzenreiter (Nashville: Abingdon Press, 1991).

7. This foundation for Christian understandings of justice is particularly prominent in the tradition of Catholic social teaching. For a succinct expression, see the pastoral letter on the U.S. economy, *Economic Justice for All*, ch. 2 (Washington, D.C.: USCC, 1986).

8. A particularly eloquent discussion is found in Francis Young and David Ford, *Meaning of Truth in Second Corinthians* (Cambridge: Cambridge University Press, 1987), pp. 166ff.

9. Which is not to say that there is one vision of justice upon which all Christians agree. See, for example, Karen Lebacqz, *Six Theories of Justice* (Minneapolis: Augsburg Press, 1986), which includes three distinct views with Christian theological foundations.

10. On the communal foundation of morality in the Old Testament, see Bruce Birch, *Let Justice Roll Down* (Philadelphia: Westminster/John Knox Press, 1991), ch. 5. Regarding the communal address and locus of New Testament ethics, a useful brief statement can be found in R. B. Hays, *The Moral Vision of the New Testament* (San Francisco: Harper and Row, 1996), pp. 196-97.

late them. The prophets rail against the acts of individuals in using fraudulent weights and measures or accepting bribes, but they also condemn broad social and economic practices. Covenant law constrains such things as lending at interest, keeping garments in pledge for debts, and the complete harvesting of produce. Even such legally permissible activities as acquiring mortgaged farms when their owners fall into hardship are condemned as unjust and contrary to God's will for righteousness and equity. This is the context of Isaiah's cry, "Woe to those who join house to house and field to field!" (Isa. 5:8). In the end, the prophets declare, the nation of Israel is dragged into exile for two cardinal sins: idolatry, and failing to observe the covenant provisions for the support of the poor and the vulnerable.[11]

Thus the Old Testament condemns not only the unjust acquisition of goods and their use for unjust purposes such as subverting judicial proceedings. It also condemns great disparities in distribution and decries ignoring the dire needs of the poor as a violation of God's will. These are an offense against God's continued claim upon the goods of the earth intended for the support of all. All of this exerts a powerful egalitarian pressure upon the concept of justice and makes it clear that justice concerns not only the elimination of force and fraud, but also the provision of basic needs on an equitable footing.

The New Testament continues this tradition. If anything, the demand for universal attention to human need is intensified as one of the hallmarks of the Messianic age. In particular, the physical needs of strangers and enemies are to be provided for as a sign of the universal love of God, and the care of the sick is expressly one of the tests by which fidelity to the Kingdom is to be judged. To put it a little more provocatively, those of us who present ourselves as beggars at God's door, asking for a mercy we have no claim on, had better be very careful about how we respond to the beggars at our own doors, whether at home or in the hospital. Overall, the Bible makes it clear that equity in treatment, procedural equality, and just distribution of life's necessities are all aspects of God's reign over the world, and are obligatory for God's people.[12] What does such a tradition about the meaning and the scope of justice do to shape Christian reflection about the meaning of justice in health care?

11. For a treatment of the Old Testament understanding of justice, see Birch, *Let Justice Roll Down*, pp. 153-82.

12. An excellent overall discussion is Stephen Mott, *Biblical Ethics and Social Change* (New York: Oxford University Press, 1982), ch. 4.

Justice in Health Care

All discussions of justice in health care in the United States must founder on the reality that, nearly alone among the industrialized nations of the world, the United States does not provide universal access to basic health care for all its citizens. Every other mention of just policies and equitable procedures for providing treatment must be qualified by the acknowledgment that millions of Americans have little or no recourse for treatment unless they reach a public hospital in a condition so poor that death is imminent without care.[13] The unlucky ones die anyway; the others get whatever treatment the hospital can afford to give them and are released as soon as their condition is stable. The fact of those excluded from the U.S. health care system hangs like a shadow over all subsequent discussion of what constitutes just treatment for those who make it in the door. There is no theoretical answer to this problem, because the lack of universal health care is not a problem of theory, but one of political will in this democracy. In the absence of a readiness to pursue this difficult social and political goal, all discussions of justice in health care have a touch of unreality about them.

Nevertheless, most people in the more developed nations, including the U.S., *are* insured through one mechanism or another. Most have access to basic care or more. However, questions remain about how we allocate the resources we have among the patients we do treat. What are justifiable bases on which such decisions can be made?

In sketching the history that has brought us to our present quandaries, I have tried to suggest that economic viability and efficient distribution of resources are themselves moral concerns, matters of moral prudence and responsible stewardship. But this raises a basic question: How do we pay attention to those things without violating each other's trust in the seeking and giving of care? We have noted the narrow focus of the traditional model of justice in health care, which ignores the broader social dimensions of justice to focus only on the interpersonal dimensions. But this too raises a question: How do we widen the scope of our concerns from the doctor-patient dyad without abusing the intimacy and power of the privileged relationship between physician and patient?

Our first task is a conceptual one. Christian commitment to the

---

13. Estimates of the uninsured range from 30 to 40 million citizens. There is also a much larger number of those who have insurance so inadequate that their access to basic care is restricted.

basic equality of all persons compels us to examine our procedures and our standards — to root out as much as we can of the biases and distortions which characterize our culture and deform our own judgment. We live in an age that values economic productivity almost to the exclusion of other goods, in a culture that worships youth and beauty and is prepared to engage in some flat-footedly utilitarian calculus about whose life is worth saving. Against such temptations Christians must declare that *all* persons are cherished by God, and all have an equal intrinsic claim on lifesaving resources.

To honor that equal claim we must distinguish more clearly and reliably between medical and nonmedical criteria for treatment eligibility or for priority in receiving scarce resources. There is, however, some vagueness to the distinction between these two types of criteria, as when candidates for treatment are judged in terms of the quality of benefit or the degree of social support they are likely to receive. Such judgments are not simply clinical, as they cannot be cleanly separated from beliefs about what constitute valuable life activities, or what kinds of relationships represent adequate social support. Because of such ambiguities, using criteria of this kind risks involving us in indefensible judgments about the worth of other people's lives, judgments we have neither the authority nor the wisdom to make. Nevertheless, responsible use of scarce resources requires that they not be wasted. If they cannot provide substantial benefit or be effective in a given situation, justice dictates that they be used elsewhere. This is a way of respecting life by assuring that resources which could be used to save lives are not expended uselessly.

When we are examining criteria for making decisions about which one of several patients receives a life-saving resource, we are addressing micro-allocation. This level of decision-making must be vigorously protected from the crude cost-benefit analysis that is prepared to make an individual's survival contingent on what ultimately comes down to market value: how much their care will cost vs. how much they contribute — which in our society comes down to a rough estimate of their future earning power. It is unsupportable to make comparative judgments about the worth of individual lives the basis for the distribution of treatment, because it is both inimical to the fundamental commitments of medical practice and an offense to God's sole sovereignty over life. We are simply not authorized to make such judgments about one another. Against them stands the warning, "Who are you to judge the servant of another?" (Rom. 14:4).

But this is not to say that all forms of cost-benefit analysis, including

72

cost-effective analysis, are inherently immoral. At the level of macro-allocation, the society decides how much of its research funds to expend in what area, or which kinds of treatment to provide with limited public resources, or how much of its resources to devote to health care as opposed to some other social good such as education or environmental protection. Here it is entirely appropriate to look at what benefits can be expected from a given expenditure: how many lives can be saved or improved, with what degree of certainty, and for how long. Such decisions can be wrenching and difficult, and they certainly constitute judgments which are moral in character. Still, they remain in the broad and general area of social policy. What we must resist is the temptation to make judgments comparing the value of John's life to Mary's. And finally, whatever decisions we may be forced to make in the allocation of resources that are inherently scarce, good palliative care as well as human support and companioning in the face of death is always an obligation. As doctors, as nurses, indeed as Christians, we may never abandon the sick. To do so is to court the fatal judgment of Matthew 25:43, "Depart from me, you accursed . . . for I was sick, and you did not visit me."

Rationing Health Care:
A Case of Justice Denied

Arthur J. Dyck, Ph.D.

Rationing is a practice or policy of intentionally creating scarcity. With respect to health care, rationing is the intentional denial of interventions known to be medically appropriate, beneficial, and available. Typically, this now occurs for the sake of limiting expenditures, and increasingly for the sake of being profitable. An example of rationing to reduce costs was that of routinely limiting women who had given birth to a hospital stay of 24 hours. So egregious and unjust was this practice that the federal government intervened to establish a minimum of 48 hours in the hospital. This is but one of many instances of rationing by for-profit managed health care in the United States, prompting 40 states to pass laws to limit abuses by 1996, and spawning malpractice suits.[1]

Disturbing as this quest for profits may be, one can take no comfort from the practices of governments around the world. The acceptability of rationing has eroded the quality and availability of medical care in countries lauded for providing universal access to health care. In Canada, for example, governments, federal and provincial, do not provide enough money to meet actual medical needs.[2] Waiting lists for care are dangerously long. Emergency care has become scarce enough to result in deaths

---

1. See Janet Michael's essay in this volume.
2. See, for example, B. Brown, "How Canada's Health System Works," *Business and Health* (July 1989): 28-30; and Adam L. Linton, "The Canadian Health Care System: A Canadian Physician's Perspective," *New England Journal of Medicine* 322 (3) (18 January 1990): 197-99.

previously preventable. In Great Britain, individuals over 65 are denied care from which many could benefit.[3] Again, this is done largely because of limits placed on expenditures. Rationing, as a matter of government policy, means that even where access to health care is universal, actual care, including life-saving care, is sometimes denied and sometimes unavailable.

Rationing was also inherent in the health care plan put forward by the Clinton administration. One example of this was the formula proposed to keep all insurance premiums uniformly low. Subsidies for a state like New York, with its considerable populations of needy individuals and groups, would be phased out in five years. In five years, New York was slated to have the same low insurance premiums as a state like North Dakota. During the time health care reform was being advocated in Washington, proposals in the literature generally condoned rationing. Many spoke of guaranteeing some kind of decent minimum of health care.[4] This way of thinking takes for granted that health care should not be exclusively based on medically diagnosed needs. Rather, medical costs should be limited by withholding or making unavailable some medical care, however efficacious. Rationing health care is a direct repudiation of the moral traditions that have guided Western medicine for nearly two thousand years. How could this be happening? Why now? What can and should be done about rationing health care, this new injustice and threat to sustaining a health care ethic worthy of the name?

To address these questions, it is necessary to discuss and analyze: (1) the traditions that undergird the moral imperatives of health care practice; (2) the changes that subvert these moral imperatives; and (3) the practical and ethical alternatives to rationing health care.

Before taking up these topics, a brief word of clarification is in order. Rationing refers only to the deliberate creation of scarcity. Health care resources are otherwise scarce in a number of ways. To accommodate patients, it is routine to schedule appointments for non-emergency care. In a national disaster, or even a single accident, some individuals may die or suffer permanent harm because a sufficient number of physicians and/or nurses and/or medical supplies may not be assembled quickly

---

3. Henry Aaron and William B. Schwartz, "Rationing Health Care: The Choice Before Us," *Science* 247 (26 January 1990): 416-22.

4. See, for example, Tom L. Beauchamp and James F. Childress, *Principles of Biomedical Ethics* (New York: Oxford University Press, 1994); and Norman Daniels, *Am I My Parents' Keeper* (New York: Oxford University Press, 1988).

enough to treat everyone in time. In emergency rooms, those most immediately at risk of dying may have to be treated while others wait. So long as the criteria reflect medical need, such exceptional deviations from queuing do not violate justice, given the unavoidable scarcities involved. None of these practices constitute rationing as I am using the term. It would be a case of rationing if, for example, a hospital administration or legislative body would knowingly underfund and/or understaff emergency care in a particular hospital or region. Now we turn to consider the ethical traditions of medical practice as they arose in the West — traditions from which have emerged some of the most important moral imperatives guiding health care practice.

The Moral Imperatives of Health Care Practice: A Blend of Greek, Jewish, and Christian Traditions

At around the fifth century B.C.E., there is evidence that the healing art began to break with its roots in religious practices. Skilled tradesmen, with growing knowledge and skills to maintain health and cure diseases, offered their services in the marketplace for a fee. Citizens received better services than slaves. Abortion and assisted suicide were widely accepted practices. Excellence in performance was the standard that governed these healers.

At the same time, however, a school of thought and practice developed that bore the name of Hippocrates, a leading physician of that time. Not only did the Hippocratics increase empirical knowledge in medicine but they also developed an explicit medical ethic. Excellent skills were not enough; skills can be used for good or evil. The Hippocratic Oath prohibited abortions and providing poisons to end life, and called upon physicians to be just, avoiding all harms to patients.[5]

Christian physicians adopted this oath, except for the references to the Greek gods, the promise to give medical education only to one's own sons, and the prohibitions against "using the knife."[6] Beyond the Oath, however, Christianity and Judaism significantly changed the moral structure of medical care and of the physician-patient relationship. The Hebrew prophets, as biblically portrayed, healed the sick free of charge. Jesus also healed without charging fees. During that time, some healers did charge

---

5. Stanley J. Reiser, Arthur J. Dyck, and William J. Curran (eds.), *Ethics in Medicine* (Cambridge: MIT Press, 1977), p. 5.

6. *Ethics in Medicine*, p. 10.

for their services. One woman had spent all of her substance seeking a cure. She needed free care desperately, and Jesus graciously obliged her.[7] Additionally, there is the biblical model of the Good Samaritan.[8] He is the good neighbor who takes the half-dead victim of robbers to an inn, giving him care there. Not only does he pay the innkeeper for additional care in his absence, but he also puts no limit on the amount and cost of the care. While paying the innkeeper, the Good Samaritan tells him: "Take care of him; and when I come back, I will repay you whatever more you spend."[9] No cap is put on expenditures; the need for care determines cost. Christian and Jewish physicians made it the norm to treat everyone, however needy and however poor. The marketplace did not dictate practice or intrude into the physician-patient relationship.

Secondly, in accord with biblical traditions, everyone with similar needs was to receive the same treatment. No one was regarded as of less worth. Medical need and medical capabilities, *not money*, were the standards for the care given and who received it.

Justice — that is, what we owe one another as human beings — as applied to medical care, consisted in at least the following moral imperatives: (1) *the responsibility to rescue*, that is, to save human life and to prevent or remove threats to it; (2) *the responsibility to nurture*, that is, to protect human life, health, and well-being; (3) *the responsibility to treat* patients on the basis of medical need and equal worth so that no one needing care fails to receive it, and receives it in the amount and quality needed to benefit the recipient.[10]

As long as these moral imperatives guided medical care as absolute requisites of its proper moral structure, the economic question was one of asking how to pay for medically indicated, beneficial care; moral responsibilities framed the question; money was not to determine what health care, how much of it, and to whom it was provided as increasingly it now does. Some of the current practices of for-profit managed care organizations are putting health care back on the road to the medical marketplace once dominant in ancient Greece when medicine was one business among others. What is driving health care backward down this long abandoned road? What is it that has shifted the imperative to care

7. Luke 8:43-48.

8. Luke 10:25-37.

9. Luke 10:35.

10. For a fuller discussion of justice in the context of providing health care, see chapter 11 in Arthur J. Dyck, *Rethinking Rights and Responsibilities: The Moral Bonds of Community* (Cleveland: Pilgrim Press, 1994).

toward the imperatives to save and make money, and to do it by rationing care? What has changed?

Changes That Tend to Erode the Moral Imperatives of Health Care Practice

There are at least four developments, largely occurring in this century, which have become increasingly pervasive in recent years: (1) third party payers; (2) costly medication and technology; (3) expensive malpractice insurance; and (4) utilitarian reasoning.

1. Third Party Payment Systems

When physicians' fees began to be paid by government and insurance companies, the payers tended to insist on similar costs for similar services. That destroyed the practice of a sliding-fee scale based on individuals' or families' ability to pay. Health care services began to be treated like goods or products. That had at least two unfortunate effects. First, services had to be priced fairly high in order to cover those who needed care but had no insurance or government aid. As the cost of services rose, it became increasingly difficult to provide for those not covered by insurance or government programs.

Secondly, having a third party pay for health care services inadvertently but seriously undermined the physician-patient relationship. When physicians accepted the responsibility to provide care to everyone, including those who could not afford care, they had to know the life situation of their patients and they were dedicated to meet more than the narrowly medical needs of such patients. Absolving the poor of the costs of health care services allowed physicians to help patients meet their other needs. Health care, for example, could mean the difference between retaining or losing the ability to work. At the same time, when the government or an insurance company pays for medical services, patients relate differently to physicians. If someone else is paying for what I ask of a physician, it takes on the character of a claim. When I am paying for a service, I relate to the physician as someone to whom I owe something. I am literally indebted to the physician. The physician is owed a living for laboring on my behalf. In turn, the physician who is not compensated by the patient has much less reason to worry about how much patients themselves can pay but rather how much their insurance companies or government will pay. It is tempting to treat companies and governments as rich, impersonal sources of revenue, and fraud does occur. Add to the mix that time spent in cultivating a physician-patient and nurse-patient relationship is uniformly undervalued and undercompensated by third party payers, and it is not difficult to discern a significant source of erosion in the quality of health care, through the erosion of the relationship of patients to their caregivers. Note, sadly, that patients are now often called *consumers* — signaling a significant departure from what should be a mutually beneficial, morally responsible relationship, characterized by gratitude, mutual respect, and altruism.

2. Costly Medication and Technology

The path from stethoscopes, to x-rays, to the latest imaging techniques is on a steep slope toward higher costs. Drugs are on this same upward slope. Whatever justification may exist for the prices charged and the profits made, those who manufacture what is used as a medical service are not conforming to the traditional moral imperatives of health care: These businesses are not attending to the ability to pay of those who need their services; these businesses do not, as a rule, share their profits with patients or the non-profit hospitals who could then better serve their uninsured or underinsured patients. The burdens of these higher costs are borne, rather, by physicians and hospitals and those who are required to pay ever increasing insurance premiums and social security taxes. Everyone in the business of health care should adopt the tradition of health care ethics that puts the needs of the sick first. By and large, that is not the prevailing norm. Again, a significant change, an erosion, has occurred in the very moral structure of health care.

3. Expensive Malpractice Insurance

It takes little imagination to figure out that the bill for surgery at Massachusetts General Hospital will be far more than most individuals can afford to pay from their own earnings and savings, when, as one surgeon reported to me several years ago, he was paying $80,000 a year for malpractice insurance. Nor will it be easy or generally feasible for such a surgeon to offer free services to those in need of them. Neurosurgeons pay even higher insurance premiums.

Consider also that lawyers charge their clients a percentage of the money recovered from a successful suit. These percentages can be high. The Clinton health plan called for a cap of one-third of the award as a fee for the lawyer's services but no cap on the amount of awards. This mode of payment obviously encourages large awards.

Lawsuits have also led to the mandatory use of expensive diagnostic tests, often in dubious or unwarranted circumstances. And so lawyers join the surging numbers of participants in the health care system who profit greatly from what they do, without adopting, for the most part, the ethic of sharing their gains with patients. I have even heard of an instance in which lawyers took 100 percent of an award because they regarded nothing less as sufficient for their efforts. The client, poor in every respect, still had a hospital bill to pay. Lawyers still do *pro bono* work but the moral imperative behind it has steadily eroded, certainly as it affects the costs of health care. In a recent work, legal scholar Mary Ann Glendon has documented the enormous diminution of one of the major purposes of legal counsel, namely to keep individuals and disputes out of the courts![11]

4. Utilitarian Reasoning

What is most threatening to the traditions that have guided health care practice, shaped its moral structure and the caregiver-patient relationship itself, is a change in the very concept of justice, of what we owe one another as human beings. Ever more pervasively, what counts as justice is being guided by utilitarian reasoning. I refer to the calculation of what ought to be done based on maximizing utility or total welfare. Rights are to be determined by what makes for the greatest good for the greatest number. The worth of life is calculable; whether it is better to live or to die depends upon an assessment of its utility, particularly its ratio of pleasure to pain.[12]

The calculations of utility are presently dominated by monetary considerations. The physician is increasingly called a *gatekeeper* and, as such, is regarded as morally bound to consider the welfare of all patients

11. Mary Ann Glendon, *A Nation Under Lawyers* (New York: Farrar, Straus and Giroux, 1994).

12. For a fuller discussion of utilitarianism, see Arthur J. Dyck, *Rethinking Rights and Responsibilities*, ch. 2.

and of society generally when deciding whether a costly service to a patient ought to be offered, particularly when the physician judges that the chances of saving or extending life appear slim, or the quality of the life preserved appears to be poor. So much for erring on the side of life! So much, also, for a relationship of shared, equal moral responsibilities on the part of both caregivers and patients for rescuing and nurturing individual life. And, if utility is to be maximized — and what has utility includes money — offering free care counts as a net cost rather than a net benefit. Free care drops out as a moral imperative altogether. Maximizing utility also militates against treating the sickest patients in need of the costliest care. So much for the inalienable right to life of every individual. So much for the equal worth of every human being.

All of this lands physicians back in the ancient Greek marketplace functioning as tradesmen, selling their wares. In Greece, physicians tended to send their sickest patients to the temple to have the priests pray for them. Risking failure and engaging in futile efforts could cost the physician customers and money, since some families were reluctant to pay for failure. It is often said that no one can turn back the clock. Nevertheless, for-profit medicine in our day is turning the clock way back in seeking to maximize profits and abandoning the sickest patients. Obviously, the practice of using money as a standard, rather than strict medical need, in effect rations care. The standard of care is no longer based solely on what is needed to heal, sustain, and/or comfort patients. Furthermore, there is no moral imperative to offer free care. When justice is understood as the maximization of utility, prohibiting care that cannot be compensated becomes the moral imperative.

The increased dominance of utilitarian reasoning in medicine, nursing, law, and business is a product of what is taught in educational institutions, including professional schools. Many students learn utilitarian reasoning; few study our biblical heritage, with its concepts of justice and the model of the Good Samaritan. Many of the students who come to study with me have read John Stuart Mill, but not John Calvin or Jonathan Edwards. I remember one student asking me how and where he could be expected to find the biblical passages I had assigned in an ethics course.

Rationing Health Care Is Not Inevitable:
Alternatives to Rationing

With utilitarian reasoning so prevalent, and with the erosion of health care ethics, books advocating rationing as an inevitable, present reality are already being published.[13] But there is no proof, nor are proofs provided, that health care has to be rationed, particularly in this extremely wealthy country. It would in any event only be possible to know whether rationing is necessary if morally justifiable cost savings were first put in place and tried — i.e., savings that do not compromise needed medical care.

One reason given for the necessity of rationing simply extrapolates this from the growth of the amount of money spent in the health care sector. The health care sector has been growing more rapidly than the rate of inflation and will inevitably become unaffordable relative to other required and/or desired goods and services. One set of statistics reads as follows:

- 10 percent of GNP in 1985
- 12 percent of GNP in 1990-91
- 15 percent of GNP in 2000, consisting of 1.5 trillion dollars, 5,000 per capita

The figure of 15 percent of GNP compares, for example, with 22 percent for governmental expenditures for the last few years.[14] In the current situation, these figures seem somewhat inflated; growth has slowed.

But why is growth viewed as a problem? We have the best available health care in the world. For other businesses, such robust employment and income opportunities would be seen as a boon! Consider the automobile industry. One could argue that there are only a finite number of automobiles that can be made, bought, and driven. One could talk of rationing. One could argue, as some now do relative to health care, that price rationing already occurs and some who need cars and public transportation lack both. There are those who call for more public transportation. But for the automobile industry, and industry generally, growth is viewed as positive.

13. Two recent examples are M. A. Hall, *Making Medical Spending Decisions: The Law, Ethics and Economics of Rationing Mechanisms* (New York: Oxford University Press, 1995); and E. H. Morreim, *Balancing Act: The New Medical Ethics of Medicine's New Economics* (Washington, D.C.: Georgetown University Press, 1995).

14. William F. Bridgers, *Health Care Reform* (St. Louis: G. W. Manning, 1992), p. 1.

Make and sell more cars, not less; grow, don't shrink! Why then is the response to growth in health care services now so different? In part, it is because some of our taxes buy health care for others; none of our taxes buy cars for others. But we do not generally notice the tax dollars that support the automobile industry — for example, the maintenance of an elaborate infrastructure including highways. Public transportation is put on a limited budget, the consequences of which are difficult to discern. But when countries cap their budgets for health care, the tragic consequences are immediate and easily documented. Indeed, the quantity and quality of health care services are definitely diminished in such countries relative to what has been achieved in the United States.[15]

Some argue that health care resources are finite while needs are infinite. One can grant that resources may well be finite but so are health care needs; they are not infinite. Most people are relatively healthy. Chronic care is limited as to incidence and duration. Everyone dies! To assert, as some do, that health care needs are infinite and resources finite is a category mistake. The ancient philosopher Zeno once contended that, to move from point 'A' to point 'B', you always have to traverse half the distance first. And before you traverse half of that distance between 'A' and 'B' you have to go half of that distance and so on *ad infinitum*. Therefore, you cannot reach 'B' from 'A', and therefore there is no such thing as motion! That is a category mistake. With respect to health care, the mistake is to treat needs as infinite and then make the obvious inference that finite resources cannot keep pace with them. If, then, there is no proof for the necessity to ration health care, it is unjust to deny care to those who require it.

Admittedly, health care has become very expensive. It is increasingly difficult for working people and employers to afford insurance, and so there are those who lack insurance altogether. Nevertheless, if there are morally justifiable ways to decrease costs without rationing services, and without reducing the quality of care and the growth of our ability to save lives and enhance health, justice requires us to test them. There are indeed at least three kinds of policies that should be tried before anyone should even contemplate rationing health care as necessary: (1) altering practices that drive up the cost of medical care; (2) promoting moral development and spiritual renewal; and (3) preserving and renewing the moral structure guiding health care.

15. Uwe E. Reinhardt, "Health Insurance for the Nation's Poor," *Health Affairs* (Spring 1987): 101-12.

1. Altering Practices That Drive Up the Cost of Health Care

In the spring of 1993, while the Clinton health care reform package was being secretly prepared without the input of former Surgeon General C. Everett Koop, Dr. Koop suggested the following ways to save money without in any way diminishing the quality or quantity of health care, and without changing its traditional moral structure:

(a) offering tax credits for reducing the administrative expenses of insurance companies, saving 100 billion dollars;
(b) conducting proper outcomes research, saving 200 billion dollars;
(c) binding mediation for malpractice claims, saving 40-70 billion dollars;
(d) creating incentives for more primary care physicians who charge less than specialists, a definite savings that could be considerable.[16]

These are the kinds of suggestions that could begin to yield dividends fairly quickly and measurably. The use of specialists is being curtailed now to save money but not always in just ways.

2. Promoting Moral Development and Spiritual Renewal

There is no question that morally irresponsible behavior costs all of us a great deal in every way, especially in the health care sector of our communities. An enormous savings in money and human tragedy would result from large reductions in the use of tobacco, alcohol, addictive drugs, and violence. All of us can and should support government efforts to combat these practices. Inattention to good nutrition, exercise, and rest take their toll as well. Poverty is correlated with all of these costly, tragic behaviors and also with much higher rates of illness.

Although the need for work to do is now being publicly asserted, much remains to be done. Not long ago, on a radio talk show addressing the problem of suicide among adolescents in the Boston area, the host read a highly articulate letter written to the *Boston Globe* by a despairing teenager. It was a plea to allow younger teens to work and so contribute

---

16. Paula Tracy, "Koop Blasts Hillary's Task Force," *New Hampshire Sunday News*, Manchester, N.H., 28 March 1993. Koop's suggestions were contained in a letter that had not been answered at the time of this article.

to their communities. Some employers called in lamenting the regulations, insurance costs, and threat of suits that prevent them from what
they would gladly do, namely teach teenagers their skills and trade. It
was heart-wrenching to learn how regulations and laws conspire to force
isolation and idleness on young people. Some Christian parents do allow
their children to do work that is technically forbidden by our labor laws.
I know personally what a joy it was for me to do adult work on fruit and
vegetable farms while still in elementary school. I have never stopped
gardening since.

Moral education is no less important to promote healthy habits.
When Nathan Pusey, a committed Christian, was president of Harvard,
he defined the purpose of higher education as twofold: to sharpen wits,
and foster moral and spiritual development. In his view, no professor
should be ashamed to speak of God in the classroom.

That brings us to a matter that deserves but does not receive headlines, namely the health benefits of religious faith and practice. It has
been empirically demonstrated that those who regularly attend worship
services in their churches are less prone to illness, live longer, and spend
less time in hospitals when they are ill.[17] The renewal and spread of our
Christian faith promotes a wholesome, healthy way of life. It affirms that
our bodies are temples of God and are to be treated as such. It has been
empirically demonstrated that prayer, and the state of our minds and
souls, promotes health and healing.[18] Atheistic governments do not work.
They have fostered deteriorating health and illness. Atheism is a failed
social experiment. We need to educate lawyers to advocate, rather than
restrict, religious freedom and religiously sponsored institutions and organizations. Certainly the courts and legislatures should not adopt official
atheism in the name of an unattainable neutrality.

3. Preserving and Renewing the Moral Structure Guiding Health Care

The core moral responsibilities that have guided health care are the
responsibilities (a) to rescue, (b) to nurture and protect life, and (c) to

17. David B. Larson and Mary A. Greenwold, "Ethical Problems in the Clinical Study
of Religion and Health," in John F. Kilner, Nigel M. De S. Cameron and David L. Schiedermayer (eds.), *Bioethics and the Future of Medicine: A Christian Appraisal* (Grand Rapids:
Eerdmans, 1995), pp. 50-67.

18. Herbert Benson, *Timeless Healing* (New York: Scribner, 1996).

respect all human beings as having equal moral worth. For medical professionals this core includes the commitment to treat everyone who has a health need they can beneficially meet, in ways that never intend the death of the patient. No one should be turned away for lack of money or insurance. Dedicated members of the Christian Medical & Dental Society model this commitment not only by upholding the time-honored Hippocratic traditions, but also by upholding Christian traditions through being "dedicated to the service of all persons regardless of the state of their economic resources or the nature of their illness." When the cost of their care is beyond a physician's own resources, the physician is pledged to "intervene on their behalf as advocates of adequate care."[19] This same dedication is very much in evidence among Christian nurses and lawyers. I experienced this firsthand while teaching medical ethics with a Christian nurse, Denise Murray Edwards. On an occasion when she had brought a panel of professionals from her hospital, a student asked one of the panelists — a financial manager — if a certain kind of patient without medical insurance could be treated by the hospital. The answer was no. That prompted a quick, quiet, but firm response from my Christian nursing colleague: "We just treated such a patient recently; we hustled and obtained the necessary financial resources." Individuals as well as organizations can make a difference.

The current situation is extremely serious and difficult for those who uphold the moral traditions of health care. Charitable institutions are literally under siege. Christian churches have founded many hospitals. Many still bear names that identify their religious, even denominational roots. The term Samaritan is still in evidence. But for-profit organizations are rapidly taking over not-for-profit hospitals, visiting nurse agencies, even hospices. And, when a single HMO president can net $990 million in a take-over deal, such take-overs can certainly be expected to continue, unless strenuous efforts to curtail them are instituted, and soon.[20] Recognizing the gravity of what is happening, Bernard Lown, who won a Nobel prize for organizing fellow physicians on behalf of peace, is once more mobilizing physicians nationally.[21] The first priority is for his own state of Massachusetts to declare "a moratorium on for-profit takeovers of hospitals, insurance plans, HMOs, physicians' practices and other

19. David Schiedermayer, *Putting the Soul Back in Medicine: Reflections on Compassion and Ethics* (Grand Rapids: Baker Book House Co., 1994), p. 134.

20. *Managed Health Care Market Report* 4 (12) (June 30, 1996):1.

21. Bernard Lown, M.D., of Harvard Medical School and Brigham and Women's Hospital, can be contacted at 21 Longwood Avenue, Brookline, MA 02146.

health care institutions . . . pending the development of comprehensive state and national policies addressing these issues." This first action, cited in "A Call to Action," is supported by over a thousand Massachusetts physicians as of May 1997. This same "Call to Action" seeks an inclusive dialogue "to formulate a caring vision true to the community roots and Samaritan traditions of American medicine and nursing."[22] The invocation of "Samaritan traditions" certainly lends great credibility to Lown's efforts to retain the ethical imperatives of medicine, and what he calls the "covenant" between patients and their physicians.

Christians, through their churches and health care professionals, are finding ways to retain the moral imperatives of medical care and remain true to their biblical underpinnings. Later in this volume, physician Alieta Eck describes how she and her husband have developed a network of care true to biblical principles. She also describes how Christian churches are networking to replace expensive insurance policies with much more affordable methods of sharing funds to provide 100 percent coverage of health care costs for individuals and families that participate.[23] Doubtless, Christian medical, nursing, and legal professionals will find additional ingenious ways to persist in healing the sick, as Jesus did, regardless of their ability to pay. Christian support for the healing ministry has never been more urgently needed.

It would help greatly to educate the public and the institutions involved if businesses or professions contributing in any way to health care would be guided by the traditional moral imperatives of health care. That means, among other things, finding ways to share profits with patients and reduce costs as much as possible for technology, legal services, and the like.

In conclusion, we should not forget that when medicine is practiced as it should be, it is in itself cost-effective and efficient. Professional moral standards are incompatible with unnecessary surgery and with faulty and excessive resort to antibiotics or other medication. Encouraging morally and religiously responsible behavior is a powerful way to prevent illness and the stress that triggers illness. Christians should affirm and live out the moral responsibilities that sustain the moral structure of health care. We should not allow ourselves to be trapped into the utilitarian reasoning that sanctions the rationing of health care for the sake of saving or making

22. The Ad Hoc Committee to Defend Health Care, "For Our Patients, Not for Profits," *Journal of the American Medical Association* 278 (21) (December 3, 1997): 1733-34.
23. See Alieta Eck's essay in this volume.

money, or for any other reason. It is still true: *No one can serve both God and Mammon.* May we commit ourselves to live in the manner articulated long ago by Joshua as he warned the Israelites against following false gods, "As for me and my house, we will serve the Lord."[24]

---

24. Joshua 24:15.

ECONOMIC ENCROACHMENT

Managed Care's Financial Incentives

Scott E. Daniels, Ph.D.

The debate about health care distribution and financial incentives has produced a spectrum of positions between two competing perspectives that are based on valid ethical principles. McArthur and Moore characterize these perspectives as two cultures, professional and commercial.[1] On one end of the continuum is the traditional physician, whose primary interest is the welfare of the patient. This professional perspective seems to prefer a traditional, unfettered fee-for-service financing system, in which the physician exerts complete professional autonomy and faces few restrictions on use of resources or cost of services. At the other end is the emerging profit-oriented health maintenance organization (HMO) or insurance company that uses sophisticated cost-managing controls with contracted physicians to reduce health care expenditures through the efficient use of medical services.[2] Several intermediate positions exist between these two perspectives, each offering some compromise to one side or the other. The present volume

---

1. John H. McArthur and Francis D. Moore, "The Two Cultures and the Health Care Revolution: Commerce and Professionalism in Medical Care," *Journal of the American Medical Association* 277 (12) (March 1997): 985-89.
2. While this perspective does not have as widespread a defense in the literature as the other, more defenders are emerging. For example, David Eddy argues that cost considerations should be incorporated "formally and explicitly in decisions about treatments." See his "Balancing Cost and Quality in Fee-for-Service Versus Managed Care," *Health Affairs* 16 (3) (May/June 1997): 172.

illustrates that a range of perspectives, *within limits*, is compatible with a Christian outlook.[3]

Each of the two polar positions turns on the hotly-contested debate over financial incentives directed at altering the physician's testing and referral practices involving specialist and hospital services. More specifically, the two polar positions reflect different ethical sensitivities. This chapter explores the key ethical issue at the heart of the debate: the use of financial inducements to alter physician-practice patterns. The methods that managed care organizations (MCOs) use to compensate physicians can be very complicated. Accordingly, the present chapter will present three levels of analysis: a schema for MCOs, a description of how MCOs compensate physicians, and an assessment of the effects of those compensation methods on quality and trust. Technical background on financial incentive mechanisms comes from *The Managed Health Care Handbook*[4] and the Physician Payment Review Commission report.[5] A literature review was conducted to identify studies addressing the effect of financial incentives on quality and trust. In line with typical managed care terminology, the term "providers" will sometimes be used for physicians — though it is recognized that "provider" language may imply a level of commodification that needs to be critiqued from a Christian perspective.

Managed Care Organizations

Managed care organizes services and financing arrangements very differently from the fee-for-service arrangements traditionally used by insurance plans. Inglehardt describes managed care as "a system that, in varying degrees, *integrates the financing and delivery of appropriate medical care* through contracts with selected physicians and hospitals that provide comprehensive health care services to enrolled members (or subscribers) for a predetermined monthly premium. Most forms of managed care represent attempts to control costs by modifying the behavior of doctors,

---

3. See, for example, Edmund Pellegrino's defense of the traditional model and Kenman Wong's support for a more business-oriented perspective.

4. P. R. Kongstvedt, *Managed Health Care Handbook*, 3d ed. (Gaithersburg, Md.: Aspen Publishers, 1996).

5. M. Gold, R. Hurley, T. Lake, and R. Berenson, *Arrangements Between Managed Care Plans and Physicians: Results from a 1994 Survey of Managed Care Plans* (Washington, D.C.: Physician Payment Review Commission, 1995), p. 80.

although they do so in different ways (emphasis added).[6] Characterizing the distinctive features of various MCOs has become harder as those selling the products have blurred their distinguishing marks to remain competitive in today's health care market. It is probably still useful, however, to think of MCOs as progressing along a continuum, moving from least structured (e.g., managed indemnity) to most structured (e.g., health maintenance organization or provider sponsored network).[7] The following list describes the different types of entities with selected distinguishing features:

- Managed Indemnity Plans provide limited management of care. They generally involve utilization review strategies such as determinations of medical necessity prior to authorization of hospital admission.
- Preferred Provider Organizations (PPOs) offer members the most comprehensive package of benefits if they receive care from providers who participate in the plan's "preferred provider" network. Patients can choose to seek care from providers outside of the network, but the PPO then gives less comprehensive benefits. In-network-providers typically receive discounted reimbursement from the insurer in exchange for higher patient volumes.
- Point-of-Service (POS) plans are a recent response by managed care organizations to offer enrollees a greater choice of providers. Unlike the traditional HMO, the POS option allows members to receive services from providers outside the network without prior authorization at the point the service is desired — for a higher premium, co-payment, deductible, or a combination of all three.
- Health Maintenance Organizations (HMOs) are the most structured form of managed care. HMOs arrange for all health care services for their members. The traditional HMO (1) uses primary care providers (PCPs), so-called "gatekeepers," to coordinate care; (2) establishes a closed network of providers for members with no benefit coverage for services rendered outside the network without prior authorization; and (3) pays for health care services using a fixed-fee structure called capitation (see below) rather than paying for services individually.[8]

6. John K. Inglehardt, "Health Policy Report: The American Health Care System — Managed Care," *New England Journal of Medicine* 327 (10) (September 1992): 742.

7. *Managed Care Handbook*, pp. 33-45.

8. Capitation is generally paid to primary care physicians and ancillary providers such as a laboratory. Some HMOs also capitate specialists.

There are several varieties of HMOs that share these three features. A group-model HMO is a physician-owned multi-specialty practice that contracts to provide services for the MCO. A staff-model HMO is a multi-specialty practice owned or totally controlled by the MCO which only sees patients of the HMO. An Independent Practice Association (IPA) is a group of physicians who practice in their own offices but are organized into a legal entity. A network model HMO is similar to an IPA, but the physicians are not organized into a legal entity.

- Provider Sponsored Organizations (PSOs) involve formal affiliations among providers. They are organized and operate as integrated networks of providers. Carriers, such as HMOs, may contract with a PSO for services to covered members.
- Provider Hospital Organizations (PHOs) are jointly formed and owned by one or more hospitals and physician groups to provide health services to members.

Payment and Incentive Structure

MCOs pay physicians in a variety of ways. These generally fall within one of three categories: fee-for-service, capitation, and salary. All of these methods can be modified by the use of "withholds" and bonuses (see below).

Fee-for-service

The term "fee-for-service" refers to the traditional mechanism that reimburses physicians for each service performed. In this system, physicians' compensation varies with the volume of services they perform (i.e., the more they work, the more they will get paid). This form of compensation, which is utilized by "indemnity plans," is frequently criticized because it lacks incentives to control volume. However, when MCOs compensate a physician via a fee-for-service mechanism, they often pay a discounted fee, a predetermined amount that is less than the physician's usual charge.

Capitation

Capitation is a payment mechanism in which physicians or hospitals receive a predetermined, prepaid amount of money (dispersed on a per member per month basis) to take care of an enrollee's health needs for a specific amount of time. In this system, physicians assume some risk because the amount of money that they receive is unaffected by the frequency or cost of the services rendered to enrollees (i.e., they will receive no additional money if enrollees require services in which costs exceed the amount of money already paid). Since physicians who are compensated through capitation are prepaid, the cost of every service they perform comes out of their pockets. Therefore, physicians will keep more money already paid to them by providing only medically necessary care.

The risk that physicians assume through capitation can be limited in several ways. One way to limit risk is to share it (e.g., through a group practice). Although sharing risk makes it safer for the individual provider, it also makes it more difficult for individual physicians to benefit financially because benefits are shared as well.

Risk can also be limited through the use of "carve-outs." Carve-outs refer to covered services that are not factored into the capitation prepayment. A service would be "carved-out" if it were not subject to discretionary utilization. For example, the medical guidelines for administering immunizations are clear. Since there is little risk for over-utilization, these costs often are not included in the capitation payment, as the goal of capitation is to reduce unnecessary utilization. Physicians are paid a contracted fee for each carved-out service they provide.

Reinsurance and stop-loss pools can also be established to limit the degree to which a provider is at financial risk. After a provider loses a certain amount of money in providing services to a patient, continued losses are curbed by funding from these pools.

Salary

This form of compensation involves paying a provider a set annual amount in return for providing care to a panel of patients, rather than compensating physicians on a per treatment or per member basis. In its basic form, no financial risk is assumed by the physician.

Countervailing and Mitigating Factors

Fee-for-service, capitation, and salary can be modified through the use of "withholds" and bonuses. Withholds refer to the practice of MCOs keeping a certain percentage of the fee or salary (typically 5-20 percent) until the end of the fiscal year. Withholds are used to pay for any cost overruns that may be incurred. Residuals are then disbursed. The assumed benefit of having physicians take on additional risk is that physicians will be motivated to control costs so that they will receive payments that are due to them. Alternatively, MCOs can use bonuses as a way of attempting to control costs. In MCO plans that use bonuses, physicians are rewarded for effectively controlling costs.

Certain compensation mechanisms are typically used in specific settings, especially for primary care physicians (PCPs).[9] Table 1 shows data from a 1994 survey of 138 managed care plans in 20 U.S. metropolitan areas (107 responses).[10] Group/staff model HMOs generally use salaries as the predominant method for compensating individual primary care physicians. Network plans, such as independent practice associations (IPAs), primarily use capitation, while PPO plans more often use discounted fee-for-service.

The picture changes slightly with regard to specialists who contract with MCOs. Typically, specialists are compensated via fee-for-service; however, there is a growing trend toward capitating specialty services in addition to primary care services. Although group/staff model HMOs use salaries as their predominant method for compensation for both primary care physicians and specialists, a significant minority of plans (31 percent) use fee-for-service to compensate their specialists. Although network/IPA plans use capitation as the predominant method of compensating primary care physicians, a majority of network/IPA plans use fee-for-service to compensate specialists. PPO plans use fee-for-service as their predominant method of compensating both specialists and primary care physicians.

---

9. Group situations add another dimension of complexity in that capitated groups have the option of compensating their physicians via fee-for-service or capitation.

10. M. R. Gold, R. Hurley, T. Lake, T. Ensor, and R. Berenson, "A Natural Survey of the Arrangements Managed Care Plans Make with Physicians," *N Eng J Med* 333 (1995): 1678-83.

Table 1. Basic Physician Payment Methods by Plan Type (1994)

Predominant Payment Method Used in Sole or Largest Product	n=107 All Plans	n=29 Group/Staff	n=49 Network/IPA	n=29 PPO
PRIMARY CARE PHYSICIANS				
Fee-for-service	43%	3%	37%	93%
With withholding or bonuses	12%	0%	24%	3%
No withholding or bonuses	31%	3%	12%	90%
Capitation	37%	34%	57%	7%
With withholding or bonuses	29%	24%	44%	7%
No withholding or bonuses	8%	10%	12%	0%
Salary	19%	62%	6%	0%
With withholding or bonuses	11%	34%	4%	0%
No withholding or bonuses	8%	28%	2%	0%
SPECIALISTS				
Fee-for-service	70%	31%	78%	100%
With withholding or bonuses	19%	7%	35%	3%
No withholding or bonuses	52%	24%	43%	97%
Capitation	18%	31%	20%	0%
With withholding or bonuses	7%	7%	12%	0%
No withholding or bonuses	11%	24%	8%	0%
Salary	11%	38%	2%	0%
With withholding or bonuses	6%	21%	0%	0%
No withholding or bonuses	6%	17%	2%	0%

Effectiveness of Incentives

Several studies have found that the use of MCO financial incentives are effective in reducing the number of hospitalizations and overall health care costs without decreasing certain outcomes such as death when compared to traditional fee-for-service plans.[11] However, this data on utilization and mortality does not give any information about whether the quality of services provided was better, worse, or remained the same. Critics of MCOs argue that quality decreases because physicians are

11. Alan L. Hillman et al., "How Do Financial Incentives Affect Physicians' Clinical Decisions and the Financial Performance of Health Maintenance Organizations?" *N Eng J Med* 321 (2) (July 1989): 86-92.

rewarded for withholding care from enrollees. Supporters argue that quality is improved because physicians are motivated to contain costs by ensuring that enrollees are healthy through the provision of preventive services, which are cheaper than treatment for advanced conditions (e.g., surgery).

Research directly investigating the effects of financial incentives on quality of care is sparse. One study, a GAO report,[12] cautioned that financial incentives may reduce quality of care in HMOs. This report was criticized by Hillman and his colleagues because its conclusions were based on subjective evaluations of the contractual arrangements in only 19 HMOs.[13]

Another study, a survey of HMO managers conducted by Hillman and his colleagues, addresses the quality issue indirectly.[14] Managing directors of HMOs were asked their opinion of the effectiveness of financial incentives in influencing primary care physician behavior (e.g., their discretionary use of outpatient laboratory tests and specialist referrals, elective hospitalizations, and other influences that mitigate or intensify financial incentives). The research focused on withhold accounts and bonuses used to augment physician payment. A majority of managers felt that withholds or bonuses would have to be over 5 percent of physicians' income to motivate individual physicians to be more cost-effective. They also found that most of the managers would begin to worry about the appropriateness of individual physicians' judgments if withholds were greater than 15 percent. A majority of managers believed that pooling at least six to ten physicians together to share risk would offset any adverse effects of withholds on decision making. Thus, it may be the intensity of the incentive and not the presence of an incentive itself that has the effect. However, more research needs to be conducted to verify this hypothesis. Similarly, the fact that HMO managers have concerns about physician behaviors in certain incentive arrangements indicates that more research is needed on the effects of financial incentives on quality of care.

12. U.S. General Accounting Office, *Physician Incentive Payments by Prepaid Health Plans Could Lower the Quality of Care* (Washington, D.C.: U.S.G.P.O., 1988).

13. A. L. Hillman, M. V. Pauly, and C. R. Martinek, "Data Watch: HMO Managers' Views on Financial Incentives and Quality," *Health Affairs* 10 (1991): 207-19. For a general discussion of research problems and a presentation of the trends in the outcome data associated with the effect of capitation on quality, see also Donald M. Berwick, "Payment by Capitation and the Quality of Care," *N Eng J Med* 355 (16) (October 1996): 1227-31.

14. Hillman, Pauly, and Martinek, "Data Watch."

The impact of financial incentives on the trust between physicians and enrollees is another issue that needs more research. There may be reason for patients to distrust physicians as HMOs provide incentives to limit some forms of services. Although there have been no studies to assess this, Mechanic has discussed various aspects of patient trust with regard to financial incentives.[15] He recommends that managed care plans rather than physicians should be required to disclose financial arrangements, that limits be placed on incentives that put physicians at financial risk, and that professional norms and public policies encourage clear separation of interest of physicians from health plan organization and finance.

Even before research data become available addressing the influence of financial incentives on quality of care, physician behavior, and patient trust, the potential dangers are identifiable. There is much in the medical literature that is helpful in this regard, both for and against the use of financial incentives. The thrust of this literature will be summarized here, and the following chapters will subject these matters to a more explicitly Christian critique.

Bridging the Ethical Impasse Confronting Physicians

Traditionally, physicians have focused on what is best for the patient and disregarded the cost. With increased societal pressure to contain medical costs, they have been forced to be more cost conscious, but have still been reluctant to conflate medical assessment with cost-assessment. Angell, in an essay entitled "The Doctor as Double Agent," illustrates the tension of compromised loyalties and states that it is inappropriate to impose on physicians an obligation to "weigh competing allegiances to patients' medical needs [and] monetary costs to society" as a response to the haphazard development of an inherently inflationary system of health care financing.[16] Likewise, Pellegrino views this commingling of clinical judgment and cost-containment as an erosion of the ideal of the medical profession.[17] Some

---

15. David Mechanic and M. Schlesinger, "Impact on Patients' Trust in Medical Care and Their Physicians," *JAMA* 275 (1995): 1693-97. See also David Mechanic, "Changing Medical Organization and the Erosion of Trust," *The Milbank Quarterly* 74 (2) (1996): 171-89.

16. Marcia Angell, "The Doctor as Double Agent," *Kennedy Institute of Ethics Journal* 3 (3) (1993): 279-86.

17. Edmund Pellegrino, "Interests, Obligations, and Justice: Some Notes Toward an Ethic of Managed Care," *Journal of Clinical Ethics* 6 (1995): 312-17.

physician observers, however, are less troubled by the interplay between clinical judgment about individual patient care and cost considerations.

Opinions in the literature also reflect a concern that managed care exacerbates these dangers, which are inherent in the commingling of financial and clinical considerations. The AMA Council on Ethical and Judicial Affairs (CEJA) recognizes that financial incentives exist in both fee-for-service and capitation payment arrangements. However, they believe that the former are less troublesome because they are compatible with meeting patient needs.[18] They conclude that financial incentives in a managed care system are more problematic than in a fee-for-service plan for three reasons: (1) they exploit the financial motive of the physician, making his or her self-interest indispensable for the success of the MCO; (2) they are less likely to coincide with the patient's interests because patients generally prefer the risk of too much care to the risk of too little; and (3) they are less likely to be noticed by patients.

Some, however, challenge the AMA's contention that financial incentives are more problematic in managed care. Concerning the first reason offered by CEJA, Hall contends that those few dishonest physicians who place their own financial interests above patient welfare will find a way to cheat any economic system.[19] Regarding their second point, Franks and colleagues list numerous adverse outcomes associated with over-treatment allowed by the economic incentives of the fee-for-service system.[20] With respect to the Council's third reason, Hall maintains that the trust issue is greatly exaggerated by opponents of financial incentives systems. He asserts that a patient's trust in his or her physician is based not merely on knowledge of the physician's personal characteristics, but on a broader trust in the ethical strength of the medical profession as a whole. This trust in the profession, along with informed consent for treatment, allows a patient to trust an individual physician. In contrast to the position of either CEJA or these detractors, Emanuel maintains that the use of

---

18. AMA Council on Ethical and Judicial Affairs, "Ethical Issues in Managed Care," *JAMA* 273 (4) (1995): 330-35.

19. M. A. Hall, *Making Medical Spending Decisions: The Law, Ethics, & Economics of Rationing Mechanisms* (New York: Oxford University Press, 1996), ch. 5.

20. P. Franks, C. M. Clancy, and P. A. Nutting, "Gate-keeping Revisited — Protecting the Patients from Overtreatment," *N Eng J Med* 327 (6) (1992): 424-29.

21. E. J. Emanuel, "Medical Ethics in the Era of Managed Care: The Need for Institutional Structures Instead of Principles for Individual Cases," *Journal of Clinical Ethics* 6 (4) (1995): 336.

financial incentives in a fee-for-service system and in a capitated system are ethically equivalent.[21]

In summary, some believe that adding cost considerations to clinical judgment compromises the professional ethic, but others disagree. Some assert that managed care exacerbates this potential danger, but others disagree. There would thus seem to be three positions on the question of the ethics of financial incentives in managed care: they are unethical; they are ethical; or they are ethical if certain conditions exist.

Financial incentives are unethical

Pellegrino believes that financial incentives of any sort in managed care (bonuses, withholds) are unethical because they create conflicts for the physician's fiduciary duties. His central objection is that "managed care . . . deliberately set[s] out to change physician behavior by incentives and disincentives according to the theory that if each of us serves his or her self-interest, the interests of all will be served."[22] He goes on to point out that ethical problems also occur in a managed care environment when fiscal incentives that delay or interfere with patient care create conflicts with obligations to self, family, and the patient. Drawing a similar conclusion, Rodwin states "[a]ll such incentives, however, create conflicts of interest: physicians have an incentive to reduce services even when it is in the patient's interest to receive them and their responsibility as fiduciaries to provide them."[23]

Financial incentives are ethical

Hall challenges the absolute prohibition against financial incentives on the basis that incentives only induce physicians to avoid expensive care that is of slight or no benefit. His rebuttal is that "properly informed insurance subscribers may rationally agree to a set of strategically crafted incentives that induce doctors to act as both their medical treatment and

22. E. D. Pellegrino, "Words *Can* Hurt You: Some Reflections on the Metaphors of Managed Care," *Journal of the American Board of Family Practice* 7 (6) (1994): 507-8.

23. M. A. Rodwin, "Conflicts in Managed Care," *N Eng J Med* 332 (1995): 605. See also *idem, Medicine, Money & Morals: Physician's Conflicts of Interest* (New York: Oxford University Press, 1993).

24. M. A. Hall, *Making Medical Spending Decisions*, ch. 5.

their economic purchasing agents."[24] Since the force of his argument involves patient consent, it prohibits undisclosed or extremely corrupting incentives. Hall's position is compatible with that of Eddy, though the latter's appeal to informed consent extends beyond the patient to society at large. Eddy's rejection of society's "cost taboo" involves an obligation of professional societies to "make it clear to physicians, patients, the press, and the courts that cost/quality trade-offs are not only appropriate, but are necessary and ethical."[25]

Financial incentives are ethical IF . . .

This middle position assumes that when financial incentives surpass a certain threshold, or risk is concentrated on an individual physician, the traditional professional ethic may be compromised. Alternatively, when incentives are below that threshold, or the risk is distributed among several physicians, this ethic is not compromised and such arrangements are therefore ethical. Emanuel and colleagues state that financial incentives should be encouraged which spread risk over the performance of many physicians and focus on significant health outcomes rather than utilization review.[26] He further argues for limits on the percentage or amount of withholds and bonuses.

To conclude, there is no universal agreement among physicians, researchers, ethicists, or policy makers that financial incentives have either a positive or a negative impact on quality of medical care. It may not even be possible to determine if capitation alone has a causal effect on quality of care. Common sense, however, would suggest that if capitation and other financial incentives are used to modify physician behavior, they should be set at modest levels, and their effect should be directed toward promoting quality improvements in care rather than merely economic savings.

25. D. M. Eddy, "Balancing Cost and Quality in Fee-for-Service versus Managed Care," *Health Affairs* 16 (3) (1997): 172.

26. Emanuel, "Medical Ethics in the Era of Managed Care." See also E. J. Emanuel and N. N. Dubler, "Preserving the Physician-Patient Relationship in the Era of Managed Care," *JAMA* 273 (4) (1995): 323-92.

The Good Samaritan in the Marketplace: Managed Care's Challenge to Christian Charity

Edmund D. Pellegrino, M.D.

Sooner or later all of us will enter a physician-patient relationship. It is the final common pathway through which any system of care reaches those whom it is presumed to serve. How that relationship is conducted will determine whether patients will be beneficiaries or victims. The moral integrity of any system of care, therefore, must be judged by the way it shapes the moral center of health care — the relationship between health professionals and those who seek their help. This is of crucial concern for Christians, whose model must be the Good Samaritan and not economics or commerce.

Today the dominant influence on the way patients are treated in the United States is the ideology and the ethos of the marketplace. Increasingly the metaphors and methods of competition and "free" markets are determining the price, availability, accessibility, quality, and distribution of health care. Healing and helping human beings is now a "product," a commodity to be regulated by the forces of profit, self-interest, and a fictive "freedom" of consumer choice. The credo of the marketplace is that through the operation of the "invisible hand" of the market, efficiency will prevail, productivity will be increased, unnecessary care eliminated, and more people served — all while quality is preserved.

These assumptions have yet to meet the test of empirical verification. But any test of the moral integrity of managed care must acknowledge that the rules of the marketplace are unforgiving; they are not designed to care for "losers." Most assuredly, they are not congenial to Good Samaritans. In this essay I wish to examine the assumptions and the current operation of the market model in managed care from the point of view of the Christian ethic of care which emerges from the Samaritan ethos of the Gospels.

To pursue this line of inquiry it is necessary to outline the elements of a Christian ethic of care for the sick, then to show how this ethic is challenged by the market and commercial models, and finally to suggest the response the Christian community and caregiver might offer to the economic imperatives within a context faithful to the Samaritan ideal.

Economics, Markets, and Christian Ethics

A Christian ethic of healing begins with full awareness of the natural phenomena that give ethical shape to the patient-physician relationship.[1] By the natural phenomena I mean those observable facts about the clinical encounter and the healing relationship ascertainable by ordinary observation and reflection. Christian ethics places these phenomena in a context set by the revealed truths of the Hebrew and Christian Bibles. These sources tell us that men and women are created in God's image; that all humans equally possess an intrinsic dignity; and that this dignity cannot be lost in illness, suffering, or disability. We see repeatedly how solicitous Jesus was for all who suffer. As Christians, we must always strive to comfort, to cure, and to care for those who are ill.

In the parable of the Good Samaritan we learn that solicitude for our neighbor's suffering is an obligation of all Christians. We are all exhorted to do as the Good Samaritan did (Luke 10:37) — i.e., to make ourselves neighbors of the sick. Christ himself charged the twelve disciples to heal the sick in every town that received them (Luke 10:8-10). For some of us, this is our vocation, a calling from God to which we must respond as our life's work, our way toward salvation.[2] It is our ministry, our apostolate, and our evangelical duty. The Christian health professional is called to do nothing less than to imitate Christ, Christ the Healer — *Christus Medicus*.[3] Our model is an ineffable model, a model

---

1. E. D. Pellegrino and D. C. Thomasma, *For the Patient's Good: The Restoration of Beneficence in Health Care* (Oxford: Oxford University Press, 1987).

2. Germain Grisez, "Health Care as Part of a Christian Vocation," delivered at the International Conference "Issues for a Catholic Bioethics" (Linacre Center for Health Care Ethics, Cambridge, 1997): 1-11.

3. Chrysologus, St. Peter, Collectio Sermonum, CL 0227+M, SLL, Sermoso, Linea 61.

of perfection but one nonetheless that we are called to emulate. In this way a naturally good life — one lived in accord with medical ethics — becomes a spiritually good life, one in eternal accord with God's will.

Even in the loosest interpretation of these Gospel teachings, healing and curing can never be primarily a commercial enterprise. Health care cannot be a commodity. Nor can the availability or accessibility of care be left to the fortuitous operation of the marketplace.[4] If the parable is taken seriously, even for the believer such a command seems almost too much to ask. It challenges our human weakness. It is a command that can only make sense within the logic of the glorification of humanity.[5]

There is no way this message of the Gospels can be compatible with a "provider-consumer" relationship. The commercial model has no place for the vulnerable, the marginalized, the poor, the persons who have neglected their health, the uninformed, or the uneducated.[6] These are the "non-players" who cannot even enter the market. They do not possess, or have squandered or lost, their resources. Rather than being rejected, on the Christian view, they have a preferential claim on all of us. In health care, as in other dimensions of human life, Christian ethics is a scandal to the well-off, the self-satisfied, and the men and women of practical affairs.

Therefore, looked at from the point of view of a Christian ethics of medical care, managed care conceived as it is today as a commercial enterprise is incompatible with Christian ethics of care. This does not mean that a Christian ethic of care condones inefficiency, low productivity, unrestrained expenditures, or irresponsibility for the care of one's own health. These are responsibilities incumbent on health professionals, patients, and institutions. But the driving force of a Christian ethic is not profit-making nor cost-containment per se. Rather, an efficient and pro-ductive, waste-free system is a moral obligation because it is essential for optimally meeting the needs of the sick. A Christian ethic imposes responsibilities on patients to care for their bodies, but it also recognizes our human weaknesses and stands ready to help and heal all — including those who have neglected their responsibility for their own health.

4. John Paul II, Encyclical Letter, Centesimus Annus, *Origins*, May 16, 1991, vol. 21, no. 1, at (39)(40)(42)(48).

5. Jean-Marie Lustiger, "Liberty, Equality, Fraternity," *First Things* 76 (Oct. 1997): 44-45.

6. Charles Marwick, "Patients' Lack of Literacy May Contribute to Billions of Dollars in High Hospital Costs," *Journal of the American Medical Association* 278 (Sept. 24, 1997): 971-72, cites the National Adult Literacy Survey which estimates the functionally illiterate population in the U.S. to be 40-44 million.

What a Christian ethic cannot condone, and what many Christians involved as managers, physicians, or investors in managed care seem to ignore, is the means whereby managed care achieves its "successes." I refer here to how the books are "balanced," and profits reaped — by the denial of claims, cutting of payments to physicians and hospitals, erecting new barriers to care, disenrolling patients and physicians who cost too much, and refusing grievances and appeals by redefining medical necessity and experimental therapy in terms favorable to the managed care organizations. I refer, too, to the legitimation of self-interest and profit-making on the part of physicians, investors, and managed care organizations.

To whom do the assets and surpluses achieved by these means justly belong? Entrepreneurs and investors assume they belong to the organization to be used as capital and counters in the frenetic game of mergers and buyouts. We must recall that nominally not-for-profit managed care organizations like Blue Cross were chartered for the benefit of the public they are presumed to serve. They were subjected to regulation to assure they served this need. But now, as they effect mergers with other organizations, across state lines and beyond the populations from which their assets were accumulated, managed care organizations take these assets as their own. This raises a question of justice, in that a misappropriation of funds is involved.

A Christian ethic of health care is consistent with a system of managed care when its aim is to improve the quality, availability, and quantity of health care and when the means employed to this end are in themselves just. The Christian community has a collective obligation to foster and participate in managed care whose purpose is the betterment of the quality of care provided to all who need it. It is not the concept of managed care that is at fault. It is the use of market forces to achieve its ends that is morally offensive.

A Christian ethic of care, moreover, is consistent with the idea of a good society built on the conception of human solidarity and the dignity of all humans as children of the same Creator.[7] In such a society, economics is not a self-justifying system for the distribution of goods and services. In a Christian social order, economics serves as a means of satisfying human need in accordance with the Gospel principle of charity. Ethics thus precedes economics; it does not deny the reality of economics, but it locates it in proper relationship to the good for humans.

7. The Pastoral Role of the Diocesan Bishop in Catholic Health Care Ministry. A statement of the Administrative Conference of the National Conference of Catholic Bishops, March 1997, National Conference of Catholic Bishops, Washington, D.C.

As Aristotle, Xenophon, and Cicero in the ancient world saw it, economics was the science of running a household *(oikos* plus *nomos)*. But ethics rather than economics tells us whether the household we run is a morally good one or not.[8] If we take a broader view of economics, it more closely resembles a behavioral science than a moral philosophy. "Humanistic" economies can explain profit-making and market behavior but these are not per se normative. In any case, for the Christian and especially for the Christian physician and nurse, it is the transformation of the traditional ethics of their professions by Gospel teachings that matters. The aims of an enlightened economics of secular humanism can never substitute for the call of the Beatitudes.

In a Christian ethic of care, the natural principles and virtues of medical ethics that derive from the nature of medicine are transformed by the Gospel message.[9] The natural virtues are raised to the level of grace.[10] Beneficence becomes charity, the unselfish love of our fellows exemplified in Jesus' life; autonomy becomes respect for the dignity of the patient because he is created in God's image; justice becomes charitable justice, justice "without the blindfold" — "giving and forgiving in imitation of the Father's generosity not simply giving strictly what is due."[11]

In the end, Christian ethics always reduces to the virtue of charity around which the whole life of Jesus was centered. We cannot love a person and treat that person unjustly, or maleficently, or without regard to her wishes. Charity is a principle as well as a virtue because it is the most fundamental norm of the Christian life. Christian ethics is agapeistic ethics; it brings God's benediction to every healing encounter in the life of the professional. The task of health professionals — doctors, nurses, social workers — is to actualize the virtue of charity in their daily encounters with the sick. It is at the bedside that the commercial and the agapeistic models collide and pose the most serious challenges for the Christian physician, nurse, social worker, or chaplain.

8. Aristotle, *Economics*, trans. E. S. Forster, Bk. III by G. C. Armstrong in *The Complete Works of Aristotle*, Jonathan Barnes (ed.), (Princeton: Princeton University Press, 1984), vol. 2, pp. 2130-2151 at 1343a, 9.

9. E. D. Pellegrino and David C. Thomasma, *Helping and Healing: Religious Commitment in Health Care* (Washington, D.C.: Georgetown University Press, 1997).

10. E. D. Pellegrino and D. C. Thomasma, *The Christian Virtues in Medical Practice* (Washington, D.C.: Georgetown University Press, 1996).

11. Servais Pinckaers, *The Sources of Christian Ethics*, Sr. Mary Noble (trans.) (Washington, D.C.: Catholic University of America Press, 1995), p. 31.

Corporate Ethics and the Christian

The incongruity of Christian ethics with the corporatization of the physician-patient relationship has sometimes been neglected in the ethical analyses of managed care. Corporate ethics focuses on the obligations of managers, boards of directors, and investors, all of whom are at a distance from the sick person; they do not make the immediate clinical decisions that might affect a patient's care unfavorably. But, because health care organizations are moral agents and display their character in the actions of all who are part of them,[12] those in charge cannot escape complicity in the harms that might result.

Closest to the patient administratively are the "managers," particularly the medical directors. They must pre-certify hospital admissions for certain treatments, and they must evaluate claims and grievances. They are the "gatekeepers' gatekeepers" — the ones who make sure the physician gatekeeper does not open the gates of access too widely. Further removed are the members of boards of directors who make the policies, negotiate the mergers and acquisitions, and determine the price and marketing strategies that have their ultimate impact at the bedside. Furthest removed are the investors who never encounter the persons from whose misfortunes they profit.

In an effort to compete or to survive, some sectarian hospitals are selling out to managed care organizations for profit, or merging with them while trying to retain their religious characters. Some Catholic hospitals believe they have successfully negotiated agreements that enable them to remain faithful to Catholic moral principles. How these will work out over the long haul, especially when the profits shrink as they will in the future, is problematic at best. In any case, board members and the professional staff of hospitals committed to serve Christ have a serious obligation to avoid networking or merging with institutions in which principles of Christian health care may be compromised.[13]

Corporate participants cannot distance themselves morally if harm comes to patients or the Christian identity of their institutions. They are part of a collectivity responsible for the moral behavior of its parts even

---

12. E. D. Pellegrino, "The Ethics of Collective Judgments in Medicine and Health Care," *Journal of Medicine and Philosophy* 7 (1) (Feb. 1982): 3-10.

13. The Pastoral Role of the Diocesan Bishop in Catholic Health Care Ministry. A Statement of the Administrative Committee of the National Conference of Catholic Bishops, March 1997, National Conference of Catholic Bishops, Washington, D.C., 8-11.

if they do not make the adverse decisions themselves or even know about them. They either make a profit, gain a salary, or receive bonuses from the results of cost-containment or profit-skimming. On any considered application of the doctrine of cooperation, they bear moral responsibility for harm done.

When the corporate actors are physicians or other health professionals, their participation as investors or corporate officers is especially suspect. The reality of conflict of interest cannot be avoided, especially in those managed care organizations wholly owned, organized, and operated by the same group of physicians who provide the care. Whether for-profit or not, these arrangements expose the patient's vulnerability to exploitation, under the guise of efficiency or public service. It is illusory to think that physician-administered plans will be more respectful of patient welfare. Whether capitation operates at the level of individual physicians, a group of physicians, or the plan, conflicts of interest cannot be eliminated. Physician administrators by the very nature of their functions are soon engulfed by the system itself. When this occurs, patients lose their last advocate against the system.

Pointing out these ethical issues in corporate and managerial ethics is not meant to impugn the good faith of those who work in managed care organizations. It is intended to suggest that even persons of good will can be corrupted by a system of care which is designed as a commercial, competitive, and market-driven enterprise. George Bernard Shaw's biting remark that the medical profession constitutes a conspiracy against the public is too genuine a possibility when health care is provided in a competitive, cost- or profit-driven system. Careful, critical, prayerful reflection on these ethical perils is an obligation of every Christian health professional, institution, and church-sponsored organization engaged in health care.

Close attention must be paid to the quiet but profound revolution perpetrated, consciously or not, by the managed care movement as it exists today. Power and authority for decisions about patients have been transferred in large part from the physician to the purchaser and the "industry." Conversely, the risks have been shifted from the purchaser to the physician. Physicians, however, remain legally liable for providing the standard of care but not for the decisions that determine how and when to provide that standard. Morreim suggests that this incongruity can be solved by excusing the physician from the obligation of effacement of self-interest.[14] She would

---

14. E. Haavi Morreim, *Balancing Act: The New Medical Ethics of Medicine's New Economics* (Washington, D.C.: Georgetown University Press, 1995), pp. 64, 145-47.

substitute adherence to a managed care definition of the standard of care. Others have voiced variations of this theme of accommodation and submission to economic exigency.[15]

This would be an intolerable degree of moral capitulation. It deprives patient and physician of legal and moral challenge to unjust policies or recovery of damages resulting from that policy. Such a policy further robs the physician of any sense of professional integrity. More importantly, it re-enforces the managed care usurpation of clinical authority to an alarming degree.[16]

Conflicts at the Bedside

The most urgently felt ethical conflict for the conscientious physician and nurse, secular or religious, is the erosion of the primacy of commitment to the welfare of the individual patient and person in a system of managed care.[17] This primacy is compromised by the fact that health professionals in a managed care organization are employees. As such they receive compensation from the organization; de facto they owe allegiance to the organizational goals they are paid to pursue. These goals may or may not concur with the needs of their particular patients. These obligations to the organization can conflict with the antecedent duty of acting in the patient's best interests. This puts the physician inescapably in a position of double agency, which pits the patient's needs against those of the organization, the other patients in the same plan, and the physician's own self-interest.

In a managed care system, emphasis shifts from the ethics of service to a particular patient to a population-based ethic. Physicians become responsible for taking into account the effect of their clinical decisions not just on the welfare of their patients but also on that of all the other patients enrolled in the system and even of society at large. This is to

15. L. H. Thurow, "Learning to Say No," *New England Journal of Medicine* 311 (1984): 1569; B. Gray, *The Profit Motive and Patient Care: The Changing Accountability of Doctors and Hospitals* (Cambridge, Mass.: Harvard University Press, 1991).

16. E. D. Pellegrino, "Altruism, Self-Interest and Medical Ethics," *JAMA* 258 (14) (1987): 1939-40; N. J. Levinsky, "The Doctor's Master," *N Eng J Med* 311 (1984): 1573.

17. D. P. Sulmasy, "Physicians, Cost Control and Ethics," *Annals of Internal Medicine* 116 (1992): 920-26; E. J. Emanuel and N. Dubler, "Preserving the Physician Patient Relationship in the Era of Managed Care," *N Eng J Med* 332 (1995): 604-7; M. A. Radwin, "Conflicts in Managed Care," *N Eng J Med* 332 (1995): 604-7; J. P. Kassirer, "Managed Care and the Morality of the Marketplace," *N Eng J Med* 333 (1995): 50-52.

say nothing of the investors whose capital is at risk as well as the physician's own legitimate self-interests.

Fee-for-service medicine, of course, also involves conflicts of interests and obligations. In the past, this conflict all-too-frequently resulted in unnecessary treatment. This is one of the reasons why managed care has been so avidly promoted by many. The major temptation in a fee-for-service system is that physicians earn more the more they do for their patients, even if the care is unnecessary. In managed care, the opposite is true: physicians are penalized if they do "too much," i.e., provide care not "covered" by the plan. Financial penalties or bonuses for productivity, cost savings, or conservation of resources are deliberate manipulations of the physician's self-interest against the patient's. In a fee-for-service system physicians are the identifiable miscreants. In managed care they share the blame. They share their acts of injustice with the organization that legitimates their actions. The other miscreants are the managed care administrator, the board of directors, and the investors, all of whom are faceless and unknown to the patient.

Managed care that makes cost-containment or profit-taking as its end, at the expense of meeting legitimate needs of sick persons, threatens the most elementary notion of Christian ethics. It makes price, availability, accessibility, and the quality of medical care a function of free-market determination or negotiation. It grants the doctor or the managed care organization a presumed proprietary right over medical knowledge. The justice of the business contract requires the physician or the organization to deliver nothing more than is owed by the conditions of the contract with the plan. If a patient at a young age opts unwisely for a cheaper plan with fewer or the wrong benefits, this is too bad.

Nor is it a concern of the managed care organization or the physician if patients do not have the wherewithal to become "players" in the market. No provision is made for those who have no insurance or inadequate insurance. Nor is there any solicitude for the many totally or partially illiterate members of American society who cannot understand an insurance plan to say nothing of being able to choose one over another. Yet these people too become ill. They present themselves often as emergencies. No physician in good conscience can refuse to treat them even if no plan is willing to pay for the costs of their care.

Managed care makes the physician the "gatekeeper" whose duty it is to prevent patients from too easy access to specialists, hospitals, or laboratories.[18] When these restrictions result in denial of truly unnecessary care — that is, care that does not change the natural history of the disease in some effective way — they are morally justifiable — even mandatory. This is "managed care" in its best sense. Unfortunately, managed care as it is presently organized is just as likely to result in deprivation of needed care. It is "managed" not for patient benefit but investor interests.

A Christian ethic of care focuses first on the sick person, the one in need, now presenting herself to the physician or nurse. The sick person is Christ himself seeking help. Some significant degree of effacement of self-interest is an inescapable obligation of physicians who see health care as a vocation and a form of ministry. For Christians the practice of medicine is an obligation of the stewardship the physician exercises over medical knowledge.

As Ecclesiasticus tells us: "Healing itself comes from God the Most High like a gift received from a King."[19] "He has also given some people knowledge so that they may draw credit from his mighty works."[20] On the Christian view, medical knowledge is knowledge held in trust. It is knowledge God has built into nature which humans may exploit to help and to heal one another. To be sure, physicians are entitled, and indeed, obliged to provide for themselves and their families. But this cannot be the primary motivation for a Christian apostolate of healing.

As noted above, the most serious conflict of loyalties occurs in those arrangements in which the physician or group of physicians become the insurers as well as the gatekeepers by assuming all of the financial risks but also all of the profits. In this arrangement patients lose their most important advocates in the system. Physicians are simultaneously judge and jury. They are no longer simply employees of the managed care organization. They *are* the organization.[21] Patients who are unjustly treated no longer have an advocate since their physician is now identified with the system that denied their need for care in the first place.

---

18. E. D. Pellegrino, "Rationing Health Care: The Ethics of Medical Gatekeeping," *Journal of Contemporary Health Law and Policy* 2 (1986): 23-45.

19. Ecclesiasticus 38:2.

20. Ecclesiasticus 38:6.

21. S. Woolhandler and D. Himmelstein, "Extreme Risk — The New Corporate Proposition for Physicians" (Editorial) *N Eng J Med* 333 (25) (1995): 1706-8; J. G. Apple, "Who Bears the Risk When Physicians Are Also Insurers?" *Minnesota Medicine* 78 (5) (1995): 23-28.

Physician Responses to Managed Care

Physicians are taking a variety of steps to respond to the shift of authority to managed care organizations and risk away from these organizations. Physicians troubled by this power shift understandably might want to regain some of that power. But the ways this is accomplished must be scrutinized from the perspective of Christian ethics. Two of these responses deserve attention: unionization and so-called equity HMOs.[22]

Unionization of physicians is not morally illicit per se if it is used as a device for collective bargaining.[23] Since physicians are employees in the managed care world they should not be denied the rights accorded other workers in any system of Christian social justice. Obviously, the strike mechanism could not be justified because this would entail compromise of patient welfare for the benefits of physicians. Even a strike to gain improvement in care violates the primary orientation of medical ethics to patient welfare. More subtle and more dangerous are the temptations to abuse of power inherent in any mechanism devised solely to gain more power. Finally, the union metaphor has connotations antithetical to the effacement of self-interest peculiar to the professional life.

Equity HMOs are equally attractive and even more susceptible to abuse and defection from the physician's obligation of advocacy.[24] In equity HMOs, physicians own shares in the organization and assume the risks themselves in return for dividends and power over policies. In doing so, however, there is no net increment of control over individual clinical decisions. Indeed, the collective impetus to avoid or share risks and to make a profit are just as dangerous to patient welfare as they are in a non-physician-owned HMO. They operate under the same aegis of competition and survival in the marketplace.

The major source of power for physicians is moral power — the sense of a communal responsibility as a profession for the welfare of those who seek their help. To compromise this power or trade it for political power is to make a Faustian compact with its inevitable loss of soul. The same is true of "gaming" the system by deceptive repre-

22. Christopher Wang, "Unions and Equity HMOs: Two Sources of Physician Power in a World of Managed Care," *Family Practice Management* (Feb. 1996): 21-27. See also the discussion of unionization in the chapter by Mary Adam later in this volume.

23. D. Mangan, "Will Doctor Unions Finally Take Hold?" *Medical Economics* 72 (14) (1995): 115-20.

24. Wang, "Unions and Equity HMOs," pp. 21-27.

sentation of diagnoses or severity, even if it might serve the patient's interests. Some physicians have resorted to "paper strikes" — refusing to fill out forms as a form of protest. But if such a tempting move results in delays in patient care, refusal of claims, or patient harassment, it cannot be justified.

Responsibility for Cost-Containment

The fidelity of Christian physicians to a Christian ethic of healing does not excuse them from a responsibility for cost-containment. Rather, it is an obligation of that ethic to use the patient's and society's resources wisely and well. When two treatments are equally effective, the less costly may be chosen. Treatment that is not indicated by the best medical practice, over-treatment at the end of life, and treatment that is futile are infractions of medical ethics, secular and Christian.[25] Only those treatments should be used that are effective in changing the natural history of the disease to the benefit of the patient and in which the burdens are proportionate to the benefits. Over-treatment is not in the patient's best interests. Over-treatment can be a maleficent act since it may produce burdens, side effects, and costs without proportional benefits. Rational, effective medicine is the most significant contribution physicians can make to cost-containment. Good medicine de facto eliminates unnecessary care and for the right reasons — not because it is expensive but because it is harmful to the patient.

When physicians are bonded in a covenantal trust relationship with a patient, they cannot be double agents. They must act in the interests of the patient presenting to them. They cannot simultaneously be agents primarily of social good or fiscal parsimony. When these goals conflict it is the good of the patient that must prevail. The current urging of physicians to abandon ethics of the person for ethics of the population is a violation of the covenant of healing, which requires the physician to act in the interests of the sick person. "Social ethics" practiced at the bedside places the needs of unidentified persons whose risks are uncertain

25. Hippocrates, *On Joints*, *V.III*, with an English translation by W. H. S. Jones (Cambridge, Mass.: Loeb Classical Library Vol. III, Harvard University Press, 1968), p. 339; Hippocrates, *The Art*, with an English translation by W. H. S. Jones (Cambridge, Mass.: Loeb Classical Library Vol. II, Harvard University Press, 1986), p. 193; Hippocrates, *On Diseases*, *V.III*, with an English translation by W. H. S. Jones (Cambridge, Mass.: Loeb Classical Library Vol. V, Harvard University Press, 1988), p. 113.

and somewhere in the future ahead of persons presenting themselves now in actual need. This is a disordered priority of obligations even in secular ethics. In Christian ethics, it is to yield the virtue of charity to the abstract demands of utilitarianism. It is as if the Good Samaritan were to pass by the stranger because there might be someone sicker at the next turn of the road.

When they are not in trust relationships with particular patients, Christian physicians can, and should, take steps to advance the health of the community using the most economical way consistent with Christian ethics. After the practice of effective, rational, evidence-based medicine, the physician can, indeed is obliged to, contribute to the optimal use of societal resources. This can be done in a variety of ways consistent with the ordering principles of Christian charity.

First, the Christian physician must encourage and support empirical studies to ascertain the relative effectiveness and benefits of treatments. These studies can legitimately focus on cost/effectiveness ratios. This is a rational way to avoid unnecessary treatment. It is the indispensable guide to scientific, evidence-based medicine to which the Christian physician like every other conscientious physician owes allegiance.

Christian physicians thus have a duty to act as technical experts providing reliable and objective data to their colleagues and to policy makers who must decide which treatments to support and which not. The temptation to advance one's own specialty or treatment interest must be resisted. The antidote is research carried out objectively, rigorously, and cooperatively in properly designed clinical tests.

A second obligation is to take leadership in advocating reforms to provide for the health care needs of the poor, the uninsured, the chronically ill, the aged, and the handicapped — all those whom managed care plans find unwelcome or unacceptable enrollees. These are the heavy users of medical care. They are most vulnerable in a market economy that favors young, healthy enrollees who will pay their premiums on time and not need the services of the system.

A third obligation is to educate one's own patients to the dangers — physical and fiscal — of unnecessary treatment. We must acknowledge that pressures for useless, dubious, or futile measures often arise from patients and their families. In addition, education in preventive medicine is crucial to avoid catastrophic illness and the high costs of "rescue" from preventable crises. Education in advance directives, anticipating and preparing for end-of-life decisions, and accepting one's finitude are necessary correlates. Christians particularly have an obligation to identify and draw on spiritual resources to blunt the illusion of immortality that high-technology medicine can unfortunately stimulate even when the illness has become untreatable.

A fourth obligation is to avoid entering contracts with for-profit organizations, with those who offer financial rewards, bonuses, or stock, or with those who require a gag rule or have other barriers to disclosure. A neglected sector of the moral life of today's physician is the sector in which one ought to say "No!" The idea that there are things which should never be done is becoming foreign territory to many contemporary bioethicists. If Hitler's Nazi physicians had said "No!", it is highly unlikely that Auschwitz, its many counterparts, and the Holocaust itself would have been possible.[26] There may well be times in this era of commercialized medicine when all physicians, nurses, and especially those who are committed Christians will have the responsibility of collective refusal to serve the plan.

Christian physicians must be prepared to define those ethical abuses of the relationship beyond which the erosion of the trust relationship is so clear that the individual and the profession must say no. Knowing when to refuse is essential. Physicians cannot escape moral complicity for harms to their patients resulting from their cooperation in a morally defective plan. After all, they write the orders; they can cooperate or protest. The final stewardship is theirs.

The burden of conscience placed on the individual physician who wishes to practice in conformity with Christian ethics within managed care is very great. Simple self-righteous condemnation of others is hypocrisy. Yet how far one may cooperate with a morally dubious system is a matter of conscience. We cannot expect individual physicians to bear the whole burden. They each must balance their other responsibilities to family, community, and religion. The moral obligation not to cooperate with any plan that is injurious to patients is a communal and collective responsibility of the entire profession. The profession must take leadership, support its members, and seek alliances with nurses and other health professions as well as the public in advocating reform.

---

26. Robert Jay Lifton, *The Nazi Doctors* (New York: Basic Books, 1996); Michael Burleigh, *Death and Deliverance: "Euthanasia" in Germany c. 1900-1945* (Cambridge: Cambridge University Press, 1994).

The Christian Community

Helping, healing, caring, and curing were so much a part of the life of Jesus that no Christians can absolve themselves of responsibility for the health care system their nation adopts. All Christians share responsibility for working towards a societal ethic of care that is imbued with the spirit of Christ's love for the sick. Without the support of the entire Christian community, it will be ever more difficult for Christian health professionals to resist the injustices of commercialization.

In the end, the kind of health care we tolerate reflects the kind of society we are or want to be. The bedside reflects back to all of us where our treasure lies. While physicians, nurses, and administrators have the immediate responsibility, they can only operate within the parameters society sets for them. If our system of "care" denies care, none of us can deny complicity. If the health care system Christians tolerate is itself a violation of Christian teaching on care of the sick, Christians cannot avoid complicity.

Managed care and its commercialization are part of the larger question of a national health care system replete with ethical incongruities. On the one hand, American medicine is, for those who can afford it, the most proficient care available; the U.S. economy at the moment is better than it has been for a very long time; U.S. institutions and health care personnel are in sufficient supply. On the other hand, these resources are denied to the poor and the underinsured, and resources are increasingly more difficult to get without harassment by the middle classes. In the face of plenty, U.S. medicine is frantically cutting costs and downsizing in imitation of American business and the ideology of markets and profits. How does all of this measure against the Christian ethic of concern for the sick and the poor?

Christians of all denominations must ask themselves some very serious questions — especially those Christians who have accommodated to managed care as "inevitable" or excused themselves by blaming "the system," or profiting periodically by cost-shaving. This is not the place to outline how Christians, joined to others of good will and social conscience, can mobilize to fashion a just and human health care apparatus. Tough resource allocation decisions may be necessary, but before accepting rationing as inevitable there are questions those of us living in the U.S. must ask ourselves:

Are we practicing rational, effective medicine that reduces unnecessary care to a minimum? Have we counted the administrative costs of

117

our complicated, multi-insurer system? What are the non-dollar costs in harassment, in delays of care, in grievance and appeal procedures, in confusion and misleading advertisements? Have we exhausted all measures short of rationing? Have we examined our enormous discretionary expenditures on amusement, spectator sports, etc? Have we considered the obligation of Christians to make sacrifices of some of their excess to provide for the needs of those less fortunate? Have all Christians, and especially Roman Catholics who have the largest system of health care institutions in the U.S., asked how they can cooperate and merge their resources to provide care that is not profit-oriented but, rather, based on Christian ethical principles?

Managed care per se is not inherently antithetical to Christian ethics of care. Indeed, properly organized around the improvement of quality and more equitable distribution of care, it is a moral obligation. However, as it is operated today, as a commercial enterprise, market-driven and insensitive to the needs of the sick, managed care diverges daily from the Gospel conception of charitable justice. For the Christian the response is not accommodation to the so-called "new" medical ethics.[36] What is needed is a bold reassertion of the Christian meaning of healing and the vocation — not the occupation — of health professionals. Accommodation to the ideology of a market-driven, commercialized health care system can only end in capitulation, danger to the patient, and a repudiation of the Christian ethic of healing and caring for the sick.

36. Morreim, *Balancing Act.*

When Health Care Becomes a Commodity: The Need for Compassionate Strangers

Patricia Benner, R.N., Ph.D.

Mounting shadows darken our calling and threaten to transform healing from a covenant into a business contract. Canons of commerce are displacing dictates of healing, trampling our profession's most sacred values. Market medicine treats patients as profit centers. The time we are allowed to spend with the sick shrinks under the pressure to increase throughout, as though we were dealing with industrial commodities rather than afflicted human beings in need of compassion and caring.

"A Call to Action"[1]

There is something radically wrong with treating health care as one more product in a free-market economy. It is unrealistic to expect patients to be consumers who will aggressively hunt for the best bargain and be wise in their "product choice." Viewing health care as a commodity to be bought and sold does not work in many situations. For example, if we

1. Ad Hoc Committee to Defend Health Care, Cambridge, Mass., "For Our Patients, Not for Profits," *Journal of the American Medical Association* 278 (21) (Dec. 3, 1997): 1733.

This essay was sponsored in part by The Alloway Bioethics Lectureship, Center for Bioethics, University of Toronto.

119

are frail elderly persons, children, busy adults seeking to make a living for our family, in an automobile accident, under anesthesia, able to speak English only as a second language, or poor and uninsured, we are in no condition to be alert, smart consumers, protecting our investments and demanding our rights. We are at the mercy of our fellow citizens who we can only hope will be wise and compassionate strangers.

Health care based on profit guidelines estranges patients from health care workers. Furthermore, in the current market-based reorganization of health care, the real buyers are employers and the government. The sellers are the insurance companies. For-profit health care systems insist that they will cut costs by focusing on preventive care rather than curative systems (that act after disease or accident has struck). However, prevention is very expensive and difficult to commodify to individual buyers. Prevention takes community effort and public health measures. Highly technical medicine is much easier to buy and sell. Consequently, insurance companies attempt to limit highly technical procedures as much as possible, while cutting the costs for these procedures by reducing essential supportive care.

Creating a Dialogue Between Lifeworld and System

Public systems are designed to extend access to goods and services to as many individuals as possible. Mass societies work to arrange transactions between strangers who have different cultural backgrounds, or lifeworlds. Large public institutions base their ethics on thin theories of the *good*, such as assurance of rights, justice, and equal access to societal goods (e.g., education, health care, public safety). Consequently, public systems organize around standardized public procedures and rights.[2] Public systems endeavor to minimize costs and maximize efficiency. However, health care has increasingly moved from public institutions to private for-profit health management organizations. The health care system in the United States has rapidly shifted to using market forces to control escalating costs. Insurance companies assumed that health care delivery could be treated like any other market, and that privatizing to create competition between health care institutions would provide the best control. A flurry of for-profit health care management corporations developed with attempts to create large conglomerates that could cut costs and increase profits through creating large economies of scale.

2. R. Dworkin, *Taking Rights Seriously* (London: Duckworth, 1977).

As a result of this shift, much of the nursing workforce shifted from hospitals to home care as hospitals closed. This rapid wholesale change disturbed, and even silenced, dialogue between the lifeworld of caregiving work and large-scale bureaucratic systems. The lifeworld side of organizations animates, coordinates, and creates the necessary social integration and vision for delivering health care. For example, the moral imagination for our health care system has depended on the multiple lifeworld traditions being bound up with the condition of our fellow human beings. In a pluralistic society, notions of good from multiple lifeworld traditions have contributed to the vision of our health care system. For example, there is the Christian tradition of the compassionate stranger who cares for the ill and injured, and the Jewish and Enlightenment traditions which contribute the moral quest to alleviate suffering.

While lifeworlds use economic exchange as a means of valuing and supporting lifeworld concerns, the concerns of the lifeworld govern the principles and style of economic exchange. In contrast, the regulatory functions of free-market economies make the buying and selling of commodities for profit the central organizing principle. Large-scale bureaucratic systems include the regulatory functions of the market and organizational structures of efficiency of scale as regulatory devices for cutting costs and enhancing profits. Max Weber[3] warned of diminishing roles of moral and sentient concerns of the lifeworld in public life by increased rationalization and creation of economies of scale in ever larger markets. Emile Durkheim predicted the dangers of *anomie* — the loss of a sense of belonging in mass societies designed only for markets.[4] Durkheim's prophetic warning about market interests fits the disturbances created by regulating health care by market forces alone.[5] Durkheim calls into question the market as a just and stable source of social integration. He notes that economic interests alone are transitory. At most there is an exchange contract, with the agents continuing to exist as outsiders to each other. The links are external; there is always a question of gains and losses in the exchange. Each party is expected to act in its own best interests in such a relationship. In strictly economic transactions, adversarial relationships are a constant background possibility.

3. M. Weber, *The Protestant Ethic and the Spirit of Capitalism* (New York: Charles Scribner & Sons, 1958).

4. P. Benner and J. Wrubel, *The Primacy of Caring: Stress and Coping in Health and Illness* (Menlo Park, Calif.: Addison-Wesley, 1989).

5. E. Durkheim, *The Division of Labor in Society* (New York: 1933), p. 39.

Durkheim asserts:

If we look further into the matter, we shall see that this total harmony of interests conceals a latent or deferred conflict. For where interest is the only ruling force each individual finds himself in a state of war with every other since nothing comes to mollify the egos, and any truce in this eternal antagonism would not be of long duration.[6]

The ethos of sales is that the seller not sell defective products and that the seller turn a profit for the business enterprise. Sharpe,[7] drawing on the work of Pellegrino and Thomasma,[8] argues for a fiduciary relationship (i.e., a special relationship of responsibility and trust) between health care professionals and patients:

The health care provider's duty to "do no harm" is grounded neither in the authority of the Hippocratic tradition nor simply in the "common morality" but, rather, in the fiduciary nature of the healing relationship. To abandon medical ethics to the marketplace would be to abandon the meaning of illness and the trust on which healing is based.[9]

Such a fiduciary responsibility has been upheld in the courts. For example, Justice Cardozo in Schloendorff v. Society for New York Hospitals wrote:

many forms of conduct permissible in a workaday world for those acting at arm's length are forbidden to those bound by fiduciary ties. A trustee is held to something stricter than the morals of the marketplace.[10]

In contrast to business exchanges, the caregiving work of health care requires that health care workers respond to the needs and suffering of others. Care of embodied, sentient persons is a fragile practice. This chapter focuses on the Christian tradition of the compassionate stranger, though the spirit of the compassionate stranger can be found in many "dispersed forms of goodness," as O'Neill[11] points out. Thus Christians

6. Durkheim, *The Division of Labor in Society*, p. 204.
7. V. A. Sharpe, "Why 'Do No Harm'?" in *The Influence of Edmund D. Pellegrino's Philosophy of Medicine* (Dordrecht: Kluwer), pp. 197-215.
8. E. D. Pellegrino and D. C. Thomasma, *For the Patient's Good: The Restoration of Beneficence in Health Care* (New York: Oxford University Press, 1988), chs. 2-4.
9. Sharpe, p. 204.
10. Quoted in Sharpe, p. 204.
11. O. O'Neill, *Towards Justice and Virtue: A Constructive Account of Practical Reasoning* (Cambridge: Cambridge University Press, 1996).

may work together with like-minded people from many different lifeworld traditions.

Two recent studies of the caring practices of critical care nurses contain many encouraging reports of protecting vulnerabilities, of providing comfort and safety, and of attentiveness and beneficence.[12] But this societally important work is being threatened by rapidly changing work environments.[13] The discouragement and demoralization of nurses who are asked to do more than is possible and who are not given the time to do their caregiving work is alarming (as reflected in Barbara White's study discussed in the Introduction to this volume). When nurses are not given the time to be attentive, large-scale health care systems become dangerous places.

Habermas points out that when things are working well there is little need for articulating the background understandings and practices of the lifeworld:

> It is only in those rare moments when culture and language fail as resources that they develop the peculiar resistance we experience in situations of disturbed mutual understanding. Then we need the repair work of translators, interpreters, therapists . . . as they try to incorporate elements of the lifeworld that are operating dysfunctionally — incomprehensible utterances, opaque traditions, or at the limit, a not-yet-decoded language — into a common interpretation of the situation.[14]

It is not always possible to come to a common interpretation of the situation, but we can create public health care systems where all voices and needs are heard. Habermas points to the importance of narratives for creating a dialogue between the lifeworld and system:

> In adopting the narrative form, we are choosing a perspective that "grammatically" forces us to base our descriptions on an everyday concept of the life-world. . . . A narrator is already constrained grammatically, through the form of narrative presentation, to take an interest in the identity of the persons acting as well as in the integrity

---

12. P. Benner, C. Tanner, and C. Chesla, *Expertise in Nursing Practice: Caring, Clinical Judgment and Ethics* (New York: Springer, 1996); and P. Benner, P. Hooper-Kyriakidis, and D. Stannard, *Clinical Wisdom and Interventions in Critical Care: Thinking-in-Action* (Philadelphia: Saunders, in press).

13. Benner et al., *Clinical Wisdom*, ch. 11.

14. J. Habermas, *The Theory of Communicative Action*, vol. 2, *Lifeworld and System: A Critique of Functionalist Reason*, T. McCarthy, trans. (Boston: Beacon Press, 1981, 1987), p. 134.

of their life-context. When we tell stories, we cannot avoid also saying indirectly how the subjects involved in them are faring, and what fate the collectivity they belong to is experiencing. Nevertheless, we can make harm to personal identity or threats to social integration visible only indirectly in narratives. . . . In coming to an understanding with one another about their situation, participants in interaction stand in a cultural tradition that they at once use and renew. . . . The symbolic structures of the lifeworld are reproduced by way of the continuation of valid knowledge, stabilization of group solidarity, and socialization of responsible actors.[15]

Engineering approaches to organizational design have emphasized productivity over quality and reliability. Considering work as a collection of part tasks does not adequately consider the worker's problem-solving, knowledge, and attentiveness. In health care, where attentiveness and relationship are central to effectiveness and reliability, adding profit incentives to "process" patients more quickly further undermines the moral arts of attentiveness and care.

Dominant views of morality that focus on autonomy as the condition for free moral choice tend to ignore the need for care, and the skill, knowledge, and time required for care:

Vulnerability has serious moral consequences. Vulnerability belies the myth that we are always autonomous, and potentially equal, citizens. To assume equality among humans leaves out and ignores important dimensions of human existence. Throughout our lives, all of us go through varying degrees of dependence and independence, of autonomy and vulnerability. A political order that presumes only independence and autonomy as the nature of human life thereby misses a great deal of human experience, and must somehow hide this point elsewhere. For example, such an order must rightly separate public and private life. . . . Care's absence from our core social and political values reflects many choices our society has made about what to honor. These choices, starting as far away as our conceptions of moral boundaries, operate to exclude the activities and concerns of care from a central place. Through that exclusion, those who are powerful are able to demand that others care for them, and they have been able to maintain their positions of power and privilege.[16]

15. *The Theory of Communicative Action*, pp. 136-37.
16. J. C. Tronto, *Moral Boundaries: A Political Argument for an Ethic of Care* (New York: Routledge, 1993), pp. 135, 179.

The modern helper tends to think of the moral self as that which is "owned" by the self. In such a view of the self, care, responsiveness, and interdependence are signs of a moral lapse and are sources of embarrassment or shame. Caring for our neighbor can be seen as one more set of choices, until of course, we find ourselves in the position of caring or needing care.[17] Care always implies situated or bounded choice. When one is vulnerable or incapacitated, choices about being cared for are constrained.

Do We Still Need Compassionate Strangers?

The care ethic given to us in the Christian tradition has been marginalized in the current market model of health care systems. Market arrangements are developed for autonomous strangers or customers to meet and buy goods and services. The market model overlooks the many ways we are not prepared to be astute and assertive consumers when we are most in need of health care — in times of vulnerability and danger.

In this book that honors the Christian tradition's contributions to health care ethics, I want to revisit the New Testament story of the Good Samaritan. A lawyer wanting to get it right and to inherit eternal life asked Jesus: "Who is my neighbor?" and the answer ushered in a new moral imagining of our interrelatedness and responsibility for one another.

Luke 10:25-37:
And behold, a certain lawyer stood up and put him to the test, saying, "Teacher, what shall I do to inherit eternal life?" . . .

And he [the lawyer] answered and said, "You shall love the Lord your God with all your heart, and with all your soul, and with all your strength, and with all your mind; and your neighbor as yourself."

And he said to him, "You have answered correctly; do this and you will live."

But wishing to justify himself, he said to Jesus, "And who is my neighbor?"

Jesus replied and said, "A certain man was going down from Jerusalem to Jericho; and he fell among robbers, and they stripped him and beat him, and went off leaving him half dead.

"And by chance a certain priest was going down on that road, and when he saw him, he passed by on the other side.

17. C. Taylor, *Sources of the Self* (Cambridge: Cambridge University Press, 1989).

"And likewise a Levite also, when he came to the place and saw him, passed by on the other side.

"But a certain Samaritan, who was on a journey, came upon him; and when he saw him, he felt compassion, and came to him and bandaged up his wounds, pouring oil and wine on them; and he put him on his own beast, and brought him to an inn, and took care of him.

"And the next day he took out two denarii and gave them to the innkeeper and said, 'Take care of him; and whatever more you spend, when I return, I will repay you.' Which one of these three do you think proved to be a neighbor to the man who fell into the robbers' hands?"

And he said, "The one who showed mercy toward him." And Jesus said to him, "Go and do the same."

Robert Wuthnow, in his study *Acts of Compassion,* found the story of the Good Samaritan to still be a major moral source in American society. But he found that the modern person usually imagines being the Samaritan rather than the person left half dead.[18] This switch in our moral imagination has profound implications. The self-assertive modern person imagines being a heroic helper, a moral ideal closer to autonomy and control over one's own destiny. I confess that I, too, would prefer to think of myself as the Good Samaritan rather than the person on the roadside in need of help. But imagining the suffering of others as separate from our own common human vulnerability and community is a poor starting point for bioethics. Taking only the vantage point of the helper creates a false sense of immunity from vulnerability. Identifying only with the helper and not the one helped spawns discourses about who is entitled to help. Too easily the abled and dis-abled become disparate and even adversarial. Thirty-four percent of every health care dollar is spent on administrative costs, and a good portion of those costs goes into determining entitlements to care.

The story of the Good Samaritan suggests that the starting point in health care ethics should be the universal human reality of vulnerability and suffering. Moral worth and respect is to be accorded to all fellow human beings. Therefore, we are to be compassionate strangers to those who fall outside our own communities and kinships. Suffering and vulnerability are the common fates of finite embodied human beings. We each might need a fellow human being to respond with compassion to our needs for protection and comfort.

18. R. Wuthnow, *Acts of Compassion: Caring for Others and Helping Ourselves* (Princeton: Princeton University Press, 1991).

Wuthnow points out that, in our modern individualistic society, we also interpret the story of the Good Samaritan as a story of individual virtue and overlook the institutional and community supports required for virtuous behavior:

> We are drawn to the story of the Good Samaritan with special magnetism because it is essentially, in our modern view, a story about individual virtue. We do not interpret it as a story about the impossibility of living according to divine law. We forget that Jesus told it to a man who had just answered that keeping the law of God perfectly was the only way to inherit eternal life. Nor do we pay much attention to the role of the inn or the symbolism of the two coins, the oil, and the wine. We do not ask the listener to identify with the injured man or show him becoming a part of a community that collectively supports charitable behavior. Instead, we think of the story as a moral lesson. The person who cares with compassion is the person who goes and does likewise. He simply gives help because it is the right thing to do. We fail to ask what sort of upbringing or social support or institutional resources that person may need to perform acts of compassion.
>
> We also fail to see institutional connections with the kind of care that is given. Despite the fact that social services often require organized efforts, we still dwell on the Samaritan sitting there alone on the Jericho road pouring oil on the injured man's wounds. . . . For most of us the story remains an illustration of individual compassion. We let it reinforce our individualism because we neglect even the institutional focus it once had historically.[19]

Nursing practice has a lively tradition of caring for and meeting the other in suffering and vulnerability. But this tradition is increasingly challenged, particularly in the U.S., by managed care. Contracts between third party payers and employers have created new styles of commodification. The market has become the central integrative mechanism for health care — fostering a system of money changers in a not-so-holy temple. For-profit insurance companies have placed incentives in the health care system for decreasing contact with patients and families, which encourages health care professionals to respond as the priest and the Levite. Stringent gatekeeping and disincentives for basic nursing care and social services overlook the fact that few incentives are needed for avoidance and neglect. Avoidance and neglect are very real human temp-

---

19. Wuthnow, *Acts of Compassion,* pp. 176-77.

tations in the face of suffering. The moral and emotional work of meeting and caring for the other in situations of need and vulnerability are required for justice and care. We cannot do without the language and the ethical moorings of justice. Justice and mercy cannot be separated. A just society will create structures for the safety, protection, and nurturance of all citizens. The work of compassion requires just institutions structured for its work. However, justice is a minimal requirement. In the face of vulnerability and suffering, it is not sufficient. Mercy, generosity, hope, and even love are required. At the very least, real relationships, where the other is met and known, are required if we are to avoid the ethical violence of neglect and abuse in the face of vulnerability and suffering.

In establishing hospitals, we understood that life-threatening illnesses are often too much for family members to bear. Even health care workers with technical know-how are not expected to provide direct care to their loved ones in times of great danger or urgency. The difficulties family members experience in assisting ill family members and in bearing witness to their loved one's suffering are increasingly overlooked, as more and more of the burdens of caregiving are shifted to family and friends. We are in danger of overlooking the role of the compassionate stranger to shore up and support families and friends caring for their loved ones. Even when families do their caring work in the best tradition possible, they too need assistance and support when their loved one is seriously ill or injured.

From the biblical story of Job, we get a vision of the possibility of arguing with God, pleading for more justice, and we get a good description of inept helping from Job's comforters. The Old Testament story of Job and the New Testament story of the Good Samaritan demonstrate notions of good. They teach us about being for the other, standing alongside, standing in for, and giving others a voice. These are all forms of advocacy also found in the role of the Holy Spirit in the New Testament, where we are given visions of the Divine Comforter who stands alongside, who advocates for, who substitutes for and meets the other.[20]

---

20. P. Benner, "Caring As Knowing and Not Knowing," in S. Phillips and P. Benner, (eds.), *The Crisis of Care: Affirming and Restoring Caring Practices in the Helping Professions* (Washington, D.C.: Georgetown University Press, 1994), pp. 42-62.

Relational Ethics: Meeting and Responding to the Other

In one of my classes, nursing students write first-person narratives about clinical situations that have taught them something new about practice. Invariably they tell stories about meeting the other in times of suffering. In a recent class, there were five stories from neonatal and pediatric intensive care nurses about caring for infants who had died. In their stories these nurses were the ones who came to know the infant, often more intimately than the parents, and therefore they were in the position of helping the parents come to know the child. These nurses asked questions spawned by their sense of loss and vulnerability after the infant's death: "Did I cross boundaries of involvement that I should not have professionally crossed? Did I get over-involved because I felt the loss of the child so keenly when the child died? Was it reasonable to expose myself repeatedly to loss? How could I protect myself?"

From a strictly defined list of moral duties, no one could ever demand that these nurses care for an infant to the point of suffering over the loss of the child. Such involvement can never be mandated by duty. The most we can ask is that the nurse be gentle, attentive, and respectful of infants and parents, from a strictly ethical perspective. We cannot demand that they love these little strangers. It would be a supererogatory demand, a demand above the call of duty. And yet an ethical violence is created if nurses do not ever become involved to the point that they know the infant in his or her particularity. The consequence of such relationships is that the particular child matters to these nurses and they therefore experience loss when the infant dies. In our modern hospitals there would be no social traces left of the infant if nurses did not come to know, and even love, the babies as they coach the parents in coming to know their infants in the strange environments of neonatal intensive care units. Within a rights and justice framework, we cannot mandate that nurses care for these infants, and yet a great ethical violence is created if nurses do not care. Neglect instead of responsiveness to the infant will occur. This responsiveness is based on an embodied and relational ethic that creates the conditions or ground of being human and living in a human world for infants, children, and adults. The sorrow of the nurses as compassionate strangers is pale by comparison to the parents' grief, but the nurses bear witness to the parents' loss and form part of the community of memory for the infant.

It is telling that the questions of personal loss only come up for these nurses after the death of the child. In the immediacy of the relationship, and the situational demands of responding to the suffering of the infants and parents, the nurses all did "what had to be done." They did not, while *in the relationship* and *in the situation,* ask moral questions about duty and personal costs. Also, they did not imagine that they had been heroic helpers with omnipotent powers to alleviate suffering. However, it is evident from their stories that their compassion and connection to the infants meant a great deal to the parents and to the infants. Being in relationship with another opens up possibilities. This is similar to being an engaged parent, who does not count the tasks or ask bureaucratic questions about hours on duty or breaks. The Good Samaritan also does not appear to have wasted any time rationalizing about personal costs or moral duty. He simply responded to a fellow human being's suffering and did what needed to be done.

Yet, from outside the situation and from a strictly contractual perspective, the nurses or the Samaritan cannot be mandated to care. Once the situation has passed, the nurses ponder how they were able to give themselves so completely to the infant, and only then do they evaluate the costs of their care. Articulating a social and personal ethic of care and compassion that cannot be mandated or legislated, but the absence of which creates the ethical violence of neglect, mis-recognition, and abuse, is a challenge in any era. However, it is especially challenging in this era of economism, individualism, and commodification of health care. We require renewed moral imagination and enchantment with the possibility of loving our neighbor as illustrated in the story of the Good Samaritan.

I worry that Christians have been too caught up in entitlement discourses about who deserves care. This is a deadly form of moralism that does not belong in the trenches where the injured may be found, half dead. It also does not belong in discussions about who deserves access to care. How can the U.S. as a wealthy nation have a health care system that fails to fully include 41 million people? How can we neglect basic public health to our children?

The Danger and Incoherence of Providing Highly Technical Medical Care Without Adequate Support Services

One study of critical-care nursing practice records many examples of breakdown and gaps in the provision of adequate basic nursing care and social services for patients who had received highly technical medicine.[21]

21. Benner et al., *Clinical Wisdom,* ch. 11.

For example, a teenage girl from a poor and unsafe home was placed under the care of her 21-year-old cousin by Child Protective Services after she had incurred extensive injuries due to an automobile accident. This young girl had multiple fractures including a fracture of her tibia, which was pinned. She was wheel-chair bound and receiving a medication to prevent blood clots from forming in her legs. Home Health Care funds were running out and her cousin, who had three young children, was unable to take her to the clinic for follow-up visits. The nurse practitioner pointed out that it was dangerous to take her off the medication to prevent blood clots, and dangerous to leave her on the medicine without adequate medical supervision. The patient had no way to get to the clinic some fifty miles from her foster home and was taken off the medication. She then was lost to follow-up medical care. In other words, expensive surgical repair was provided, but the supportive care needed to render that care safe was not funded. If the young girl develops clots in her legs, the outcome could be fatal, or would at least require a longer and more expensive hospitalization. Being left on the medication without adequate monitoring of blood clotting times is also dangerous. The nurse practitioner found it impossible to bridge the gaps in the services offered and was left with no moral options for the care of this young girl.

In another situation, a 43-year-old former school teacher with early AIDS dementia was discharged to the streets to an almost certain injury or death. His HMO insurance provides no social services and had reached the limit of skilled nursing care provided by the HMO. He was without family or friends who could step in and care for him. He was too functional to be placed on a psychiatric hold and yet was no longer competent enough to advocate for the care he needed. The nurse, in defeat, stated, "sometimes you just have to let the system fail." But of course it is not just a "system failure" for the endangered former school teacher. It is his life. Working in such a failed system is demoralizing, forcing health care workers into immoral choices between equally untenable options. Mohr and Mahon[22] have written about such dilemmas in the current destabilized health care system as the "dirty hands" moral dilemma, because the agent is constrained to choose between two bad alternatives:

> These situations differ from most moral dilemmas in that those commonly encountered are cases in which there is no right act open to the

22. W. Mohr and M. Mahon, "Dirty Hands: The Underside of Marketplace Health Care," *Advances in Nursing Science* 19 (1) (1996): 23-37.

agent; every option is simply wrong. Dirty hands cases are those instances in which one agent is morally forced by someone else's immorality to do what is, or otherwise would be wrong. A key element of dirty hands situations is not only the choice between two options, but also the role of immorality in creating situations that necessitate and justify acting with dirty hands.

Compassionate, safe, just health care cannot be mandated or managed by distant, profit-driven systems, controlling the services offered. Almost daily, newspapers provide examples of distant rationing decisions being made by insurance companies about when and which provider can provide service regardless of the incovenience and even risk of the patient and family. Compassionate, safe, and just health care requires the political will of the society to demand safe and reliable health care as a basic good and a human service. It also requires health care workers who have a clear moral vision and a call to be worthy, compassionate strangers who seek to act with justice and mercy. Health care professionals must be able to work in systems that do not provide incentives for under-treatment or over-treatment. The economic structures need to restore the moral contract for protection of vulnerability, for justice and mercy between providers and patients, rather than economic deals between employers and insurers to increase profits. Our health care and educational systems are based on fundamental social contracts between citizens. When our health care fails to be humane and compassionate, our most basic social contract and connections are broken. Our most basic social contract — to be a civil society where citizens' lives demand respect and care — is being undermined and broken daily in the current market-driven health care system.

Our psychological age has taught us to articulate more clearly the many aspects of caring that can go awry, such as burnout, co-dependency, and heroic helping, or as in the case of Job's helpers, shaming and blaming the marginalized. The work of Danish theologian Knud Logstrup[23] and that of nurse philosopher Kari Martinsen[24] hold the position that caring for one another is a natural response to the gift of life, of being a part of the created universe. In Logstrup's creationist theology, one must have a reason *not* to care, *not* to experience joy, *not* to express oneself, *not* to

23. K. Logstrup, *The Ethical Demand*, T. I. Jensen, trans. (Philadelphia: Fortress, 1971).

24. K. Martinsen, *From Marx to Logstrup*, in press. Translation, National League for Nursing.

trust in response to the gift of life. Care, joy, self-expression, and trust are sovereign manifestations of being part of a created universe. Logstrup is not blind to our rather dark human history, but as a theologian/philosopher wants to point out how blind and unnatural it is not to care for fellow human beings. He states:

> People are bound to one another, among other things, through love, sympathy, and solidarity. By love and friendship they are bound together in a spontaneous way, whereas in solidarity they are bound together more through cooperative endeavor and common circumstances. But whether these ties are formed spontaneously or socially, it is these ties which constitute a person's existence. The more intensely and comprehensively a person binds himself to other people spontaneously and socially, the more he will see that a selfish life lived at the expense of others is empty and unsuccessful and the more he will refrain from that kind of life.[25]

Unfortunately there are many reasons that block persons' sociability. For example, in current health care settings, work overload and rapidly changing systems make it harder to meet the other with kindness and respect. However, it is misleading to think that there was once a perfect system or a utopian time when meeting the other was easy. Meeting those who are suffering presents an ethical challenge regardless of the environment and circumstances. However, unjust systems and distressing conditions make compassionate responses less likely.

The Challenge and Opportunity Before Us

Logstrup's position that it is natural to respond to the suffering of other human beings is a controversial and provocative philosophical stance, especially in societies riddled with violence or war. It seems to overlook the perverse rationalizations we make about not being called to help our neighbor, and the rampant selfishness and greed. Complex bureaucracies, violent behavior, too many demands, and viewing the "other" as wholly other (outside one's own community and even outside of humanity) are all sources of dehumanization that prevent persons from seeing the other's suffering and trying to help. But what if we, as a society, stopped focusing on the "reasons" why we cannot respond to others'

25. Logstrup, *The Ethical Demand*, p. 133.

suffering and focused on alleviating that suffering and violence in our society?

O'Nora O'Neill points out that community development inherent in caring labor requires attentiveness and work.[26] This work is central to communities and families and to our public caregiving institutions such as health care systems and schools. It is so basic that it is overlooked as the very fabric that holds together the possibility for acting in a social world.

One might wonder whether caring for and meeting the other as a compassionate stranger is possible in unjust institutions. In fact, nurses ask themselves this question daily in a market-driven health care system that has systematically cut the caring and support services required for highly technical medical interventions.[27] O'Nora O'Neill points out that while care cannot compensate for unjust and neglectful systems, it becomes even more necessary, though insufficient, in such systems:

> The directly expressed social virtues are particularly important, and their neglect peculiarly undermining, when public institutions are bitterly unjust or destitution extreme. Although no amount of virtuous action can compensate for injuries of injustice, it can make some difference. Although nobody can care for and help all others, so that any obligation to do so must be selective, and more selective still under the yoke of unjust or corrupt institutions, or in harsh poverty, the very fact that virtue can best be embodied in individual character, and hence exercised in dispersed forms, means that at times it survives when justice does not. Then, as in easier times, nobody can show concern or care for everybody, but some people may be able to show some care or concern for some others, and so forge and sustain forms of solidarity or friendship which ease the pain of poverty and injustice, even if neither can be mitigated. Sometimes dispersed acts of solidarity and support also have cumulative public effects: this is the power of the powerless even in hard times.[28]

There are many reasons nurses and physicians cannot meet the other with kindness in an unjust health care system where the safety of patients is being undermined by extreme staffing cuts. Zigmunt Bauman

26. O. O'Neill, *Towards Justice and Virtue.*
27. Benner, "Caring As Knowing and Not Knowing."
28. See V. Havel, "The Power of the Powerless," trans. P. Wilson, in Jan Vladislav (ed.), *Living the Truth* (London: Faber and Faber, 1986), pp. 36-122.

traces our slide from a social polity of a sense of shared responsibility for individual weal and woe:

> The welfare state, wisely, institutionalized commonality of fate: its provisions were meant for every participant (every citizen) in equal measure, thus balancing everybody's privations with everybody's gains. The slow retreat from that principle into the means-tested focused assistance for those who need it has institutionalized the diversity of fate, and thus made the unthinkable thinkable. . . . Altogether different principles are embodied in, say, a child benefit for every parent, and child benefit for indolent parents alone. The first makes tangible the bond between public and private — community and individual — and casts the community as the pledge of the individual's security. The second sets the public and the private against each other, and casts the community as the individual's burden and bane.[29]

We have to face up to the injustices in our health care system, as well as the way these social structures and meanings create different pathologies of caring. The possibilities of caring relationships play out differently based on the background social meanings for caring practices. The heroic helper who gains manipulative power over the other through "helping" — or an unliberated view of the victimized, overburdened helping martyr — have built into them social injustice. A society that commodifies care at every turn has every reason to be cynical.[30]

We tend to forget what a cultural innovation we have in the Christian tradition of hospitality and the Good Samaritan. We would do well to revisit the premodern understandings of this parable. Logstrup's notion of meeting the other — in the sovereign life expressions of trust, openness, and mercy — suggests moral sources that could create new understanding of the possibility of meeting and responding to others, even in the midst of suffering. The possibilities opened up in direct caring relationships and in concrete situations of need are different from those we imagine for ourselves outside of particular relationships and situations. Situated in caring relationships and concrete situations of need, one usually "does what needs to be done." Christians have much to add to a more community-oriented vision of nurturance and relationships. If we are to leaven the society these caring practices must be disbursed throughout our public institutions.

29. Z. Bauman, *Post-Modern Ethics* (London: Blackwell, 1993), p. 243.
30. Bauman, *Post-Modern Ethics*, p. 243.

Guidelines for Gatekeepers:
A Covenantal Approach

Gregory W. Rutecki, M.D.

One might describe the current economic predicament of U.S. health care in terms of a pressing need to cut costs while substantially preserving quality. To attain what arguably may be unattainable, numerous reforms have been implemented, and one — hereafter designated under the rubric of gatekeeping — has captured the fancy of third party payers. Gatekeeping is defined as the practice of controlling access to "pricey" specialty interventions by means of primary care physicians who are strategically located at the entry point into the health care system. Although this practice has become increasingly common in health maintenance organizations (HMOs), the impact of such a strategy on health care costs and on the quality of care rendered remains controversial.[1] Further scrutiny of gatekeeping from the perspective of the Christian-Hippocratic tradition is necessary.

In the past, the role of gatekeepers in American medicine was accepted transiently but with a healthy skepticism. The committees who selected patients for dialysis in the late 1960s and early 1970s were equated by at least one author with the *gauleiter* of concentration camps,

---

1. E. Ginzberg, M. Ostow, "Managed Care: A Look Back and a Look Ahead," *New England Journal of Medicine* 336 (1997):1018-20; and J. P. Kassirer, "Is Managed Care Here to Stay? *N Eng J Med* 336 (1997): 1013-14. Ginzberg and Ostow observe, "Moreover, the rapid expansion of enrollment in managed care has *not* prevented the estimated overall spending for health care in 1995 from increasing by 5.4% . . . if one considers the period from 1980 to 1995, the decade and a half in which managed care grew very rapidly, overall health care outlays quadrupled, from $250 billion to 1 trillion."

literally deciding life and death for others.[2] The gatekeeper concept has been resurrected within a health care system undergoing a transformation driven by pressures to lower costs. Enrollments in HMOs have increased tenfold since 1976.[3] Congress has recently signed legislation that will give Medicare patients strong financial incentives to enroll in managed care plans.[4]

Today's gatekeeping model in such a cost-conscious environment has linked physician income to proficiency in limiting tests and referrals.[5] Financial arrangements may take several forms including financial penalties for resource "spendthrifts," rewards for "efficients," or savings through capitation. The fundamental motivation for this approach is an almost universally held but untested theory which holds that specialists provide more costly and expendable services than do generalists. Thus, an increase in the utilization of primary care physicians who control access to specialty interventions and expensive testing should decrease health care costs.

However, a potential side effect of this gatekeeping is that limiting access to specialty interventions may sometimes compromise outcomes, resulting in an ominous "trade-off" for the money saved. Because quality concerns have been raised about this gatekeeper model, the role of the physician gatekeeper could create an ethical dilemma for Christian health care workers.

Gatekeeping, Acute Coronary Syndromes, and Beyond

One way to test the theory underlying the current gatekeeper model is to look at the potential effect of gatekeeping on a prevalent and serious condition. Coronary artery disease is a common cause of hospitalization, it results in substantial mortality, and its treatment has yielded data

2. B. D. Kahan, "Organ Donation and Transplantation: A Surgeon's View," in *Organ Transplantation: Meanings and Realities*, ed. S. J. Youngner, R. C. Fox, L. J. O'Connell (University of Wisconsin Press, 1996), p. 137.

3. J. E. Ware, M. S. Bayliss, W. H. Rogers, M. Kosinstei, A. R. Tarlov, "Differences in 4-Year Health Outcomes for Elderly and Poor,Chronically Ill Patients Treated in HMO and Fee-For-Service Systems," *Journal of the American Medical Association* 276 (1996): 1039.

4. D. P. Sulmasy, "Physicians, Cost Control and Ethics," *Annals of Internal Medicine* 116 (1992): 9210.

5. Group Health Association of America, *Patterns in HMO Enrollment* (Washington, D.C.: Group Health Association of America, June 1995).

suggesting that specific interventions reduce morbidity and mortality. In 1990 there were 525,000 admissions for unstable angina, resulting in 2.9 million hospital days.[6] Myocardial infarction continues to be the leading cause of death in the United States, accounting for nearly 700,000 hospital discharges annually.[7] Because of their economic and human toll, coronary syndromes have become a major target of health care reform.

Management of acute coronary syndromes has become standardized enough that Clinical Practice Guidelines have been suggested by the American College of Cardiology and the American Heart Association.[8] Age-adjusted mortality rates from coronary syndromes have fallen by approximately 40 percent over the last two decades — a result of large-scale clinical trials which have proven the efficacy of several interventions. Therapeutic benefit has been established for beta blockers, calcium channel blockers, aspirin, heparin, cholesterol-lowering agents, and thrombolytics, as well as for angioplasty and coronary artery bypass grafting.

Jollis and coworkers examined mortality from acute myocardial infarction (MI) in 8,241 Medicare patients from four states during a 17-month period beginning in 1992.[9] They specifically looked at the specialty of the admitting physician. They applied proportional hazards regression models to determine survival up to one year after an MI. In addition, to determine the generalizability of the findings, they examined insurance claims and survival data of all 220,535 patients for whom Medicare claims were made for hospital care necessitated by an acute MI during the study period. After adjustments were made for patient characteristics, it was demonstrated that patients with an acute MI who were admitted to the hospital by cardiologists were 12 percent less likely to die within one year than those admitted by primary care physicians (p < 0.001). The authors concluded: "Health care strategies that shift the care

6. E. J. Graves, "Detailed Diagnoses and Procedures," National Hospital Discharge Survey (1990). National Center for Health Statistics. Vital Health Statistics 1992; 13: 113.

7. E. J. Graves, *1991 Summary: National Hospital Discharge Survey* (Hyattsville, Md.: National Center for Health Statistics, 1993). (DHHS publication no. [PHS] 93-1250).

8. R. M. Gunnar, P. D. V. Bourdillon, D. W. Dixon, "Guidelines for the Early Management of Patients with Acute Myocardial Infarction: A Report of the American College of Cardiology/American Heart Association Task Force on Assessment of Diagnostic and Therapeutic Cardiovascular Procedures," *Journal of the American College of Cardiology* 16 (1990): 249-92.

9. J. G. Jollis, E. R. DeLong, E. D. Peterson et al., "Outcome of Acute Myocardial Infarction According to the Specialty of the Admitting Physician," *N Eng J Med* 335 (1996): 1880-87.

of elderly patients with myocardial infarctions from cardiologists to primary care physicians lower rates of resource utilization but they may also lead to decreased survival."

In an article entitled "Do Cardiologists Do It Better?" Nash and coworkers reviewed the Pennsylvania Health Care Cost Containment Council Report on 40,684 hospital admissions for myocardial infarction in the state during 1993.[10] These data demonstrated that patients cared for by cardiologists had a lower risk-adjusted mortality than patients cared for by either general internists (risk ratio 1.26) or family practitioners (risk ratio 1.29). If all 12,960 patients who were treated by internists had been treated by cardiologists instead, it was calculated that 285 fewer deaths would have been anticipated. Had cardiologists cared for the 6,971 patients of family physicians, 174 fewer patient fatalities would have been expected. These authors concluded that "there is enhanced value in the care provided by cardiologists for patients with acute MI and this calls into question the growing trend toward reliance on generalists instead of specialists."

Why are there striking differences between the outcomes produced by generalists and specialists in their care of patients with acute coronary syndromes? A number of studies have documented that both a knowledge of appropriate therapy and a tendency to apply interventional techniques may significantly impact patient survival. Ayanian and colleagues demonstrated by a survey of 1,211 cardiologists, internists, and family practitioners that internists and family practitioners were less aware and less certain about key advances in the treatment of myocardial infarction than were cardiologists.[11] The knowledge gap involved the use of thrombolytic therapy, prophylactic lidocaine, aspirin, and beta blockers, as well as the use of diltiazem in non-transmural infarctions. The survey data was expanded to actual practice by Schreiber and colleagues who demonstrated that internists were less likely than cardiologists to use aspirin or beta blockers and more frequently used exercise testing but avoided catheterization for unstable chest pain.[12] In unstable angina, the mortality rate

10. I. S. Nash, D. B. Nash, V. Fuster, "Do Cardiologists Do It Better?" *Journal of the American College of Cardiology* 29 (1997): 475-78.

11. J. Z. Ayanian, P. J. Hauptman, E. Guadagnoli et al., "Knowledge and Practices of Generalist and Specialist Physicians Regarding Drug Therapy for Acute Myocardial Infarction," *N Eng J Med* 331 (1994): 1136-42.

12. T. L. Schreiber, A. Elkhatib, C. L. Grines et al., "Cardiologist versus Internist Management of Patients with Unstable Angina: Treatment Patterns and Outcomes," *Journal of the American College of Cardiology* 26 (1995): 577-82.

was 4.0 percent for general internists and 1.8 percent for cardiologists. The authors concluded that "patients with unstable angina treated by internists were less likely to receive effective medical therapy or revascularization procedures and experienced a trend to poorer outcomes. This study does not support a positive gatekeeper role for generalists in the treatment of unstable angina."

Are diseases other than coronary syndromes adversely affected by the managed care approach? Ware and coworkers compared the physical and mental health outcomes of chronically ill adults, including elderly and poor subgroups, treated in HMOs versus fee-for-service (FFS) systems.[13] Two thousand thirty-five patients 18-97 years of age with hypertension, noninsulin dependent diabetes, recent acute MI, congestive heart failure, and depressive disorders were analyzed. In comparisons between HMO and FFS systems, Medicare patients declined in physical health more frequently in HMOs (54 percent versus 28 percent; p < .001). The authors concluded: "During the study period, elderly and poor chronically ill patients had worse physical health outcomes in HMOs than FFS systems . . . current health care plans should carefully monitor the health outcomes of these vulnerable subgroups." It appears that both acute diseases requiring potentially costly interventions and chronic diseases requiring complicated management strategies have poorer outcomes in an HMO approach to health care.

Finally, lest one assume that generalist/specialist disparities are unique to either a select disease or an age range, similar trends have been demonstrated in the management of asthma and diabetes mellitus.[14] Asthma is a disease prevalent in a younger cohort and asthmatic patients experience adverse outcomes when they do not have access to specialty care.

13. J. E. Ware, M. S. Bayliss, W. H. Rogers et al., "Differences in Four-Year Health Outcomes for Elderly and Poor, Chronically Ill Patients Treated in HMO and Fee-for-Service Systems," *JAMA* 276 (1996): 1039-47.

14. R. S. Zeiger, S. Heller, J. H. Mellon et al., "Facilitated Referral to Asthma Specialist Reduces Relapses in Asthma Emergency Room Visits," *Journal of American Clinical Immunologists* 87 (1991): 1160. See also W. M. Vollmer, M. O'Hallaren, K. M. Ettinger et al., "Specialty Differences in the Management of Asthma: A Cross-sectional Assessment of Allergists' Patients and Generalists' Patients in a Large HMO," *Archives of Internal Medicine* 157 (1997): 1201. See also E. Ritz, A. Stefanski, "Diabetic Nephropathy in Type II Diabetes," *American Journal of Kidney Diseases* 27 (1996): 186-87.

Formulating a Christian Paradigm
in the Era of Managed Care

George Lundberg, in coining the term *"caveat aeger"* or "let the patient beware," has compared the recent philosophical shift in contemporary medicine to a "rocking horse" — with physician professionalism on one end and business interests on the other.[15] He expresses grave concern that medicine's rocking horse has rocked to one extreme — that medicine has become fixated on business interests. His apprehension, as well as that of others, stems from the all-too-real ethical conflicts inherent in managed care.[16] For example, although physicians have been traditionally viewed as moral agents who act in their patients' best interests, they have now emerged as contracted employees of managed care organizations. The financial constraints inherent in these contracts create conflicts of interest for physicians with the potential to foster estrangement as well as to compromise care. Typically, when managed care organizations utilize primary care physicians as gatekeepers, monetary incentives are provided to decrease specialty referrals. If these incentives lead physicians to withhold services that would be in their patients' best interests, the rocking horse has truly tilted away from a traditional ethic. In addition, the gatekeeper approach disguises the real rationing of decision-makers; it rations by "class" rather than in general; it places physicians in an environment of moral stress; and it threatens the trust so necessary in the doctor-patient relationship.[17]

From a Christian perspective, William May has characterized the physician-patient relationship as a covenant.[18] A covenantal outlook is different from the contractual understanding of the physician-patient relationship increasingly influential in contemporary medicine. A proper covenant is tripartite, involving two partners and God. Substantially more

15. G. D. Lundberg, "Countdown to Millennium — Balancing the Professionalism and Business of Medicine: Medicine's Rocking Horse," *JAMA* 263 (1990): 86.

16. Group Health Association of America, *Patterns in HMO Enrollment*. See also M. A. Rodwin, "Conflicts in Managed Care," *N Eng J Med* 332 (1995): 604-7. I am indebted to the author for comprehensively identifying the ethical pitfalls of managed care. See also D. Buckley, "Gatekeeper Ethics: The Primary Care Physician in the Era of Managed Care," *Ethics and Medicine* 132 (1997): 39-42 for a Christian perspective.

17. Group Health Association of America, *Patterns in HMO Enrollment*. See also Rodwin, "Conflicts in Managed Care."

18. W. F. May, "Code and Covenant or Philanthropy and Contract?" in *Ethics in Medicine: Historical Perspectives and Contemporary Concerns*, ed. S. J. Reiser (Cambridge, Mass.: MIT Press, 1977), pp. 65-76.

is required of covenanting partners than is necessarily required by a contract. A covenant involves the notion of a change in being, a so-called ontologic change in those covenanted. A covenanted people is a people changed utterly by the covenant. A covenant involves a permanent commitment, not just a limited agreement for the duration of a contract. A covenant relationship continues even while eating, sleeping, working, praying, and through all facets of doctor-patient interaction. In May's words, Christian physicians are altered "pervasively" in their being by the covenant.

Comparing the requirements of covenant relationships with the business interests of managed care (especially its gatekeeper model) reveals certain critical differences. First, a covenanted physician must be ready to cope with the unexpected. Services that exceed those anticipated within the financial constraints of contract may be required. Whereas contractual capitated funding or referral algorithms may deny expensive but efficacious interventions, covenant relationships demand better patient access. Second, the covenant relationship continually builds up the doctor-patient relationship. When health care is delivered primarily as a commodity, negative consequences will ensue, leading to estrangement within what should be a sacred relationship. Third, a covenantal outlook must remind the professional community that it is not sufficient for only the doctor to be in a covenant with the patient; institutions must be also, whether they are hospitals, HMOs, PPOs, or other varieties of practice. Incentives that benefit two of the three key partners in managed care plans — i.e., the gatekeeper and provider — but exclude the patient, are inconsistent with a covenant. The "triangular relationship" of Hippocratism involving doctor, patient, and God is disturbed by the intrusion of business priorities that take precedence over patient needs.

Finally, covenant entails promises of faithfulness and truthfulness that go beyond agreements explicitly affirmed. Being a doctor in covenant is more than telling truths; it also requires an unswerving commitment to any promises made and even to those unmade that are intrinsic to the purposes of medicine. The promise of care excludes the withholding of any therapy that is in the patient's best interest, if that withholding is solely for the purpose of maximizing profit.

How should the Christian physician respond to those aspects of gatekeeping that are in conflict with covenantal medicine? A number of preliminary guidelines may be deduced from the previous discussion. First, monetary incentives designed to reduce specialty referrals, and aimed at cost-cutting to the exclusion of benefit, are inconsistent with

Christian-Hippocratic practice. Cost-savings aimed at unnecessary tests or unnecessary referrals are acceptable and just, and should be differentiated from savings that negatively affect morbidity and mortality. Second, covenant truthfulness requires full physician-to-patient disclosure of any constraints or limitations on specialized procedures that are part of the managed care guidelines. Third, gatekeepers are obligated to identify areas of medicine wherein specialty efficacy exceeds that of primary care. There is little question that generalists provide some types of essential care better than specialists. Outcomes research can help identify which group — i.e., generalist or specialist — should manage specific diseases.

Finally, Christian specialists affirming the covenantal model of medicine may be obligated to capitate charges at a level substantially lower than at present, while at the same time permitting reasonable access to expensive technology for those who cannot pay. Prohibitive charges for specialty expertise are as unacceptable as the lack of a referral. There is evidence suggesting that patterns of specialist practice create a whole new set of conflicts with Christian-Hippocratic practice. Data have demonstrated that African-American, Hispanic, poor, uninsured, and public hospital patients receive necessary cardiac catheterization less often than other patients.[19] Such instances represent another pernicious variety of gatekeeping already occurring with the consent of subspecialists. Safeguards for patients in a post-Hippocratic era are increasingly becoming necessary.

Daniel Sulmasy has trenchantly observed a temporal convergence between the interest in managed care and managed death.[20] His physician soliloquy describing the care of a patient with amyotrophic lateral sclerosis (ALS or Lou Gehrig's disease) involves an array of possible medical interventions: bladder control by catheter, ventilator support if necessary, comfort care and/or assisted suicide if it is legalized. In essence, assisted suicide as a medical option is a specter that could irreversibly corrode the already troubled ethics of managed care. The gatekeeper would enter a maelstrom of unspoken costs and conflicting interests while actually

19. M. Laouri, R. L. Kravitz, W. J. French et al., "Underuse of Coronary Revascularization Procedures: Application of a Clinical Method," *Journal of the American College of Cardiology* 29 (1997): 891. See also E. D. Peterson, L. K. Shaw, E. R. DeLong et al., "Racial Variation in the Use of Coronary Revascularization Procedures — Are the Differences Real? Do They Matter?" *N Eng J Med* 336 (1997): 480.

20. D. P. Sulmasy, "Managed Care and Managed Death," *Archives of Internal Medicine* 155 (1995): 133-36.

receiving financial rewards for well-timed euthanasia. Sulmasy's hypo-
thetical patients with terminal disease would cost managed care less if
their needs for health care — i.e., they themselves — are eliminated. In
Sulmasy's words, "real care is about people in all their unfathomable
mystery. Care breaks through the boundaries of practice guidelines. Care
stands over the carrot-and-stick approach of financial incentives. There
are even those who believe that, in the end, it is only the mystery of care
that can subsume the mystery of death." Never has there been a day
when clarity is more needed regarding the proper role of the physician.
A Christian-Hippocratic covenantal model has much to offer.

For Patients and Profits: Business Ethics for Managed Care Organizations

Kenman L. Wong, M.B.A., Ph.D.

The rapid emergence of managed care medicine, particularly when delivered by for-profit organizations, has raised growing concerns about the clash between the divergent goals of business and medicine. In a number of recent situations, patients have allegedly been given substandard care or denied specific treatments altogether as a result of cost-cutting practices, ostensibly implemented in the quest for greater profits.[1] As a result of such incidents, it has become evident that there is a pressing need for a set of ethical norms from which moral responsibilities and social policies can be developed to govern the activities of managed care organizations.

However, the development of such standards is a difficult task. These organizations are in the perplexing position of attempting to function simultaneously as both traditional businesses with obligations to return financial gains to shareholders, and as medical providers with duties to

---

1. See, for example, David R. Olmos, "Cutting Health Costs — or Corners?" *Los Angeles Times*, 5 May 1995, pp. A1, 22-23.

I am extremely grateful to William W. May of the University of Southern California and Scott B. Rae of Talbot School of Theology, Biola University, for their extensive comments on earlier versions of this paper. The preparation of this paper was made possible, in part, by the generous support of a faculty development grant from Biola University, where I served on the faculty until May 1997.

uphold the primacy of patient health. Thus, standards that apply to one function do not necessarily apply to the other.

Consequently, numerous commentators have summarily dismissed the usefulness and applicability of norms developed through the lens of business ethics in favor of those formulated through traditional medical ethics. For example, Wendy Mariner makes the observation that in their commercial functions managed care organizations can act like "ordinary business organizations with no moral obligations or, at least, obligations that have little to do with traditional medical ethics."[2] More poignantly, she states that when "an MCO's financial goals conflict with its service methods, little in the field of business ethics argues for giving subscribers priority."[3]

While the sentiments expressed in statements such as these make intuitive sense, they erroneously overlook the value of business ethics for managed care arrangements. Business and medicine, and their respective ethical standards, have much more in common than a cursory examination would accurately indicate. In fact, a number of insightful authors have pointed out that the perceived dichotomy between these two arenas is largely overstated.[4] Medicine, they argue, is not nearly as altruistic as commonly portrayed, and business is not nearly as greed-driven.[5]

Based in part upon the recognition of similarities between the two arenas, the primary aim of this paper is to contribute to the important task of constructing guidelines that account for the dual nature of these organizations. In so doing, I will show the relevance and applicability to managed care organizations of norms derived from business practice and the field of business ethics. Furthermore, I will make the argument that the use of standards informed by business ethics is not only possible, but may in some ways be preferable to a traditional medical model, given the current fiscal limits of the new health care environment.

One of the primary benefits of utilizing business ethics, to be de-

2. Wendy K. Mariner, "Business vs. Medical Ethics: Conflicting Standards for Managed Care," *Journal of Law, Medicine & Ethics* 23 (1995): 236-46.

3. Mariner, p. 238.

4. See Andrew Wicks, "Albert Schweitzer or Ivan Boesky? Why We Should Reject the Dichotomy Between Medicine and Business," *Journal of Business Ethics* 14, no. 5 (May 1995): 339-51; and Nancy Jecker, "Managed Competition and Managed Care: What Are the Ethical Issues?" *Clinics in Geriatric Medicine* 10, no. 3 (August 1994): 527-40; and Uwe Reinhardt in Arnold Relman and Uwe Reinhardt, "An Exchange on For-Profit Health Care," Institute of Medicine, *For-Profit Enterprise in Health Care* (Washington, D.C.: National Academy Press, 1986).

5. Wicks, pp. 348-49.

scribed later, is that managed care organizations may respond better to norms developed with business-oriented terms and concepts. These organizations do function, in part, as commercial enterprises, with responsibilities for shareholder interests. Although many physicians and the broader public may not be comfortable with the idea, it is likely that these institutions will be the dominant model of health care delivery for some time to come. Thus, it is helpful for patients, physicians, and policy makers to be equipped with ideas and concepts from business ethics in order to hold managed care organizations to appropriate levels of responsibility.

To be clear, the argument here is not that business ethics offers a perfect or seamless paradigm, as there are some medical obligations which may not fit too easily with business functions. However, norms stemming from business ethics should not be readily dismissed, for they add substantially to the discussion.

In the conclusion of this paper, some examples of the ethical responsibilities that can be assigned to managed care organizations based upon business ethics will be described. These responsibilities are consistent with both the medical and business functions of these institutions.

Reassessing the Differences Between Business and Medicine

Much of the objection to the participation of shareholder-owned business organizations in managed care stems from concerns over the challenges raised by the profit motive. Simply put, it is believed that there will be inevitable and irreconcilable conflicts in mixing business with medicine. The traditional "good" for medicine, embodied in the Hippocratic Oath, has been the health of the patient, while the "good" for business has been and continues to be profit.[6] For instance, Lonnie Bristow, President of the American Medical Association, recently stated that:

> We now have health care being controlled by MBA's rather than by physicians committed to the Hippocratic Oath . . . once health care becomes corporatized . . . then its major commitment is to Wall Street

6. I am indebted to William W. May for stating this in such a poignant and insightful fashion. See William W. May, paper presented at the American Academy of Religion, panel on "Managed Care: Insurers, Values, and the Bottom Line on Care," New Orleans, 25 November 1996.

and the stockholders to maximize profits, rather than to give the best possible patient care. Business principles are introduced that unfortunately put patient care second to corporate profits.[7]

While statements to this effect have become common, they do not adequately frame the relationship between these two arenas. To begin with, a reexamination of medicine reveals that it has always had a strong "business" dimension to it, and physicians are not nearly as charitable as has been portrayed.

Unlike priests, doctors do not take vows of poverty. Despite claims to the contrary, medicine continues to be a very well-paying profession, notwithstanding the recent downward trend in income brought about by managed care, especially in those specialties that have had an overabundance of providers. Moreover, self-serving abuses such as fee splitting, self-referrals, kickbacks from hospitals, and other activities in which physician actions are intimately tied to their own financial interests have also been well documented.[8] It is also well known that most physicians are concentrated in wealthy geographic areas, while poor rural regions often suffer from a dearth of available providers.

While many physicians are motivated by more altruistic concerns, the above considerations should temper the view of medicine as a profession devoid of self-interest (and selfishness). However, it is important to point out that health care delivery prior to managed care was also riddled with financial conflicts of interest. Economic incentives under fee-for-service arrangements functioned in a manner that led physicians to overtest and overtreat.[9] While overtreatment may at first appear to be less harmful than the potential for undertreatment resulting from managed care arrangements, overtreatment is not always benign. Iatrogenic harm is well documented in the medical literature. Moreover, even if no physical harm is ever suffered by individual patients, overtreatment contributes to the rising cost of care, which in turn exacerbates the problem of lack of access to formal health care coverage by millions.[10]

In light of these examples, it seems evident that there has always

7. Bettijane Levine, "He Might Have the Cure for Medicine's Ills" (Interview with Lonnie Bristow), Los Angeles Times (18 July 1995): E1.

8. See Mark A. Rodwin, *Money, Medicine and Morals* (New York: Oxford University Press, 1992); Dan Brock, "Medicine and Business: An Unhealthy Mix?" *Business and Professional Ethics Journal* 9, nos. 3 & 4 (1990): 21-37; and Dan Brock and Allen Buchanan, "The Profit Motive in Medicine," *Journal of Medicine and Philosophy* 24 (1987).

9. To be sure, the litigious environment also contributes a great deal to this situation.

10. Wicks, p. 342.

been a close connection between business and medicine. In addition, the current strain on macro-level resources is increasingly forcing a closer relationship between these two arenas. In a context of resource constraints, physicians can no longer operate under a system that has often encouraged inefficient and wasteful practices.

Toward an Enlightened Business Ethic

Dismissals of the usefulness of business ethics in medicine rely upon the assumption that commerce is solely concerned with profit maximization. This assumption needs further scrutiny. Such negative conceptions of commerce have intuitive appeal given common portrayals of business organizations and the actors within them as being immoral, or at a minimum, amoral.[11] Without a doubt, some economists of the neo-classical school of thought have done much to advance this notion.[12] For example, in his oft-cited essay, "The Social Responsibility of Business Is to Increase Its Profits," Milton Friedman, the leading advocate of the "custodian of wealth" model of business, argues that a corporation fulfills its ethical duties by simply maximizing the wealth of shareholders within the parameters set by explicit legal guidelines. He further argues that for managers to act "socially responsible" in a manner that is above the law and does not contribute to profit, is tantamount to stealing from the owners of the corporation, the shareholders.[13]

11. Such negative depictions of business can be seen often. Scenarios in which the corporate pursuit of profit conflicts with other social interests such as full employment, public safety, individual privacy, and a host of other moral norms have filled newspaper columns and television "news magazine" segments. Almost on a weekly basis, television programs such as ABC's *20/20, Primetime Live!,* NBC's *Dateline,* and CBS's *48 Hours* feature a segment on a business-vs.-society issue. Furthermore, feature-length films often utilize themes of conspiring, evil corporations for plot lines. While films like *Wall Street, The Firm,* and *Glengarry Glen Ross* are more obvious ones, evil corporations play ominous roles (much like the CIA or "the Company" used to play) in movies such as *The Pelican Brief, The Net,* and *Jerry McGuire.* The less negative, but nonetheless questionable, amoral view of business comes in the form of assumptions that financial goals are separate from moral ones. From this perspective, ethical concerns are assumed to be mere afterthoughts to economic efficiency.

12. For a more detailed description of this portrayal and a critical assessment of it, see Robert C. Solomon, "The Myth of the Profit Motive," in *Excellence and Ethics* (New York: Oxford University Press, 1992), pp. 39-47.

13. Milton Friedman, "The Social Responsibility of Business Is to Increase Its Profits," *New York Times Magazine,* 13 September 1970, pp. 33, 122-26.

More recently, however, Friedman's "custodian of wealth" approach has been challenged by a number of alternative frameworks to business ethics and, more importantly, business practice. The most popular alternative is "stakeholder theory," which suggests that the interests of other parties such as employees, the community, and suppliers should be balanced with those of shareholders in the decisions a company makes.[14]

Although this approach sounds too idealistic to be representative of actual business practice, it may in actuality be more consistent with the stated purposes of many business organizations. For example, consider corporate mission statements that commonly contain objectives such as excellence in the delivery of the service/product, service to the community, and a *fair* rate of return for investors. Few, if any, mission statements reflect Friedman's assumptions by promising investors that everything within the extent of the law will be done in order to maximize financial return.

In addition, there is a growing body of empirical evidence that suggests that investor expectations may actually be more consistent with a more enlightened approach to business than the narrow custodian-of-wealth model. Recent research into shareholder voting patterns by Pietra Rivoli reveals that many informed and involved shareholders vote for initiatives that decrease their financial returns in favor of other social goals. Rivoli states that these patterns show that "wealth maximization is a constrained objective, and the constraints are social and ethical values."[15] Thus, Friedman fundamentally errs in his assumption about shareholder expectations.

Furthermore, real-life examples of more enlightened behavior are prevalent. The well-publicized actions of then 73-year-old Aaron Feuerstein is a good case in point. Citing his commitment to the community, Feuerstein rebuilt a burned-down manufacturing plant, which was a vital economic lifeline to the town of Methuen, Massachusetts, because it was

14. The seminal formulation of this approach is credited to R. Edward Freeman, *Strategic Management: A Stakeholder Approach* (Boston: Pittman Publishing, 1984). A well-known formulation of the model can be found in William M. Evan and R. Edward Freeman, "A Stakeholder Theory of the Modern Corporation: Kantian Capitalism," in Tom L. Beauchamp and Norman Bowie, eds., *Ethical Theory in Business* (Englewood Cliffs, N.J.: Prentice-Hall, 1988, rpt. 1993), pp. 75-93. For a discussion of the current direction of ongoing research in integrated social contracts theory as a model for business ethics, see Thomas W. Dunfee and Thomas Donaldson, "Contractarian Business Ethics: Current Status and Next Steps," *Business Ethics Quarterly* 5, no. 2 (April 1995): 173-86.

15. Pietra Rivoli, "Ethical Aspects of Investor Behavior," *Journal of Business Ethics* 14 (1995): 265-77.

"the right thing to do," despite the fact that he could have simply retired on the insurance money. Other shareholder-owned corporations, such as Herman Miller, Starbucks, Johnson & Johnson, and many others, function as values-oriented stakeholder enterprises that view their social commitments as being perfectly consistent with their financial success.[16]

Andrew Wicks cites the pharmaceutical giant Merck as a good example of this dynamic at work in a health care related business. A number of years ago, Merck found itself in a curious dilemma. A company scientist discovered that one of its veterinary drugs could be adapted to cure the horrible Third World disease of river blindness. The discovery of the cure was great news, but the problem for Merck was that none of its potential "customers" could afford to pay for it since the disease mainly struck in rural areas of poor countries. After failing in its efforts to secure external funding for the manufacture and distribution of the drug, Merck decided to allocate $20 million per year in order to give away the drug to any country that asks for it, forever. The reason they did so was mission driven.[17] One of the core components of Merck's corporate philosophy is: "We try never to forget that medicine is for the people. It is not for the profits. The profits follow, and the better we have remembered that, they have never failed to appear. The better we have remembered it, the larger they have been."[18]

While such practices may seem like anomalies in the world of commerce, they are actually more consistent with the spirit of the writings of Adam Smith than are those driven by a profit-maximization ethos. The traditional interpretation of Smith is inaccurate. Patricia Werhane notes that when Smith's more widely known *Wealth of Nations* is read in conjunction with his *Theory of Moral Sentiments*, it is evident that, for Smith, greed *impedes* rather than enhances a free-market economy.[19]

For Smith, enlightened self-interest, as opposed to selfishness, was the engine of capitalism. He drew a sharp distinction between greed and legitimate self-interest, which is consistent with Paul's advice in Philippi-

16. Wicks, p. 346.
17. Quoted in Wicks, p. 345.
18. Quoted in Wicks, p. 345.
19. For further discussion on this reinterpretation of Smith's writings and his contributions to modern business ethics, see Patricia Werhane, *Adam Smith and His Legacy for Modern Capitalism* (New York: Oxford University Press, 1991). For a specific application of Smith to the business of medicine in managed care see Werhane, "The Ethics of Health Care as a Business," *Business and Professional Ethics Journal* 9, nos. 3 & 4 (Fall-Winter 1990): 15.

ans 2:4, where he says, "look out not only for your own interests, but also for the interests of others." In support of this distinction, Michael Novak states that there can be virtuous forms of self-interest in addition to neutral or evil compositions of it. For example, he cites the desire to develop one's talents, or to develop self-mastery and control, as examples of forms of self-interest that are not inherently evil.[20]

More importantly, Smith assumed that ethics and self-restraint play critical roles in the proper functioning of the market and everyday commercial transactions. Practical evidence for the truthfulness of Smith's beliefs can be seen in the daily affairs of the economy. Without values like fair play, respect for others, trustworthiness, keeping of promises (contracts), truth telling, and so on, an economic system would look like the system that now exists in the former Soviet Union.[21]

In line with Smith's writings, an enlightened business model such as the stakeholder approach challenges the assumption that corporate business must be conducted for the exclusive purpose of profit maximization. The stakeholder approach is a great improvement over the traditional narrow conception of business activity since it legitimates broader moral considerations. Thus, while it is true that some firms operate on the "greed is good" philosophy, characterizing this as *the* "business ethic" is both descriptively inaccurate and an internal contradiction.

To be certain, the conduct of some managed care organizations does reinforce the notion that they are solely interested in profit at the expense of patient well-being. However, through the lens of a reconceptualized understanding of commercial activity, it can be stated from a *business* perspective that these organizations have been acting unethically in their pursuit of financial gain. By extending a reconceptualized model of business to the realm of managed care, we as a society have much less reason to believe that the solution to ethical problems in medicine *must* come with the eradication of business values.

20. Michael Novak, *This Hemisphere of Liberty* (Washington, DC: AEI Press, 1992), p. 41; and *The Spirit of Democratic Capitalism* (Lantham, MD: Madison Books/University Press of America, 1991), pp. 92-95.

21. Philip Boyle, "Business Ethics in Ethics Committees?" *Hastings Center Report* (September/October 1990): 37. For a detailed discussion of the trust necessary for an efficient economy, see Francis Fukuyama, *Trust: The Social Virtues and the Creation of Prosperity* (New York: Free Press, 1995).

Possible Shortcomings in the Extension
of a Business Model to Medicine

Clearly, there are several possible shortcomings in the application of business ethics to medicine. The most significant challenge is that under any business-based model, no matter how "enlightened," profit is still a central component of the "good" to which commercial activity aims. Thus, even a restrained pursuit of profit is still perceived by some to be at odds with an ethical approach to medicine. For example, Edmund Pellegrino acknowledges the distinction between legitimate self-interest and selfishness. However, he states that:

> by code or by covenant, the physician promises to serve the interests of the patient, not to exploit the patient or take advantage of the patient's vulnerability. It is the obligation to suppress even *legitimate* self-interest in this way that characterizes medicine and other professions.[22]

Partially based upon this view, he concurs with numerous other observers who argue that profits from health care should be placed back into the system rather than distributed to shareholders.[23] As such, he favors the exclusive use of non-profit provider organizations.

This concern is understandable. Non-profit organizations have their place, and altruistic behavior should be encouraged. However, he appears to be aiming his criticism toward a narrow conception of business activity. An enlightened business model would not support the exploitation of patients or capitalizing on their vulnerabilities in the name of *legitimate* self-interest.

Furthermore, it remains to be seen how the expectation to suppress even acceptable forms of self-interest could be systematized in a workable fashion. As noted earlier, profit in health care is not something that has been newly introduced by managed care organizations. Physicians have and continue to earn high levels of income. Consequently, it is quite natural to ask why it is acceptable for doctors to profit from their work, especially when their training is heavily subsidized by the public, while it is not legitimate for investors to earn a reasonable return for their

---

22. Edmund D. Pellegrino, "Toward an Ethic of Managed Care," *Journal of Clinical Ethics* 6 (1995): 314. Italics mine.

23. Pellegrino, "Toward an Ethic of Managed Care," p. 316. Also see Kate T. Christensen, "Ethically Important Distinctions among Managed Health Care Organizations," *Journal of Law, Medicine & Ethics* 23 (1995): 223.

contributions.[24] Shareholders clearly create value by risking their capital for research, expansion, and the acquisition of facilities, equipment, and technology. While there are legitimate concerns that returns on investment will be too high, and will thereby subtract too greatly from available medical resources, the overall amount of revenue that leaves the system as "profit" has been well overstated by critics.

Needless to say, individual organizations can pay inappropriately high executive salaries or over-emphasize profit. However, a commonly cited profit figure among for-profit managed care organizations in general is 30 percent. Even a cursory examination of the data in California, the state in which managed care has made its greatest inroads, reveals that this is grossly inflated. Data from the 1994-95 Knox-Keene Report Summary reported that no plan reported a figure anywhere close to 20-30 percent in profits. The highest reported figure for the years 1992-94 was Aetna Health Plans of California, Inc., which reported a profit of 13 percent in 1994. By comparison, one *non-profit* plan reported a profit (surplus) of 9.9 percent during the same period. Furthermore, for-profit plans with enrollments of over 20,000 reported an average profit as a percentage of revenue of only 4.6 percent for 1994, compared to 2.9 percent for *non-profit* plans, a much smaller difference than what is popularly believed. In the 1995-96 report, profit figures are even lower. No plans had more that 10.5 percent in profit. In addition, data in the newer report was also adjusted for some differences in taxation between non-profits and for-profits. In previous years, the figures for for-profits were calculated using gross instead of net income, resulting in overstated "profit" figures since taxes are not retained as profits. After taxes were accounted for, the profit figure differences between non-profits and for-profits was reduced.[25]

Indeed, non-profit organizations also earn profits (known as surpluses) and pay physicians competitive salaries. Doctors who work for these organizations can still be motivated by self-interest (and selfishness). Thus, limiting health care to non-profit organizations would hardly eliminate self-interest from medicine.

Although one could argue that normative standards (oughts) should not be developed from the way the system currently is, lest the naturalistic

24. See Reinhardt, p. 214.

25. See California Medical Association, *1994-1995 and 1995-96 Knox-Keene Health Plan Expenditure Summaries*, available from the California Medical Association, Sacramento, California.

fallacy be committed, the eradication of legitimate self-interest in medicine is a difficult, if not impossible task. The only available method to
eliminate all vestiges of the profit motive consistently would be to develop
a socialized system even more radical than the Swedish model. Doctors
would be paid set wages consistent with a social service scale. Clearly the
ramifications would be profound. Uwe Reinhardt asserts that it would be
far from certain that the same caliber of people who are currently attracted
to medicine would continue to compete so rigorously for the right to
engage in its practice.[26] Novak has suggested that a realistic appraisal of
complex motives in human behavior mandates that we construct an
"economy for sinners."[27] While his language may be too strong, his point
is well taken. The best system is one that best accounts for self-interest,
especially in the virtuous, enlightened sense of the term.

A related challenge that could be raised about the appropriateness
of business norms is that medicine is a *profession*. As such, medical
practitioners have higher behavioral expectations, such as fiduciary obligations, that are placed on them by society. Conversely, it is claimed
that business is run almost exclusively on a pure contractual model, which
extends ethical obligations only to the point of upholding explicitly made
promises.[28] Therefore, some actions that are obligatory in medicine would
be considered "heroic" in business.

These claims again rely on faulty notions of the gap between medicine and business. As a profession, medicine has never been as heroic
as it is often portrayed to be. Fiduciary-level obligations exist only after
the patient and physician are in an actual relationship, which the physician has the right to decline to enter into in the first place. In addition,
such obligations are not absolute once a relationship is established. Dan
Brock further observes that it would be naive to think that by becoming
professionals, individuals lose concern for their own interests.[29]

At the same time, these claims also rely on the false belief that
business runs on a largely amoral contractual model. In addition to growing
numbers of corporations that have adopted a more enlightened stakeholder
model of behavior, there are a number of participants in business who have
traditionally been bound by higher ethical duties. Accountants and archi-
tects are examples of "business" people who are regarded as professionals

26. Reinhardt, p. 211.
27. Novak, *The Spirit of Democratic Capitalism*, p. 95.
28. Relman, in Relman and Reinhardt, "An Exchange on For-Profit Health Care,"
p. 222.
29. Brock, p. 27.

or, at the very least, "quasi-professionals." Because of differences in knowledge, they are held to fiduciary-level obligations to their clients.[30] Although the specific nature and content of these duties may differ from those of physicians, they can accurately be characterized as going well beyond a simple contractual model. Thus, there is the possibility of assigning moral responsibilities to organizations and individuals involved in business which go well beyond honoring explicitly rendered agreements.[31]

While these concerns represent significant challenges, they do not sufficiently negate the value of extending an enlightened business model to managed care. In fact, in addition to the benefit mentioned in the introduction, standards derived from a reconceptualized *business* approach may have some other distinct *advantages* over the traditional charity-based medical model.

Advantages of an Enlightened Business Model over a Traditional Medical Model

First, an enlightened business model more accurately reflects the true connection between human motivation and ethics. Consistent with the biblical assumption (and Smith's view), a more realistic view of this relationship holds that ethics is not opposed to self-interest, but broadens its definition to include a host of other moral considerations. "Love your neighbor as yourself," as Jesus put it. In fact, many physicians serve as prime examples of this dynamic at work as they have been able to serve others without undermining their financial well-being.[32] Although service rather than the pursuit of wealth is their stated mission, doctors have traditionally "done well by doing good."

The fact that doctors can profit while engaging in service to the community gives us reason to reject the view that an ethical approach to medicine mandates the removal of a business dimension. An enlightened *business* model offers a clear advantage because it allows for a more

30. George W. Rainbolt, "Competition and the Patient-Centered Ethic," *The Journal of Medicine and Philosophy* 12 (1987): 90.

31. There are also many commentators who argue that business *ought* to be cast in more professional terms. See, for example, Michael Novak, *Business as a Calling* (New York: Free Press, 1996); and Joshua D. Margolis, "Casting Business as a Profession," paper presented at the 1996 annual meeting of the Society for Business Ethics, Quebec City, August 1996.

32. Wicks, p. 347.

comprehensive account for the mixed motives at work in both the arenas of business and medicine.

Second, a more enlightened understanding of business allows us to consider greater areas of overlap with medicine. This can have the practical benefit of moving us away from some of the simplistic "business bashing" that has permeated the current discussion and towards a place where a more realistic assignment of moral responsibility can take place. Consistent with the earlier described narrow depiction of business, managed care organizations have often been falsely blamed for financially related treatment decisions that may have been made by another party such as an individual physician, a hospital, or a practice group.[33] As long as such false attributions continue and the wrong party is targeted for blame, workable solutions and policies cannot be developed. A more accurate appraisal of business can work towards the development of a more realistic and operational assignment of moral duties.

Third, with our current fiscal crisis, there are some other practical advantages to assessing medicine from a business perspective. The consideration of financial limits and the application of such business concepts as total quality management and organizational learning and realignment can undoubtedly improve the efficiency with which medicine is delivered. In turn, scarce resources can be saved and access can be improved for those who have no coverage at all. Excess spending is already being reduced as the number of physician specialists and length of hospital stays are on the decline.

Finally, the integration of medicine under a business model brings into sharper focus the various ethical concerns that owning and operating a business entail. These concerns remain hidden as long as medicine is viewed in terms of patient-physician relationships under the caring model, which is falsely presumed to be free from a business dimension.[34]

Organizational Responsibilities in the New Intersections of Business and Medicine

Starting from a more enlightened model of business, numerous ethical responsibilities can be developed for managed care organizations. These

33. Sandra Johnson, "Managed Care as Regulation: Functional Ethics for a Regulated Environment," *Journal of Law, Medicine & Ethics* 23 (1995): 266-72.
34. Jecker, p. 534.

entities should be held to behavioral standards consistent with the objective of service to the community through the provision of quality health care, in return for a *reasonable* profit. Such a purpose is consistent with a more enlightened model of business, if the more complex account of human nature is accepted with the realities of medicine as it has been predominantly practiced by individual physicians. Moreover, these objectives are almost always expressed outright in the mission statements and promotional materials of managed care organizations. (No such organization expresses "profit maximization through cost-cutting initiatives within legal limits" as its stated purpose.) If these mission statements are to be taken seriously, stakeholders such as patients, physicians, and the surrounding community should be important parts of the planning and decision-making process.

Consistent with the overall progression of medicine towards greater patient involvement in decision making, managed care organizations also have duties to engage in the complete disclosure of plan contract terms and to end controversial practices such as "gag orders" that limit patient access to important information.[35] There is precedent for such disclosure in some traditional business settings where the consumer must be provided with information about practices or products that have potentially adverse consequences.[36]

Paying physicians through capitation plans is another controversial practice in which ethical duties must be assigned to organizations. Many observers argue that such arrangements should be made illegal based upon the belief that when a doctor agrees to treat a load of patients in exchange for a fixed monthly sum, insurmountable temptations to skimp on care are presented since the physician's financial well-being is directly on the line. While these are understandable concerns, it must be stated that no method of payment, including salary, is completely free from the potential for a financial conflict of interest. Thus, while it changes the specific nature of the tension, capitation does not introduce a new ethical problem to medicine. Furthermore, David Orentlicher notes that in most cases these incentives will not result in insufficient care because of professional norms, the threat of malpractice, and the

35. Although there is little available evidence about their prevalence, and spokespersons for these organizations deny their existence, anecdotal evidence from physicians abounds that practices such as gag orders are used. See Robert A. Rosenblatt, "Doctors, HMO's Clash at Hearing 'Gag Rules,'" *Los Angeles Times,* 31 May 1996, p. A1.

36. Examples of disclosure requirements can be found in industrial products, food packaging, and the financial services industry.

cost effectiveness of preventative treatments that curtail higher costs later.[37]

Although capitation leaves the direct conflict in the hands of individual physicians, several ethical obligations can be assigned to managed care organizations since the institutional pressure resulting from the structure of the arrangements can serve to either enhance or reduce the degree of the tension at hand. In addition, assigning such obligations is consistent in spirit with the efforts of some business organizations in other industries which are attempting to realign compensation systems to more adequately protect consumer interests.[38]

To begin with, the amount of the payment itself is of critical importance. Consistent with claims made by spokespersons for managed care organizations, these payments must be adequate to truly cover the cost of patient care. If these amounts are in fact sufficient, physicians should be protected in advocating for their patients within these limits. Following the lead of organizations such as U.S. Health Care, catastrophic insurance should also be made available to physicians who treat sicker patient loads and exceed their actuarially set capitation amounts.[39] This would relieve physicians from the tension that may arise at the end of the fiscal period to severely skimp on patient care in order to avoid either a loss of income or removal from a provider panel.

In addition, many arrangements use bonuses and withhold "at risk" amounts until the end of a fiscal period. The amount of ancillary payment may make a difference with respect to the strength of potential conflicts of interest that may arise. In general, the larger the amount withheld, the greater the pressures will be to withhold needed care.[40] However, these ancillary payments are usually determined in conjunction with a "risk pool" that may further affect decision making.[41]

---

37. David Orentlicher, "Managed Care and the Threat to the Patient-Physician Relationship," *Trends in Health Care, Law & Ethics* 10, nos. 1/2 (Winter/Spring 1995): 21.

38. See Nancy Kurland, "Trust, Accountability, and Sales Agents' Dueling Loyalties," *Business Ethics Quarterly* 6, no. 3 (July 1996): 289-310.

39. See Arthur Leibowitz et al., "Corporate Managed Care," *New England Journal of Medicine* 334, no. 16 (18 April 1996): 1060.

40. Rodwin, pp. 139-41.

41. In capitated arrangements with smaller risk pools and/or in which physician performance is tracked individually, a more direct conflict of interest occurs. In an individualized risk pool, each prescription for a test or procedure or referral to a specialist directly affects the physician's own income. Conversely, in a pool that is made up of a larger number of physicians, and in which tracking is conducted accordingly, the costs of further tests or

Working together, the greater the amount withheld and the more individualized the risk pool, the stronger the potential for conflicts will be. It is critical then that the withheld amount is low enough and the actual risk is spread across a group of physicians so that situations in which the withholding of an expensive treatment directly results in more take-home pay are clearly avoided. Finally, specific screens must be established to ensure that physicians are not skimping on quality or preventative care procedures in order to maximize their own income.

Managed care organizations also have moral obligations to refrain from the use of certain types of claims in the persuasive advertising and promotional materials that they use to attract new members. Moreover, they should participate in initiatives with public sector institutions to establish information disclosure standards that can help enrollees differentiate between plans on the basis of real quality distinctions. This information should be made widely available to the public through the use of uniform standards. The *Fair Labeling and Packaging Act* for food products could be used as a model to help consumers understand competing claims of better care.

Curbing certain types of persuasive claims and the use of uniform information are consistent with the variable "reasonable consumer" standard which are used to regulate advertising in traditional business settings. The typical potential enrollee for managed care can be more easily misled with respect to advertisements for health care than he or she might be regarding other consumer goods — especially by claims for "better quality care" since there is broad disagreement over how this is best measured.[42] Self-imposed restrictions on advertising are by no means inconsistent with the "commercial" side of the organizations. There are precedents for voluntary restrictions in other traditional business settings. For example, the software industry recently formed a group to address the use of questionable marketing tactics by some members of its industry.[43] Wine makers have had an effective self-developed and enforced code for responsible advertising for a number of years. The health care community could do the same.

---

referrals are spread throughout the group, reducing the financial importance of individual decisions. See Rodwin, pp. 139-41.

42. Ezekiel Emanuel and Allan S. Brett, "Managed Competition and the Patient-Physician Relationship," *N Eng J Med* 329, no. 12 (16 September 1993): 879-82.

43. Allan S. Brett, "The Case Against Persuasive Advertising by Health Maintenance Organizations," *N Eng J Med* 326, no. 20 (14 May 1992): 1353-56.

Recent developments in business ethics have much to contribute to the formation of behavioral norms to guide managed care organizations. While negative reactions to the emergence of a more explicit business dimension in medicine are understandable, cursory dismissals of the applicability of business ethics have often resulted from false assumptions about the nature and scope of the differences between business and medicine. The medical profession has never been as altruistic as it is commonly thought to be, and business has been fundamentally misunderstood as being solely concerned with profit maximization.

In light of the commonalities between business and medicine, extending to managed care a morally sensitive business approach is not only possible, but also advantageous in comparison with a traditional medical model. Within such an approach, managed care organizations can be expected to honor moral duties that go well beyond the maximization of shareholder wealth. While this more enlightened framework is not a perfect paradigm for bridging the traditional gaps between business and medicine, it greatly reduces the distance between the two arenas. As a result, there are good reasons to conclude that the delivery of managed care by organizations with both medical and business obligations can be much less damaging to patients and to society than many have suggested.

Hippocrates Meets Managed Care: A Study of Contemporary Oath-Taking

Robert D. Orr, M.D.

Suppose Hippocrates were practicing medicine today. How would he respond to modern medical care in general, and to managed care in particular? The Hippocratic tradition can provide some helpful insight as we evaluate the changes in the delivery of medical care today.

The basis for medical care, ancient and modern, is the doctor-patient relationship. This relationship has been conceptualized at times in altruistic terms (e.g., as a profession, a mission, or a covenant) and at other times in legalistic terms (e.g., as a duty, a fiduciary trust, or a contract). In fact, there are some elements of all of these concepts in the ideal doctor-patient relationship. But at heart, this relationship is the encounter of one individual who has a special need and another who has specialized knowledge or skill, with a goal of meeting the specific need.

But even when we recognize the unchanging nature of this basic relationship, we must also note that this professional relationship has changed considerably over the past 100 years. The physician's role has evolved from being a physician-priest (someone who cares, but has very little to offer in the way of effective therapy) to physician-scientist (someone who could often intervene to actually change the course of illness) to physician-provider (someone who is assigned to dole out services). In addition to this evolution, the physician's role has also undergone significant dilution during this century by the introduction of specialization and team care, by the major change from solo to group practice, and by the increasing involvement of third-party payers in treatment decisions.

Much of this change has been good because it allows a group of professionals to deliver needed services efficiently to a large group of individuals. Some of the changes have been less laudable from the perspective of both patient and physician. In particular, recent changes in the financing of health care have caused some potential conflicts of interest. One physician laments, "Today two ethically incompatible cultures exist in medicine. The traditional culture (our calling to care and to heal) is now dominated by a business culture that is eroding the essence of healing relationships."[1] Clearly he is correct in one regard because medical ethics has a goal of health and is based on the needs of the individual, while business ethics has a goal of profit and is often based on efficiency, or even on mass production. But is the difference really that stark? Is the outlook really that bleak?

Rather than thinking of the dilemma here in traditional ethical categories, we would do well to consider it in terms of a potential conflict of interest. A conflict of interest occurs when there are two competing interests, but only one legitimately claims priority; the issue is to ensure that it prevails. For example, a physician who receives an emergency call while at his daughter's Little League game has two interests, each of which is legitimate in its own right. However, his personal pleasure, even his obligation as a father, is clearly outweighed by his obligation as a physician. The "dilemma" in a professional conflict of interest is to ensure that the professional obligation is accorded proper priority.

Conflicts of interest, even financial conflicts of interest, are not a discovery of the late twentieth century. Jesus recognized conflicts of interest and warned his followers nearly 2,000 years ago, "No servant can serve two masters. Either he will hate the one and love the other, or he will be devoted to the one and despise the other. You cannot serve both God and Money."[2]

In the practice of medicine, the health of patients should be the primary interest, and it takes priority. There may be several other interests competing for the physician's time, such as fortune, fame, free time, family, and a host of other things. But the patients' needs trump all these other things.

There has been much concern raised about financial conflicts of

1. M. A. Adson, Mayo Clinic Proceedings 1995; 70: 499.
2. Luke 16:13.

interest in the practice of managed care medicine. But conflicts of interest are not new in medicine. In the older fee-for-service practice, there was financial incentive to increase the utilization of medical services ("do more, get more"). With the prospective payment and capitation mechanisms used in managed care, there is now incentive to decrease utilization ("do less, get more"). In addition to this generic conflict of interest for a physician, there is the parallel but distinct conflict involving the interests of *my* patients versus those of other patients covered by the same health plan, which has a finite number of dollars to spend on all enrollees. I want what is best for my patients, but so does another physician in the same system.

The evolution of heath care financing during this century has resulted in a shift of the financial risk of illness. This risk previously rested with the patient in that he or she was charged fee-for-service by the physician, and the patient paid out-of-pocket. The introduction of indemnity insurance several decades ago shifted the risk to insurance companies. They continued to pay the physician fee-for-service, whereas the patient (or employer) was charged a fixed premium regardless of the amount of service utilized. The more recent change to capitated prospective payment has again shifted that risk, now to the physician who has become financially responsible, at least in part, for the amount of service given to a particular patient.

In commenting on this change, Edmund Pellegrino has said, "The question is not conflict of interest, or the existence of self-interest, but the obligation to suppress self-interest in the interest of others if one wishes to act virtuously. . . . By code and by covenant, the physician promises to serve the best interests of the patient, not to exploit. . . . it is the obligation to suppress even legitimate self-interest in this way that characterizes medicine as a profession."[3] Pellegrino has reminded us that medicine is a profession based on virtue, and designated by the swearing of an oath: a solemn, usually formal calling upon God to witness to the truth of what one says or to witness to the fact that one sincerely intends to do what one says. Thus, a young physician's taking an oath is an important statement of goals and intentions. Looking at the content of such oaths should help us define what is important in medicine.

---

3. E. D. Pellegrino, "Interests, Obligations, and Justice: Some Notes Toward an Ethic of Managed Care," *Journal of Clinical Ethics* 6, no. 4 (1995): 312-17.

The Use of Medical Oaths

The Oath of Hippocrates (see Appendix) is an ancient professional oath commonly attributed to Hippocrates of Cos (c. 450 B.C.E.). It was composed as a statement of virtuous practice and was probably sworn by a minority of physicians at that time, to contrast their practices with the common practitioners of the day. Those who took this oath had to do so before they were allowed to begin the study of medicine; i.e., they had to make this pledge before they became medical students. This historic oath, along with the other writings of the Hippocratic Corpus, formed the basis of what came to be called the Hippocratic ethos of ancient medicine. To this ethos, which emphasized the competence of the physician, was added another emphasis on compassion as taught by Jesus, resulting in the ethos of modern medicine that has been accepted for many centuries.[4] The Hippocratic Oath, though ancient and in some regards archaic, is often still used as a standard of comparison when an attitude or practice of modern medicine is questioned.

Medical oaths that are used today are generally taken after professional studies have been completed. And the classical Oath of Hippocrates is rarely sworn by graduating medical students today. There is a much-shortened modified version (165 words versus 335 in original) still called the Hippocratic Oath in common use, and there are a variety of other oaths in use as well. What are the oaths currently in use, what is the content of those oaths, and how does this content compare to that of the classical Hippocratic Oath? Some colleagues and I undertook a study to try to answer these questions.[5] We surveyed all of the academic deans of the 157 schools of allopathic and osteopathic medicine in the U.S. and Canada about oath-taking practices in 1993. Ninety-seven percent of the deans responded to the survey. We compared this recent usage data to similar surveys done in 1928, 1958, 1978, and 1989. We then compared the content of oaths in current use to that of the classical Hippocratic Oath using the well-accepted analysis of Leon Kass (see Table 1 for a list of content items in the Oath).[6]

The oaths in use by medical schools in North America in 1993 can

4. A. R. Jonsen, *The New Medicine and the Old Ethics* (Cambridge, Mass.: Harvard University Press, 1990).

5. R. D. Orr, N. Pang, E. D. Pellegrino, and M. Siegler, "The Use of the Hippocratic Oath: a review of 20th-century practice and a content analysis of oaths administered in medical schools in the U.S. and Canada in 1993," *Journal of Clinical Ethics* 8, no. 4 (1997): 374-85.

6. L. R. Kass, "Is There a Medical Ethics?: The Hippocratic Oath and the Sources of Ethical Medicine," in L. R. Kass, *Toward a More Natural Science* (New York: Free Press, 1985), pp. 224-46.

Table 1. Traditional Hippocratic Oath Content Items
(modification of Leon Kass's analysis)

covenant with deity	1. Sworn before gods, suggesting that the medical relationship includes a transcendental element; any mention of deity was counted
covenant with teachers	2. Original pledge of collegiality and financial support; any mention of teachers was counted
commitment to students	3. Original promised to teach those who swear oath; any mention of teaching or students was counted
covenant with patients	4. Pledge to use "ability and judgment"
appropriate means	5. Original promised to use "dietetic measures"; this interpreted to imply the use of standard of care
appropriate ends	6. "The benefit of the sick"
limits on ends	7. Delimitation, by restriction, of the ends fittingly served:
	8. Original proscribed abortion
	9. Original proscribed euthanasia
limits on means	10. Delimitation, by restriction, of the means properly used; original proscribed surgery for renal stones, by deferring to those more qualified; any mention of limits to practice based on competence was counted
justice	11. "Remain clear of all voluntary injustice"
chastity	12. Original proscribed sexual contact with patients or members of household
confidentiality	13. Will not repeat things seen or heard
accountability	14. Prayerful request that the physician be honored if oath is kept, and "may the opposite befall me" if it is transgressed or sworn falsely

be found in Table 2. In comparing this usage to the studies done earlier in this century, we found that there has been a marked increase in the percentage of schools administering an oath over the past 65 years. The graduates of 98 percent of the 150 responding schools took an oath in 1993 while only 26 percent of surveyed schools administered an oath in 1928,[7]

7. E. J. Carey, "The Formal Use of the Hippocratic Oath for Medical Students at Commencement Exercises," *Bulletin of the Association of American Medical Colleges* 3 (1928): 159-66.

**Table 2. Professional Oaths Taken by Graduates
of Medical Schools in the U.S. and Canada in 1993**

	no.	%*
Oath of Hippocrates		
classical version	1	1
modern version	45	30
modified version	22	15
unknown version	1	1
Declaration of Geneva		
1948	10	7
1983	24	16
The Osteopathic Oath	15	10
The Oath of Louis Lasagna	5	3
The Prayer of Maimonides	4	3
Other	20	13
No oath administered	3	2
Total	150	

72 percent did so in 1958,[8] 90 percent in 1977,[9] and 100 percent in 1989.[10] We determined that only one responding school used the text of the classical Hippocratic Oath in 1993, but 68 reported they used other "versions" of the traditional oath.

It may be that the increased use of professional oaths in this century is a recognition of how important it is for a new physician to make a public promise to be trustworthy. On the other hand, the importance may lie in the content of the oath rather than just the process of oath-taking. As Nuland has stated, oaths "deal with deontological concepts, concepts that arise from a sense of duty and the obligatory doing of things because they are, quite simply, the right things to do."[11] Cameron believes that current medical oath-taking focuses on process rather than content. He says, "Every one of the modern restatements of medical values has . . .

8. D. P. Irish and D. W. McMurray, "Professional Oaths and American Medical Colleges," *Journal of Chronic Diseases* 18 (1965): 275-89.

9. W. J. Friedlander, "Oaths Given by U.S. and Canadian Medical Schools, 1977: Profession of Medical Values," *Social Science and Medicine* 16 (1982): 115-20.

10. E. Dickstein, J. Erlen, and J. A. Erlen, "Ethical Principles Contained in Currently Professed Medical Oaths," *Academic Medicine* 66 (1991): 622-24.

11. S. B. Nuland, *Doctors* (New York: Alfred A. Knopf, 1988), p. 24.

cast itself in the Hippocratic form. The claim to stand within the great tradition of the old medicine is all but universal. Yet it is a claim which increasingly lacks credibility; the continuity is one of form, and can be claimed only by manipulating the substance of the tradition."[12] Thus, it becomes important to compare the content of currently used oaths to that of the classical Hippocratic Oath.

When we examined the content of each oath in current use, we discovered that although 100 percent and 86 percent, respectively, still pledge a commitment to patients and to teaching, only 43 percent vow to be accountable for their actions, only 14 percent include a prohibition against euthanasia, only 11 percent invoke a deity, only 8 percent foreswear abortion, and only 3 percent retain a proscription against sexual contact with patients. Thus, there are now significant omissions from the content of the original Oath as devised by Hippocrates and his followers.

There has been a nearly steady decline in the number of content items from the 14 found by Kass in the original Oath (see Table 3). The Prayer of Maimonides is clearly different from the others in that it is a prayer rather than an oath. With this exception, each new oath that has been developed over time has had fewer of the original content items than earlier ones. In fairness to the newer oaths, we must point out that most have added new content items such as the prevention of disease, commitments to science and learning, whole-person care, patient autonomy, gender inclusive language, etc. But if the classical Oath of Hippocrates is considered to be the first and traditional articulation of the virtues of being a physician, it is somewhat alarming to learn that recent graduates are often asked to pledge themselves to less than half of the original commitments.

It is interesting to speculate on the paradoxical findings that the administration of oaths to medical graduates has steadily increased throughout this century while the content of those oaths has steadily shifted away from the basic tenets of the original Hippocratic Oath. Perhaps we are entering the *post-Hippocratic era* in which every element of the Hippocratic ethic is under scrutiny and many are being discarded.[13] Since specialization has made the medical profession less monolithic, some might argue that it is no longer realistic to expect physicians with

12. N. S. Cameron, *Life and Death after Hippocrates: The New Medicine* (Wheaton, Ill.: Crossway Books, 1991), pp. 58-59.

13. E. D. Pellegrino, "Medical Ethics: Entering the Post-Hippocratic Era," *Journal of the American Board of Family Practice* 1 (1988): 230-37.

Table 3. Number of Content Items in Oaths

Oath	Approximate Age	Content Items
Classical Oath of Hippocrates	2500 years	14
Prayer of Maimonides	200 years	5
"Modern" Oath of Hippocrates	70+ years	10
Osteopathic Oath	60 years	9
Declaration of Geneva (1948)	50 years	7
Oath of Louis Lasagna	35 years	6

a variety of practice types and patterns to swear the same oath. Perhaps the content of the oaths has been attenuated because in a secularized, pluralistic society it is difficult to reach agreement (even within the medical profession) on all matters of content. Most oaths have preserved some content areas, e.g., a commitment to patients and to teaching. It may be that in medicine, when we no longer agree on the entire substance (content of oaths), we become even more concerned about process (taking the oaths). But as we eliminate from the oath those content items on which we cannot agree, we may be left with a very different kind of oath and a different kind of medicine. To be sure, the newer oaths include new ideas, but they omit at least four important elements: swearing to deity, protection of human life, not taking advantage of vulnerable patients (avoidance of sexual contact), and accountability.

There is one other interesting finding in the most recent survey. Although the question was not specifically asked of the deans, 11 volunteered that the graduating medical students were allowed to choose which oath they would swear. At some of those schools, the students even wrote a unique oath for their graduation. Such choice might encourage the young professionals to invest more energy and thought in the oath-taking process.[14] Recent efforts by graduating classes at Harvard and Johns Hopkins Medical Schools, however, suggest that students' modifications have produced "oaths vague in precept and betraying a self-solicitude inimical to professional maturity."[15] If there are standards of conduct expected of physicians, it ought to be within the province of the profession and medical educators to include them in oaths rather than making them optional.

14. N. Hupert, "What's in an Oath?" *Harvard Medical Alumni Bulletin* 68, no. 2 (1994): 42-44.

15. P. R. McHugh, "Hippocrates à la Mode," *Nature Medicine* 2 (1996): 507-9.

Implications for Modern Medical Practice

This attenuation of patient-centered precepts from oaths bespeaks the "postmodern" trend to denounce traditional absolutes and declare oneself the judge of the goodness or the badness of a particular action or result. However, this postmodern trend is not so new. In discussing God's wrath against humankind, Paul told the Romans, "Although they claimed to be wise, they became fools and exchanged the glory of the immortal God for images made to look like mortal people and birds and animals and reptiles. . . . They exchanged the truth of God for a lie, and worshiped and served created things rather than the Creator — who is forever praised."[16] We have declared ourselves as the judge of truth, rather than looking to the Truth of the ages.

This is not to imply that either the Hippocratic Oath or the Hippocratic tradition is God-given or sacred. It is merely to point out that the mindset of postmodern individuals is to forsake traditions and previously accepted standards in order to create our own standards. The evolution of the content of medical oaths demonstrates a significant change. Postmodern practice differs from the traditional practice of medicine, in that there is now a diminished view of the importance of patients' interests and an elevation of concern about the good of society as a whole, or at least the good of the health plan in particular.

There arguably is a new shift underway from an earlier emphasis on patient beneficence, which was prominent prior to the 1960s, to an emphasis on patient autonomy, which became dominant in the 1970s and 1980s, to a current emphasis on justice or utilitarian profit maximization. Needless to say, justice is not a bad goal or aspiration. In fact, many countries, especially the United States of America, have a rather dismal history of injustice in many spheres of life, including the allocation and availability of health care. But as soon as we lift our eyes from the needs of individual patients to consider the needs of others, we have changed our focus; we have changed our mission; we have changed our covenant. This change is especially troubling — and difficult to justify in terms of "justice" — when our new focus places as much emphasis as it does on the best interests of a for-profit health plan.

The best safeguard for the vulnerable patient seeking care is for each physician to be pledged to virtue and to be dedicated to the patient's best interests. With the decrease in professional consensus, demonstrated by

16. Romans 1:22-23, 25.

the changes in oath content, the remaining safeguard is the integrity of the individual physician; therefore, this integrity takes on even greater significance.

Managed care has been designed to save money by not over-treating, by standardizing treatment practices, and by shifting the financial risk of treatment decisions from the insurance company to the professionals providing the care. Saving money is not bad. Managed care is not inherently evil, or even unethical. But greed is inherently evil. The old ethic of *patient's needs come first* hopefully will continue to prevail when the medical indications are clear for the use of a particular test or treatment. The danger, however, is that when the indications are marginal, the new ethic of *economic interests come first* will overcome the physician's primary interest and obligation. The answer to the new ethic is the same as the essence of the old ethic — physician integrity and dedication.

Appendix

The Hippocratic Oath

I swear by Apollo Physician and Asclepius and Hygieia and Panaceia and all the gods and goddesses, making them my witnesses, that I will fulfill according to my ability and judgement this oath and this covenant.

To hold him who has taught me this art as equal to my parents and to live my life in partnership with him, and if he is in need of money to give him a share of mine, and to regard his offspring as equal to my brothers in male lineage and to teach them this art — if they desire to learn it — without fee and covenant; to give a share of precepts and oral instruction and all the other learning to my sons and to the sons of him who has instructed me and to pupils who have signed the covenant and have taken an oath according to the medical law, but to no one else.

I will apply dietetic measures for the benefit of the sick according to my ability and judgement; I will keep them from harm and justice.

I will neither give a deadly drug to anybody if asked for it, nor will I make a suggestion to this effect. Similarly I will not give to a woman an abortive remedy. In purity and holiness I will guard my life and my art.

I will not use the knife, not even on sufferers from stone, but will withdraw in favor of such men as are engaged in this work.

Whatever houses I may visit, I will come for the benefits of the sick, remaining free of all intentional injustice, of all mischief and in particular of sexual relations with both female and male persons, be they free or slaves.

What I may see or hear in the course of the treatment or even outside of the treatment in regard to the life of men, which on no account one must spread abroad, I will keep to myself holding such things shameful to be spoken about.

If I fulfill this oath and do not violate it, may it be granted to me to enjoy life and art, being honored with fame among all men for all time to come; if I transgress it and swear falsely, may the opposite of all this be my lot.

SELECTED SETTINGS

Therapeutic Relationship in Managed Mental Health Care

Stephen P. Greggo, Psy.D.

One of the last frontiers to be broached by managed care is mental health.[1] Managed care organizations have been established to control cost and ensure quality by restricting access, regulating treatment, and specifying outcomes. Such an approach has not been welcome on mental health turf. The complexities of appropriate diagnosis and suitable treatment have historically been so tied to diverse theoretical conceptualizations that to consider the application of standardized procedures has appeared to be too vast an undertaking. Furthermore, the sanctity of the therapeutic encounter has appeared to be so well protected by professional codes and supported by popular consensus that exploration by any outside parties has seemed brazen. Regardless, the steady rise in the acceptance and utilization of psychotherapeutic services has prompted an increasing awareness of their contribution to the rising cost of health insurance, especially on the part of those who monitor such costs. Additionally, informed consumers are demanding consistency in the quality of all medical services while preferring minimal co-payments and the lowest possible insurance policy costs. These trends have gradually opened the way in the wild and woolly territory of mental health treatment for the introduction of managed care.[2]

1. K. Corcoran, and V. Vandiver, *Maneuvering the Maze of Managed Care: Skills for Mental Health Practitioners* (New York: Free Press, 1996), pp. 1-24.
2. C. S. Austad and W. H. Berman (eds.), *Psychotherapy in Managed Health Care:*

A note of thanks to David Wever, my teaching assistant, for his help with the diagram on p. 187.

The application of managed care to the domain of psychotherapy to control costs and ensure quality standards has not been without considerable heated controversy. Those clinicians who currently practice have likely experienced inner turmoil as well as collegial debates regarding changes in professional identity, autonomy, practice procedures and, ultimately, pressures on the patient/therapist relationship. Certainly this author has.[3]

Herron and Adlerstein's[4] words regarding those who do not believe they can supply ethical and effective practice under managed care conditions capture well the contention in the field. They wrote that those therapists who are so opposed to managed care are either the newest *"revolutionaries or the oldest reactionaries."*[5] The next few years will help determine which label best fits. In the meantime, professionals who agree to provide services under managed care systems must address very real dilemmas. Does the title "participating provider" reflect an actual shift that has reduced the

---

The Optimal Use of Time and Resources (Washington, D.C.: American Psychological Association, 1991), pp. 3-18.

3. On June 15, 1997, this author attended the New York State Psychological Association Conference in New York City on the topic of Mental Health Services under Managed Care. The morning was filled with presentations by top-level clinical directors from four of the major mental health managed care networks. After lunch, a prominent psychiatrist spoke on the "myth of managed care" and cited the abuses of "mangled care" forced upon the American people by the new "robber barons" of health care. Early in the presentation, the speaker pounded the podium to drive home the point that for the past few hours conference participants had been learning about future trends and expectations for *providers* of mental health care. He appeared to scold the audience with biting humor for letting the managed care presenters out of the room unharmed for using that term "provider," on the basis that psychologists are professionals and therefore never mere "providers." There was loud audience applause for his rebuke. Apparently, accepting the label "provider" with its commercial overtones implies a passive accommodation to an unjust system. Due to my own transference issues, that senior psychiatrist was transformed before my very eyes into the image of my gruff, opinionated grandfather. I recalled the time he attacked my father with heavy words for selling off our three acres of land and a small house built by Dad's own hands in order to buy a half-acre parcel with a moderate sized, modern home. Dad defended his position with his hopes for the future, while Grandfather accused him of selling out his "soul" to progress. I cannot say how my own life would have been different if Dad had not made that difficult decision. In retrospect, I do not see how he had any real alternative, and in his own way he made that new home a wonderful place for our family to grow. My grandfather's angry accusations haunted me as I listened to that seasoned veteran of the anti-managed care resistance movement. I knew that I would have to address the genuine concerns raised by that speaker as well as the unconscious, accusatory attacks of my long-deceased grandfather who saw certain changes as fundamentally flawed.

4. W. G. Herron and L. K. Adlerstein, "The Dynamics of Managed Mental Health Care," *Psychological Reports* 75 (1994): 723-41.

5. Herron and Adlerstein, "The Dynamics of Managed Mental Health Care," p. 726.

professional to a technician in a corrupt business that will never be just, fair, or therapeutically effective? Is the integrity of professional therapeutic services sacrificed to secure the promise of reimbursement, as treatment plans are communicated to case managers who provide the all-important "authorization number" that makes payment possible? Furthermore, is there a place within a managed care system for the professional who desires to integrate Christian faith into the psychotherapeutic process? The Christian therapist must discern whether there is a potential to live out his/her charge to be the "salt of the earth"[6] in this changing health care system or whether the salt will lose its saltiness and become a waste product with no recycling possibilities.

This chapter focuses on just one of the many changes in the mental health area brought about by managed care, namely, the typical "intrusion" of the fourth party or case reviewer into the therapeutic process. Exploration of this issue will not comprehensively answer all of the pressing ethical or efficacy questions related to managed care. However, examining how managed care affects the central and critical contribution of the therapeutic alliance to the entire treatment process will be revealing.[7] If it is possible to conceptualize how that relationship can be preserved under managed care, there may be hope of finding solutions to the other pressures. Therefore, the first task here is an analysis of how the therapeutic relationship is shaped by the review process itself and by the restrictions on therapy that it imposes. Second, a basic model for managing these risks will be outlined. The chapter then concludes with suggestions on how the Christian therapist can understand and make good use of today's revolutionary changes in light of God's desires and purposes.

Changing Dynamics in the Therapeutic Relationship

When managed care mental health treatment is compared to traditional psychotherapy, there are differences in how the relationship is defined and developed as well as in the dynamics that shape it. In the traditional model, after structuring the boundaries of the relationship and the fee, the therapist explored the reason for treatment through some version of a diagnostic interview, with ample room for the telling of the patient's

6. Matt. 5:13.
7. A. O. Horvath and L. S. Greenberg (eds.), *The Working Alliance: Theory, Research, and Practice* (New York: Wiley-Interscience, 1994).

story. The content was problem-focused and diagnostic. Nonetheless, this surface focus was of secondary importance to the formation of the therapist-client bond, which was the essential goal in those first encounters as the therapist and client developed both a conscious and an unconscious therapeutic alliance. The safety and fidelity of the helping relationship were based upon the therapist's undivided commitment to the welfare of the client, informed consent, and the promise of confidentiality. Also key was the newly formed dyad which autonomously decided the direction of treatment, which indeed centered on the nature of the therapeutic relationship itself. The hope for healing was based upon the provision of a safe, controlled, protected setting for personal work where the therapeutic relationship was critical no matter what interventions, strategies, or methods were applied.

In the prospective utilization review of managed care, the early inclusion of a case manager who authorizes care alters the relationship in several significant ways. The entire definition of confidentiality changes.[8] The personal information gleaned through the intake/diagnostic interview is disclosed to a case manager in enough detail to demonstrate impaired functioning, yet veiled enough to protect the dignity of the no-longer-anonymous patient. This is a difficult dilemma, even when a proper release is carefully obtained, for professionals have been trained in the premise that patient confidentiality is at the core of the patient-healer relationship. The potential clash of roles — private confessor versus data gatherer for the gatekeeper — may become even more significant as new trends in the health care industry and in technology raise concerns over who owns and has access to medical records,[9] databases,[10] and the reviewer's records.

The initial review addresses the problem definition and treatment direction. The autonomy of the therapist-patient dyad to determine goals and methods is limited by the managed care organization's criteria which are enforced through this procedure. These limits may be entirely acceptable to all parties, and be consistent with best-practice protocols. In an optimum case scenario, the impact of their existence may not even be noticed. However, it is important to recognize that the review itself is a quality-control step that is a far more intensive intervention, whether

8. Corcoran and Vandiver, *Maneuvering the Maze of Managed Care*, pp. 189-217.

9. K. Corcoran and W. J. Winslade, "Eavesdropping on the Fifty-Minute Hour," *Behavioral Sciences and the Law* 12 (1994): 351-56.

10. J. R. Davidson and T. Davidson, "Confidentiality and Managed Care: Ethical and Legal Concerns," *Health & Social Work* 21 (August, 1996): 208-15.

conducted through a telephone interview or via written summaries, than the previous reliance on clinicians to use their best judgment based upon "scientifically and professionally derived knowledge."[11] When the review reveals conflicts in any of the expectations of the various parties, there is need for ongoing negotiation. In those early client encounters, the rapport-building approaches of the past are now often compressed into fleeting moments as the therapist endeavors to gather as much data as possible. The priority goal in those early sessions is no longer primarily alliance-building, but establishing the medical necessity of the treatment.

Therapists may be caught between their role as advocate for the client and as agent for the managed care company through which they are operating as participating providers or perhaps even as employees. Role conflicts arise between meeting the expectations of a company that rations care to serve a defined population while protecting profit, and the therapist's overarching commitment to a client who may benefit from therapeutic services. These role conflicts, most evident during the prospective, concurrent, and retrospective review procedures, may jeopardize the healing nature of the psychotherapeutic relationship and violate its basic integrity.

The arguments against offering managed mental health services can make for sleepless nights for astute participating therapists. They recognize that the goal of working for the welfare of the client has indeed subtly shifted to also include the need to service and meet the expectations of the entire insured client population.[12] Discerning clinicians know that obtaining truly informed consent now includes explaining a complex review procedure. They understand that the promise of confidentiality is in conflict with the managed care reviewer who will enter some portion of that personal information into a mysterious database and who will perhaps require that a copy of the treatment plan be supplied to the current primary care physician. They realize that the autonomy of the therapeutic relationship has parameters and that the outcomes of the therapy need to be assessed. Most of all, clinicians sense that the therapeutic relationship itself is at risk due to these external pressures. In order to get a better night's sleep, the professional who has signed on as

---

11. American Psychological Association, "Ethical Principles of Psychologists and Code of Conduct," *American Psychologist* (December 1992).

12. James, Sabin, "A Credo for Ethical Managed Care in Mental Health Practice," *Hospital and Community Psychiatry* 45:8 (1994): 859-60.

a provider must explore and manage the therapeutic relationship which holds the key to ultimate progress and success.

Treatment Review and the Risks to the Therapeutic Relationship

The following items are examples of potential threats to the integrity and effectiveness of a therapeutic relationship. Such threats arise out of the dominant model of micro management or case-by-case review procedures.[13]

1. The initial review may force a premature definition of the client's problem. This review establishes the focus of treatment and determines specific goals which may not be entirely appropriate or may not be targeted correctly to make substantive changes. This can occur when there is acceptance of a surface definition without exploring underlying dynamics, when there is insufficient challenge of the client definition of the problem, or when the specific goals formed at the outset become rigid guidelines that resist revision or refinement.

2. The adoption of a prototype or standardized treatment plan without enough customization or acknowledgment of individual needs can result in the therapist/reviewer alliance coercively imposing the treatment plan on a vulnerable client. Goals that communicate well to the reviewer may not be precisely understood or accepted by the client. The therapist may feel caught in the middle.

3. Reviewers make key decisions or recommendations based upon minimal information and may not spend time getting to know enough case detail. The therapist who needs to abbreviate key material for the sake of a succinct review must be aware of the potential to distort information in the interest of brevity or simplicity.

4. In the review procedure, there may be selected ignoring of Axis II or treatable long-term characterological issues. If addressed, these will inflate the number of sessions needed for this round of treatment. Both the case manager and therapist are aware that length of treatment is monitored and the mutual desire to keep the dose of

13. Steven Stern, "Managed Care, Brief Therapy, and Therapeutic Integrity," *Psychotherapy* 30:1 (Spring, 1993): 162-75.

psychotherapy as low as possible may increase the risk that the dose will not reach effective levels. Short-term therapy is the norm in managed care systems but it is not always best or even valid if the underlying issues are predictably going to resurface in the future.[14] Like the politician who knows that hard decisions need to be made but who does not want to be the one to make them during an election year, the therapist and manager in a review may select the issues to treat based upon what is plausible in the short term without sufficient prevention planning for the long term.

5. Early discussion of termination and/or the final date of service does tend to help keep the treatment briefer as it decreases dependency on the therapist. Yet, it may also create an obstacle to forming the trusting relationship patients need in order to make the necessary progress on clinical issues. Planning the termination prior to relationship development can be a "trust inhibitor."

6. Discharges may occur prematurely in order to comply with treatment plan time lines established with the case reviewer, instead of modifying the plan to fit the client's rate of progress. A projected treatment plan is a guideline that may require adjustment even after it is written and approved. In addition, clients frequently have a "breakthrough" and/or feeling of relief in the early phase of treatment which can be used therapeutically to instill hope. This could be misread as a satisfactory level of gain with a resulting move toward discharge.

7. Reviewers may increase the pressure on therapists and clients to use biological interventions. The medication option can be viewed as an end in itself and not as a way of assisting and strengthening a client to make necessary psychological and lifestyle changes.

8. Therapist anxiety surrounding panel membership can be heightened during treatment reviews. The therapist's apprehension of being labeled as uncooperative can work against the client when the therapist needs to assume an advocate role. The therapist "report card" has become a reality. Such reports on therapist activity are generated by the company's database and demonstrate provider trends broken down by diagnosis or other variables. Therapist concern over the number of sessions may lead to underserving the client.

9. Patient distrust of managed care and review procedures fueled by media controversy and knowledge of the impending decision can

14. Stern, "Managed Care, Brief Therapy, and Therapeutic Integrity," p. 169.

increase anxiety and take up precious time in therapy. On the other side, therapist resentment of the review requirements can also become a progress inhibitor. In other words, while doing therapy on a tight time line there are more, not less, feelings to sort through, process, and manage.

10. Subtle shifts in transference and counter-transference forces may occur. The patient may view the therapist as subject to the higher authority of an unknown case reviewer.[15] On the other hand, the therapist may view the client as an undesirable candidate for short-term therapy and thus maintain distance in the relationship. Add to this mix the reviewer, who by assigned role takes a skeptical view of the entire proceeding, and the elements are present to create a tangled triad rather than a therapeutic dyad, with all the complications of a triangulated relationship.[16]

11. Treatment which is medically necessary is targeted to restore baseline functioning and thus is not primarily designed to optimize one's potential for functioning. The reviewer following company standards may restrict attempts by the therapist and client to construct a plan that has the goal of self-improvement unless the preventative benefits can be demonstrated plainly. For the therapist, stabilization may feel like a short cut, while for the client, returning to the status quo may feel like being shortchanged.[17]

12. Finally, there may be little room for resolving spiritual issues as part of the treatment protocol, since spirituality may not relate to the "best" practice methods determined by the managed care company. The contents of the session are no longer private, particularly in retrospective utilization review. Clinicians may be perceived as too pastoral in their approach to therapy if spiritual matters are addressed and properly recorded in the progress notes.

In summary, therapists must face each of these potential risks in all of their permutations with great clarity as they provide therapy under the scrutiny of a managed care review. Therapists need to have a sense of purpose as they contend with these demands and diverse agendas. They

15. Fredric Neal Busch, "The Impact of Managed Care on the Psychotherapeutic Process: Transference and Countertransference," *Psychoanalysis and Psychotherapy* 11:2 (1994): 200-206.

16. Janet Pipal, "Managed Care: Is It the Corpse in the Living Room? An Exposé," *Psychotherapy* 32:2 (Summer, 1995): 323-32.

17. Pipal, "Managed Care: Is It the Corpse in the Living Room?" p. 331.

must fulfill their treatment task *using the foundation of a healing relationship.* Can therapists keep the nature and direction of their responsibilities clear and manage the risks to their relationships with their patients to a reasonable degree?[18] We can answer in the affirmative only with the accompanying clarification: *The client may be best served when a seasoned professional, with the accumulated knowledge of the nature of therapeutic alliances, fills the role of provider.* A therapist experienced, trained, and supervised in the art as well as science of psychotherapy is best suited to achieve and manage the relationship even if the treatment techniques are predictable and accessible to a technician who might be able to describe what could and should be done. In addition to acquiring the appropriate experience, a therapist must adopt operational principles to protect the fidelity of the relationship in the midst of imperfect systems.

Nearly two decades ago, Edward Bordin[19] wrote about the central importance of the working alliance as the key to the attainment of change through psychotherapy. The crisis that he noted was not identical to the one today. Bordin was concerned with the divergent and at times contradictory theoretical approaches that seemed to be proliferating at a rapid rate. Each school of therapy contained its assortment of methods and approaches, making the field appear chaotic, undisciplined, and less than professional. In order to protect therapy from becoming a practice directed only by the apparent whim of any particular practitioner, Bordin proposed a way of unifying the field using the core concept of working alliance. According to his model, a working alliance required an open collaboration regarding tasks and goals along with a live bond between patient and therapist appropriate for their personalities and the problem at hand. Since that time, this model has undergone expansion and empirical research.[20]

A Model for Maintaining the Therapeutic Relationship

The following proposed model for checking a therapeutic relationship in the midst of changing delivery systems is quite simple and is based on a basic carpenter's tool — a builder's square. This uncomplicated device

18. American Psychological Association, "Ethical Principles of Psychologists and Code of Conduct."

19. Edward Bordin, "The Generalizability of the Psychoanalytic Concept of the Working Alliance," *Psychotherapy: Theory, Research and Practice* 16:3 (Fall, 1979): 252-60.

20. Horvath and Greenberg, *The Working Alliance.*

provides a perfect right angle as a handy reference during building in order to keep corners true and precise. As the therapeutic relationship necessary to promote healing is built, a therapist can learn to check four angles intuitively to ensure that they are true to the client and the broader setting requirements. These angled corners can be labeled as follows: *content*, *contact*, *contract*, and *context*.

The *content* angle refers to what actually fills the conversation between the therapist and the client, and it includes the focus, concerns, topics, goal development, values and viewpoints of the parties involved. To maintain the integrity of the relationship, the content needs to be related to the other angles or the square will be skewed. One cannot speak of appropriate content without considering the agreement guiding the process or the treatment setting. Thus, it cannot be completely isolated from the other angles. Keeping this corner square does mean that check-ins at the outset of the session are quite brief. Each topic must be weighed carefully as every avenue of dialogue needs to lead back to the overriding concerns of the presenting problem. New themes are rapidly identified as either dead ends or potential routes to the ultimate destination. A crucial aspect of this angle is the confidentiality of the content. Patients need to know what is being shared by the therapist with the reviewer. The presenting problem, diagnosis, symptoms, approaches, and long/short-term goals are typically described in general terms during a review. Prior to the start of therapy patients are informed about these procedures through written information and person-to-person orientation.

The *contact* angle refers to the nature and quality of the human connection between the therapist and the client. The person-to-person, authentic, genuine, and purposed relationship is one of the prime ingredients in the healing process. It is based upon trust, empathy, and respect. The reason it offers such a healing effect is undoubtedly anchored in the very nature of persons created in the image of God. We are designed to relate to a Creator as well as to human beings. It is sin manifested in our nature and sinful action that distorts and destroys the very relationships that are life-giving. In a therapeutic contact, the relationship itself promotes healing because the boundaries and priorities are carefully and at times painfully constructed. The tendency to distort or to use the relationship in selfish ways is controlled to some degree. The contact cannot be clean and genuine if the therapist is working to fulfill ulterior motives prompted by the review or fears about being cut out of managed care. The aware therapist trained to sort out and be sensitive to such conflicts can work to filter out potential interferences to the relational contact.

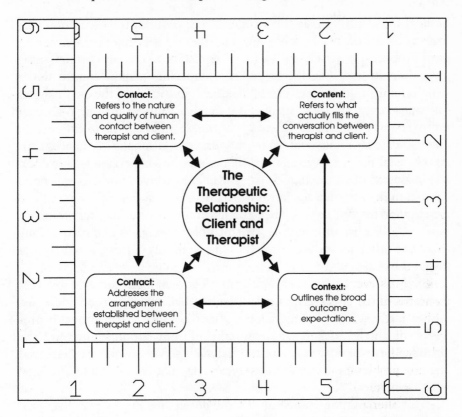

The *contract* addresses the arrangement and understanding that is established between the therapist and the client. It speaks to defined roles, expectations, anticipated outcomes and options. In current managed care procedures a case manager/reviewer is included in the contract with the client, and it is the helping professional's task to work with that player while keeping the adverse impact on the client at a minimum. In addition, the therapist must replace implicit contracts with an explicit therapeutic contract.[21] Hidden agreements can easily be struck in therapy, as clients may desire a caretaker, authority figure, companion, or permissive parent. Therapists for their own mixed motives may agree to fulfill such a counter-therapeutic function. By arriving at a mutual contract that fits the treatment request and clarifies the collaborative aspect of the relationship, there is a guide to keep therapy on track.

Finally the *context* or therapeutic frame must be square with the

21. N. Cummings, "Brief Intermittent Psychotherapy," in Austad and Burman (eds.), *Psychotherapy in Managed Health Care*, pp. 35-45.

other three areas. This is the structure that outlines the broad outcome expectations under a health plan. Therapeutic services are designed to treat and prevent psychopathology that results in impaired functioning and relates to other health concerns. This is the medical context under which therapeutic services can be rendered, but it is not the only context for counseling services. Clients still find great value in making their own arrangements for therapy outside of the insurance-system context to address desirable personal goals or pursue relationship enhancement. Another common context is the therapist who cooperates with a local pastor where the church may pay for or be involved with the services. This context may require acknowledgment of church policies and the expected outcome may be that clients eventually fulfill their ministry potential. The pastor might be informed of the progress and plan as long as the proper releases are secured. This is simply a less formal type of review procedure.

In the context of mental health treatment paid for by a medical insurance plan, client issues may be identified which can be addressed as well or better in a different treatment context. Mental health professionals should make that recommendation or option known to their clients. They should communicate that such services would be beneficial and add life value, but that such services may not be covered by patients' health plans.

Checking the relationship at these designated angles may help professionals establish a treatment relationship that accounts for each of these aspects. When we offer services as providers under a managed care plan, we acknowledge the terms, conditions, limits, and expectations of the concerned parties. A helping relationship is built in such a way as to minimize the risks that the particular frame or context creates. We must not ignore or deny those risks. Some risks will indeed need to be addressed by modifying the context itself. For example, the micro management of the case review process can be substantially altered in order to better protect the confidentiality of clients. Coding methods can be used to enhance confidentiality. In time, the close monitoring by case reviewers might be eliminated as these steps do not appear to be a helpful practice for client care, but serve more as an accountability step for the clinician. Such services may turn out to shift rather than decrease actual costs and may do little to improve quality.

In the best-case scenario, then, managed care can function reasonably well. The safety and fidelity of the helping relationship are maintained as long as the therapist remains committed to the welfare of the client. Informed consent procedures are practiced and treatment options are presented. The promise of confidentiality is maintained, yet qualified by the open acknowledgment of the review procedure. Finally, the therapist-patient dyad does have the autonomy to make choices regarding the direction of treatment even though that freedom operates within certain normative criteria and expectations.

A Christian Professional's Response

Christian therapists recognize that psychotherapy, whether focused on symptom removal or personality reconstruction, is a relational process under grace. Whether the goals are recovery or growth, management or relief of psychopathology, the work is under God's providential care. God is not limited and he is the one committed to bringing every client into wholeness for all eternity. It is for this reason that his Son became a man, suffered, died, and was resurrected. God is not bound by finite resources. He has been doing this re-creation work throughout history and will continue to accomplish it despite the changing conditions in social institutions. God brought about change in the lives of people before the practice of psychotherapy was developed, and he can still bring about those transformations either miraculously or by using many other effective means to accomplish his purpose. It is by grace that helping through the use of psychotherapy has developed in our day.

Christians engaged in the profession of psychology may offer professional services in a number of settings including taking a provider role with a managed care organization. However, we must answer not only to those who grant our license or pay our fee, but to the One who actually commissioned our ministry. Certainly it is necessary to pray for wisdom, and as we have been sent out as sheep among wolves, we therefore need grace to be as shrewd as serpents and as innocent as doves (Matt. 10:16).

The believer is born by the Spirit into a relationship not only with the Lord, but with the body of Christ, the community of believers. Although it may be difficult to experience this in our individualistic contemporary culture, the true corporate nature of our faith is richly and wonderfully portrayed in Scripture (1 Cor. 12:12-31; Rom. 12:3-8). The Christian therapist may view the clinical relationship as serving the purpose of conceptualizing and triggering change for the patient that will be realized and experienced within the church as the local body of Christ.

The Christian researcher and writer Everett Worthington, in his response to the changes in mental health care, speaks of the "catalytic" model of therapy as a useful metaphor for the therapist who offers brief therapy under managed care conditions.[22] The emphasis is on the therapeutic encounter with the contact between therapist and patient creating the site for a natural "chemical" type reaction to begin. In other words, the well defined and purposeful therapeutic relationship becomes the place where conditions are favorable for the client to experience change in a controlled setting, and this begins a chain of reactions that flow into the natural life setting. The believer can participate in the body life of the church and in the family to continue the healing process. This is not to suggest a step-down service model. Rather, the professional encounter is used as part of a divine corrective process to modify patterns and motivate change which is carried on in the community of believers. Christian therapists must keep in perspective that the One who started the work is going to bring it to completion (Phil. 1:6).

Worthington goes on to assert that the Christian therapist is in an ideal position to accept the role shift brought about by managed care systems. The therapist is removed from the all-responsible healer role and becomes a collaborator or catalyst for change.

> For Christians, one would think that this mental transformation should be easier than for those who are not Christians. Christians should know that we cannot heal anyone. We should know that the real healer is Jesus Christ through the Holy Spirit. For years, we have played by the rules of the world, which assumed that the counselor was the healer. We must give up that world-stimulated fiction.[23]

With this perspective, the therapist can find a way to use the therapeutic relationship and the built-in review procedures with a clear purpose and may not become overwhelmed by the limits of the contemporary system. In therapy with Christian clients, we can help them to identify, form, and grow in their place in the body under the shepherds that God provides in broader community. We know that our professional healing relationship can be used by the Holy Spirit to alter the client's relationship with God the Father through his Son. It is ultimately that relationship which

22. Everett Worthington, Jr., "Speculations about new directions in helping marriages and families that arise from pressures of managed mental health care," *Journal of Psychology and Christianity* 15:3 (1996): 197-212.
23. Worthington, "Speculations about new directions," p. 203.

provides healing. We are aware that there are additional relationships available to clients in the body of Christ where the believer is to function according to his gifts and calling. In clinical practice, we may use the Global Assessment of Functioning (GAF) scale to determine medical necessity and demonstrate improvement. However, it is actually the Ministry Activity and Fulfillment scale — what we might call the "MAF" criteria — that is most important for the Christian. Even in the case of the nonbelieving client, the therapist remains aware that God is at work, and the openness to change brought about by the conditions that led to therapy may be the very forces God uses to draw the individual into the kingdom. Therefore, the Christian professional has the opportunity to help with an inner sense of service to the Lord even if the context, contact, contract, and content are not such that there is direct evangelism or faith discussion.

This modest yet strong rationale for Christian therapists to participate in the contemporary managed mental health system does not answer all the charges and contentions about managed care. It is a human institution in a fallen world. Christian therapists may find themselves at odds with a system that does not provide fairly or justly for patients who are "hungry, thirsty, sick, or in prison"[24] and who do not know how to speak up for their rights.[25] Although Christian therapists may be able to provide mental health services under redefined therapeutic relationship models, there may be tension with the delivery systems and it may need to be addressed. There is indeed the potential to be the "salt" that helps preserve the healing effects of a therapeutic encounter in this redesigned system. The challenge is ongoing. May we pray for wisdom and grace as we seek to fulfill not only our professional function but our ministry calling.[26]

---

24. Matt. 25:34-36.

25. Sabin, "A Credo for Ethical Managed Care in Mental Health Practice," p. 860.

26. I recall the challenge to my professional identity brought out in a dramatic way on that June day by a critic of managed care and disguised by my own inner distortions as the voice of my grandfather. My dad, under the painful criticism of his father, brought into our modern house what was important about a home and in doing so gave what was necessary to his family. I will attempt to remember the essentials of client care via a well-defined therapeutic relationship as I move into the contemporary scene of psychotherapy under managed care with all of its inherent conflicts. May the Lord be the real "provider" and supply his grace.

Managed Long-Term Care

Richard W. Olson, M.A., C.P.A.

"Hold her Newt. She's headed for the rhubarb." It was an old farm phrase frequently used by the former vice president of finance at Covenant Retirement Communities. When the phrase resounded from his office, it signaled to all within hearing distance that the long-term care organization was experiencing some unique challenges and financial demands at that particular time. It also communicated a feeling that things could get out of control and that certain financial aspects of the mission-driven organization might experience serious difficulties. If he were alive today and given an opportunity to look over the long-term care horizon, the office walls would no doubt resonate with his often-used phrase. Indeed, the challenges and demands appear to be greater than ever.

A Dollar-Driven Mindset

The long-term care environment is becoming increasingly dollar driven. Medicare currently represents approximately 3 to 5 percent of all patient day activity within skilled nursing facilities. Eligibility for coverage is based on the rehabilitative or restorative care that follows a hospital stay. A maximum of 100 days is eligible for coverage.

Changes in the Medicare system to date have generally not focused on long-term care, but this is changing. Because the Medicare program is based on the need for rehabilitative services, actual dollars received by long-term care providers from Medicare can be quite significant. Not only is reimbursement received for routine costs (such as room and board); extensive therapy and other services are usually incurred and become a

192

significant component of the dollar amount reimbursed to skilled nursing facilities.

Medicare has begun to take several actions, all seemingly targeted at reducing overall dollar outlays to long-term care providers. For example, Medicare has started to restrict reimbursement amounts in areas such as physical therapy and has introduced a prospective payment system similar to the DRG system introduced in hospitals in the 1980s. This system will dramatically change the way skilled nursing facilities are reimbursed and most likely reduce the amount of reimbursement.[1]

The Health Care Finance Administration (HCFA) strongly encourages senior adults to enroll in Medicare Health Maintenance Organizations (HMOs). Many in the Administration and Congress view incentives to transfer coverage of senior adults from the traditional Medicare program to a Medicare HMO as a means of reducing overall dollars expended by Medicare for long-term care.

Current estimates indicate approximately 10 to 15 percent of senior adults are enrolled in a Medicare HMO. HMOs, particularly in California and Minnesota, have become quite aggressive in their marketing to senior adults, with Medicare HMO coverage offered at no additional cost. Compared to the cost of supplemental insurance, this at times looks like a bargain to senior adults. But the long-term care coverage a Medicare HMO provides may not result in the same level of benefits enjoyed under the traditional Medicare program. A fractured hip may receive four weeks of payment instead of six. The HMO may allow fewer daily therapy units than Medicare. A skilled nursing facility often faces the choice of either providing the additional care required with no reimbursement from the HMO or not providing the care at all.

In the case of a continuing-care retirement community that offers multiple levels of care (Independent Living Units, Assisted Living Facilities, and Skilled Nursing Facilities), a provider contract with an HMO is a key component in keeping residents on campus and covered by the services of the retirement community. If a continuing care retirement community does not have a contract with an HMO but the HMO has enrolled community residents, the residents, on a temporary basis, may have to go to another facility which has a contract with the HMO. Legislation passed in Florida states that the HMO has to cover the resident at the skilled nursing facility of the same retirement community. This

---

1. Deloitte & Touche LLP, *Washington Commentary: A Perspective on Health Care* (June 16, 1997).

legislation, although positive, does not determine how much payment the provider receives or what services the HMO covers.

The Medicaid program pertains to senior adults at skilled nursing facilities who no longer have financial resources to pay for their care. Within Covenant Retirement Communities, approximately 25 percent of the residents at skilled nursing facilities receive assistance from Medicaid, but other organizations may have a much higher percentage.

A budget-neutral mentality exists in most states relating to Medicaid. For example, within Illinois, the payment system is being redesigned. However, current indications are that the number of overall dollars involved will not be materially changed, just distributed differently based on a new reimbursement methodology.

Some states look at managed care as a possible way to maintain or reduce overall spending for Medicaid. Many states await approval from the Health Care Finance Administration to allow HMOs the ability to manage their Medicaid systems. Recent health care reforms indicate serious efforts to "eliminate the need for states to obtain federal waivers in order to include home and community based services in a state's optional service package."[2]

Skilled nursing facilities, in general, have experienced decreases in census even though the senior adult population continues to increase. Medicaid and other third party payers continue carefully to explore other ways to provide care, which include home health care and a greater use of assisted living facilities. "In 1990, the nation's spending on home health care was only 29 percent of what it spent on nursing home care. By 1995, it had risen to 44 percent." It seems to be an automatic assumption that home care is less expensive than care provided in a skilled nursing facility — an assumption that is highly debatable.[3]

The state of Oregon provides a good example relating to assisted living. Oregon received a Medicaid waiver from HCFA. Residents who formerly received care at skilled nursing facilities and whose care is more custodial in nature now receive care in assisted living facilities and are eligible for reimbursement from Medicaid. Meanwhile, skilled nursing facilities experience shorter stays, lower patient census, and a significant increase in the acuity level of patients. The state pays a lower rate at the assisted living level of care, hopefully resulting in fewer dollars paid in the overall system. Fewer dollars paid out for state Medicaid programs also benefits the federal government, because state Medicaid dollars are matched with federal dollars.

2. Katten, Muchin, & Zavis, *Law News: Health Care* (May 1997).
3. *Contemporary Long-Term Care* (June 1997), p. 40.

Tying Reimbursement to Quality of Care

Another major area of concern — along with a dollar-driven mindset on the part of third party payers — relates to attempts to measure quality of care and tie these measurements into payment systems. For example, there are more and more efforts being made to integrate reimbursement systems directly with acuity levels. HMOs frequently reimburse providers based on several payment levels, which factor in heavier acuity levels. The Minnesota Medicaid system has 11 acuity levels of reimbursement ranging from A to K, with K being the highest payment rate.

Patient care can easily become more standardized rather than individualized. For example, a critical pathway may say "this is the way to treat a fractured hip." Providing care for the "fractured hip" may become so involved with the standard method of treating the condition that other care concerns or issues can be missed. Caregivers might view the patient as "a fractured hip in room 101" rather than "Mrs. Jones who happens to have a fractured hip and needs help."

National efforts currently in process and tied to the implementation of the Medicare prospective payment system attempt to measure quality and outcomes in long-term care. HCFA requires each resident staying at a skilled nursing facility to have a minimum data set completed. This minimum data set (MDS) provides information in a number of areas such as activities of daily living. Pilot programs exist in about a half a dozen states for the electronic transfer of this data to HCFA. It is anticipated that all MDS data will be electronically transmitted to individual states and then from all states to HCFA beginning in the summer of 1998. New legislation will accelerate the MDS completion cycle for each Medicare resident. Collection of this information may provide measurements of quality and information relating to treatment methods and plans on a diagnosis-by-diagnosis basis. Payment methodologies would then be developed by diagnosis.

Many states are in the process of developing quality indicators and standards for assisted living facilities. These efforts generally take the form of the Oregon program; to provide "appropriate care to as many persons in need as possible."[4]

In Illinois the purpose of the Assisted Living Act:

. . . is to promote the availability of appropriate services for elderly persons in the least restrictive and most homelike environment; to

---

4. State of Oregon, Chapter 410, *Senior & Disability Services* (1995 edition).

encourage the development of assisted living that promotes the dignity, individuality, privacy, and decision-making ability of those persons; to provide for the health, safety, and welfare of residents receiving assisted living services in this State; to promote continuous quality improvement of assisted living; and to encourage the development of innovative and affordable assisted living establishments.[5]

While the above objectives may sound fine on the surface, definite concerns exist within the long-term industry regarding the availability of resources to care for senior adults adequately. Attempts are being made to identify quality indicators and to establish whether the hoped-for quality will be affordable.

Quality monitoring should be structured into the daily operations of any assisted living residence with the goal of constant improvement in clinical, functional, and quality-of-life outcomes. This system largely relies on internal quality teams to monitor performance using information from quality indicators, incidental monitors, and management experience. The goal is to identify problems and implement action plans to achieve improvement in performance outcomes. The state or its monitoring agent would adopt a largely consultative role with the goal of improving quality with all providers. Minimum standards would be used in the quality-improvement phase primarily when the provider fails to achieve an acceptable level of performance.[6]

It is not a difficult step to move from attempts to measure quality to equating quality with value-of-life considerations, particularly when overall systems become more and more dollar-driven. The following comments from Dr. Joanne Lynn, a geriatrician writing about end-of-life care, illustrate this concern.

Since . . . three-quarters of all people die in federal programs, most medical costs are managed by a bureaucracy. One consequence is that end-of-life care is not cost-effective for most doctors. "If you develop a reputation to be the best in town at providing good end-of-life care,

5. State of Illinois, 90th General Assembly, *Assisted Living Establishment Act* (1997 and 1998).

6. Alzheimer's Association, American Association of Homes and Services for the Aging, American Associated of Retired Persons, and the Assisted Living Facilities Association of America, *The Assisted Living Quality Initiative: Building a Structure That Promotes Quality* (August 1, 1996), p. 23.

you'll go out of business within a year. . . . We have to make it possible to have excellence. It has to be possible to be really good at end-of-life care and still be able to make a living. Now, we've perversely set it up so you just can't do it."[7]

It is becoming increasingly difficult to serve as an administrator of a long-term care facility. The administrator must be concerned that rates charged for care remain marketable and cover the operating needs of the organization, that employees are able to be recruited and retained, that the physical plant is maintained (and many times the physical plant needs upgrades to handle changes in care such as special care units for dementia) — all within a third-party-payer environment that is attempting to minimize and even reduce care payments. It is quite clear that there will be more compliance-reporting requirements in the future relating to the measurement of quality care combined with fewer dollars from Medicare, Medicaid, and managed care generally. It will be a challenging path to travel.

Basis for a Christian Response

Before discussing strategies to deal with these concerns, certain foundational convictions must be noted. These convictions can then provide a base for development of strategies and action plans for dealing with concerns raised by eroding financial resources combined with efforts to measure quality.

It is an awesome privilege to realize that the God of the universe created us in his image (Genesis 1:27).

> The Scriptures tell us that the universe exists and has form and meaning because it was created purposefully by a personal Creator. This being the case, we see that, as we are personal, we are not something strange and out of line with an otherwise impersonal universe. Since we are made in the image of God, we are in line with God. There is a continuity, in other words, between ourselves, though finite, and the infinite Creator who stands behind the universe as its Creator and its final source of meaning.[8]

7. *Christianity Today* (June 16, 1997): 40.
8. C. Everett Koop and Francis A. Schaeffer, *Whatever Happened to the Human Race?* (Wheaton, Ill.: Crossway Books, 1979, 1983), p. 108.

Because of sin and rebellion against God, the world needed a redeemer. God not only created humankind but also provided for redemption in the person of Jesus Christ. Jesus paid the price for human sin. He died for everyone in spite of who they are and while they were still sinners. We cannot begin to comprehend his love for humanity.

> In I Corinthians 6, Paul says that we have been purchased with a great price. The value or worth of an object is usually determined by the price one is willing to pay to purchase or redeem it.[9]

It is indeed a blessing and privilege to have the opportunity to be children of God.

In the world today, there are a number of approaches to ethics that potentially can influence views of senior adult care. Steve Wilkens has summarized a number of ethical systems, including cultural relativism, ethical egoism, behaviorism, utilitarianism, Kantian ethics, virtue ethics, situation ethics, natural law ethics, and divine command theory. A major challenge for Christian long-term care providers is to understand and resist the temptation of such outlooks and to operate from a worldview derived from Biblical principles.[10] Admittedly, according to Isaiah 55:7, it is impossible to comprehend the ways and thoughts of God. Yet, God has established definite standards and rules of conduct (e.g., the Ten Commandments) where the goalposts should not be lowered. In John 14:6, Jesus not only says he is the way and the life but also the truth. Truth is not relative. Societal standards alone should not determine morals.

Elements of a Christian Response

These foundational convictions suggest several responses to the issues raised by dollar-driven systems and attempts to measure quality. God has made us stewards of his resources — not owners, simply stewards. First Corinthians 4:2 proclaims faithfulness as a requirement of stewardship. A phrase near and dear to the hearts of financial people, credited to Mother Teresa, states, "No margin = no mission." A not-for-profit organization must generate enough cash to meet all of its obligations.

9. Josh McDowell, *The Secret of Loving: How a Lasting Intimate Relationship Can Be Yours* (San Bernardino, Calif.: Here's Life Publishers, Inc., 1985), p. 24.

10. A helpful aid for this task is Steve Wilkens, *Beyond Bumper Sticker Ethics: An Introduction to Theories of Right and Wrong* (Downers Grove, Ill.: InterVarsity, 1995).

Long-term care providers may serve as stewards of God's resources in a variety of ways.

There needs to be a willingness to be accountable. Accreditation represents one way of achieving this objective. In the long-term care industry, the Continuing Care Accreditation Commission has developed a number of standards for Continuing Care Retirement Communities in the areas of governance, finance, resident life, and health care. A peer review of these standards often serves as a source of counsel and insight. There is wisdom in counsel. Managed care organizations increasingly recognize the value of accreditation.

There needs to be a willingness to work with other providers in areas of common ground. Long-term care organizations have often wanted to do things their own way. Relationships with other providers consisted of an occasional discussion over a cup of coffee or attending association meetings together.

The last couple of years have witnessed the development of alliances within the long-term care industry. An alliance is a group of providers who band together to accomplish certain common objectives. These long-term care organizations usually represent a variety of denominations and organizational structures and backgrounds. There is no transfer of ownership or loss of control by each individual organization. A separate corporation is formed for specific purposes. From a conceptual perspective, an alliance representing a number of facilities should have far more success working with HMOs, therapy companies, pharmacy companies, and other health care vendors than a facility trying to negotiate pricing and services on its own. The objective is to provide the same or better level of service at a lower negotiated price.

The church has a variety of opportunities to fund the cost of long-term care for those without the resources to pay for their care. In addition to funding long-term care providers directly, the church can advise people to consider leaving a portion of their estate to a long-term care provider. By investing the funds when received, the provider can use the earnings from the fund to help cover the cost of benevolent care, thereby reducing dependence on third party payment sources. The earnings from a church's benevolent care fund can purchase long-term care insurance for those with inadequate financial resources. Long-term care insurance can help reduce a facility's overall dependence on Medicaid as resources for care become available on a longer-term basis.

Stewards need to know costs from a management perspective. Does the pricing structure adequately cover the costs incurred? Covenant Retirement Communities has worked hard to develop outcome measurement systems that include on a person-by-person basis a calculation of the cost of care provided. This particular computerized tool is now being compared with other outcome measurement tools within the industry. A greater negotiating power with third party payers such as managed care organizations and state Medicaid agencies may result after obtaining a better understanding of costs.

While serving as the best steward of resources possible, one must also function as a servant. According to Philippians 2, one must not only look after personal interests but also the interests of others. The description of the Lord in this passage — his willingness to be a servant — should continue to serve as our standard.

Real servants must lay aside personal turf. The different disciplines within a facility need to work closer together than ever before. Nursing, accounting and information services, chaplaincy, activities, environmental services, dietary, administration, social service, marketing, and other areas of operation must see their roles as working together to serve the residents. Teamwork is not optional.

Care providers must work hard at maintaining a "care" mentality. It is easy to have a "cure" orientation. The tendency to depersonalize patient care can naturally lead to the reduction of a sense of individual accountability and responsibility. Staff can easily fall into a task orientation that may at times clearly miss the real care needs of the residents and yet comply with all external requirements. Compliance is not the standard. Quality care is not only doing things for people. It is *being there* — listening and understanding. Quality care cannot always be quantified or measured. An ongoing review of operating structures and procedures should assure that the care provided reflects the residents' specific needs.

Surveys of patients in nursing homes reveal that they are more concerned about the kindness of their caregivers, having their own space and their own friends, and the little details of their day-to-day life, than whether or not they have a valid Living Will or have decided about receiving cardiopulmonary resuscitation. In the nursing home, the little things count the most.[11]

11. Robert D. Orr, David B. Biebel, and David L. Schiedermayer, *More Life and Death Decisions: Help in Making Tough Choices about Care for the Elderly, Euthanasia, and Medical Treatment Options* (Grand Rapids: Baker Books, 1990), p. 40.

Church-based long-term care providers need to step back and review the long-term care delivery system in terms of how, where, and what services are provided. They should focus greater attention on developing other service ministries (such as parish nursing, home health or homemaker services, hospice care, etc.) in cooperation with the local church. Care providers should look for ways to strengthen overall internal resources and ministries rather than looking to third party payers for direction.

However, even success at providing care and staying financially afloat is not enough:

- Christian long-term care providers must obtain, maintain, and model a Micah 6:8 mindset.

  > He has showed you, O man, what is good.
  > And what does the Lord require of you?
  > To act justly and to love mercy
  > and to walk humbly with your God.

- Caregiving practices of Christian long-term care providers must consistently involve pointing people to the cross.
- Those within the long-term care industry must model principles of salt and light.
- Just as the Lord placed tremendous value on each person as demonstrated by giving his life, so caregivers must demonstrate his love for others, regardless of the situation.

As an example of God's love in action, I think in particular of a highly effective activity director for an extended care floor. This woman views each patient as special — requiring individual attention and specific activity plans. A stroke victim recently admitted into the extended care facility of her church-sponsored hospital indicated he had loved to sing but now doubted that he would ever sing again. The activity director, who was determined to at least provide an opportunity, took him to a room with a piano and began to play. As she played the piano, the man once again sang. Not only did he sing, he sang beautifully and was a blessing to other patients who heard him.

As even this brief discussion of the issues facing the long-term care industry reveals, the cow is most certainly out of the barn, has gotten past the fence, and is headed toward the rhubarb. But may the way we care for people in the challenging long-term care world of the twenty-first century "sing out the glory of God."

201

The Impact of Changes in Health Care Delivery on Minority Communities

Frank E. Staggers, Sr., M.D. and
Barbara C. Staggers, M.D., M.P.H.

The changing face of health care is a global issue. Nevertheless, change is particularly pronounced today in the United States — nationally, regionally, and locally. The fee-for-service share of the market has significantly declined in the past 15 years with the massive shift toward a managed care system.[1] As this change has occurred, there has been a major emphasis on the business of medicine, including measurements of efficiency and cost/profit considerations.[2] Service agencies, health care professionals, and communities are all now dealing with this new reality.

For the minority community and the professionals who care for them, the impact of these changes in health care delivery has been quite negative. There are major obstacles in access to and delivery of health care for minorities,[3] including the existence of racial and ethnic dispari-

1. V. R. Fuchs, "Managed Care and Merger Mania," *Journal of the American Medical Association* 277 (1997): 920-21.

2. Editorial, "HMO Patients Deserve Broader Rights on Care," *Los Angeles Times*, June 18, 1997; N. A. Jeffrey, "How to Tell If an HMO's 'Quality' Promise Is for Real," *Wall Street Journal*, June 13, 1997.

3. R. S. Cooper, B. Simmons, A. Castaner et al., "Survival Rates and Prehospital Delay During Myocardial Infarction Among Black Persons," *American Journal of Cardiology* 57 (1986): 208-11; R. J. Blendon, L. H. Aiken, H. E. Freeman, and C. R. Corey, "Access to

ties in health[4] and health care,[5] the constraints of capitation reimbursement, and changes in Medicare and Medicaid — issues that affect both the caregivers and the communities they serve.

There have been some responses to this crisis from organized medicine on both national and state levels. A few local initiatives have also been started to address this injustice.

Medical Care for Black and White Americans: A Matter of Continuing Concern," *JAMA* 261 (1989): 278-81; J. S. Weissman, R. Stern, S. L. Fielding, and A. M. Epstein, "Delayed Access to Health Care: Risk Factors, Reasons, and Consequences," *Annual of Internal Medicine* 114 (1991): 325-31; L. J. Cornelius, "Barriers to Medical Care for White, Black, and Hispanic American Children," *Journal of the National Medical Association* 85 (1993): 281-88; E. Ginzberg, "Access to Health Care for Hispanics," *JAMA* 265 (1991): 238-41; E. Moy and C. Hogan, "Access to Needed Follow-up Services: Variations Among Different Medicare Populations," *Archive of Internal Medicine* 153 (1993): 1815-23; J. J. Escarce, K. K. R. Epstein, D. C. Colby, and J. S. Schwartz, "Racial Differences in the Elderly's Use of Medical Procedures and Diagnostic Tests," *American Journal of Public Health* 83 (1993): 948-54; L. R. Snowden, T. Hu, and L. F. M. Jerrell, "Emergency Care Avoidance: Ethnic Matching and Participation in Minority-serving Programs," *Community Mental Health Journal* 31 (1995): 463-73; G. Pappas, W. C. Hadden, L. J. Kozac, and G. F. Fisher, "Potentially Avoidable Hospitalizations: Inequities in Rates Between U.S. Socioeconomic Groups," *American Journal of Public Health* 87 (1997): 811-17.

4. H. W. Nickens, "The Health Status of Minority Populations in the United States," *Western Journal of Medicine* 155 (1991): 27-32; F. S. Mendoza, S. J. Ventura, R. B. Valdez, R. O. Castillo, L. E. Saldivar, K. Baisden, and R. Martorelli, "Selected Measures of Health Status for Mexican-American, Mainland Puerto Rican, and Cuban-American Children," *JAMA* 265 (1991): 227-32.

5. K. H. Todd, N. Samaroo, and J. R. Hoffman, "Ethnicity as a Risk Factor for Inadequate Emergency Department Analgesia," *JAMA* 269 (1993): 1537-39; P. A. Johnson, T. H. Lee, F. Cook, G. W. Rouan, and L. Goldman, "Effect of Race on the Presentation and Management of Patients with Acute Chest Pain," *Annual of Internal Medicine* 118 (1993): 593-601, 617-20; D. W. Baker, C. D. Stevens, and A. R. H. Brook, "Regular Source of Ambulatory Care and Medical Care Utilization by Patients Presenting to a Public Hospital Emergency Department," *JAMA* 271 (1994): 1909-12; K. L. Kahn, M. L. Pearson, E. R. Harrison, K. A. Desmond, W. H. Rogers, L. V. Rubenstein, R. H. Brook, and E. B. Keeler, "Health Care for Black and Poor Hospitalized Medicare Patients," *JAMA* 271 (1994): 1169-74; D. K. Padgett, C. Patrick, B. J. Burns, and H. J. Schlesinger, "Ethnicity and the Use of Outpatient Mental Health Services in a National Insured Population," *American Journal of Public Health* 84 (1994): 222-26; R. A. Wright, T. L. Andres, and A. J. Davidson, "Finding the Medically Underserved: A Need to Revise the Federal Definition," *Journal of Health Care for the Poor and Underserved* 7 (1996): 296-306.

Racial Disparities

There is a longstanding pattern of racial and ethnic disparity in the access to and the delivery of health care services in the United States.[6] Minority patients and poor patients are more likely to be uninsured or underinsured.[7] In addition they are more likely to have co-morbidities, chronic illness, and higher acuity of illness.[8] Minority and poor patients also have higher mortality rates in infants[9] and adults.[10] Cultural and language barriers plus unfamiliarity with the health care system often hamper access for minorities.

Numerous articles have been written documenting major disparities in health and in medical care delivery for minorities. Three landmark reports have documented and summarized the data: The Kerner Commission Report (1968),[11] the Heckler-Malone Report (1985),[12] and the Report of the AMA Advisory Committee on Minority Physicians (1994).[13]

6. Council on Ethical and Judicial Affairs (AMA), "Black-White Disparities in Health Care," *JAMA* 263 (1990): 2344-46.

7. F. M. Trevino, E. Moyer, B. Valdez, and C. A. Stroup-Benham, "Health Insurance Coverage and Utilization of Health Services by Mexican Americans, Mainland Puerto Ricans, and Cuban Americans," *JAMA* 265 (1991): 233-37; C. Halton, D. L. Wood, V. Burciaga, M. Pereyra, and N. Duan, "Medicaid Enrollment and Health Services Access by Latino Children in Inner-city Los Angeles," *JAMA* 277 (1997): 636-41.

8. R. S. Kingston and J. P. Smith, "Socioeconomic Status and Racial and Ethnic Differences in Functional Status Associated with Chronic Diseases," *American Journal of Public Health* 87 (1997): 805-10.

9. A. Kempe, P. H. Wise, S. E. Barkan et al., "Clinical Determinants of the Racial Disparity in Very Low Birth Weight," *N Eng J Med* 327 (1992): 969-73; R. J. David and J. W. Collins, "Differing Birth Weight Among Infants of U.S.-born Blacks, African-born Blacks, and U.S.-born Whites," *N Eng J Med* 337 (1997): 1209-14; J. E. Becerra, C. J. R. Hogue, H. K. Atrash, and N. Perez, "Infant Mortality Among Hispanics," *JAMA* 265 (1991): 217-21.

10. L. B. Becker, B. H. Han, P. M. Meyer et al., "Racial Differences in the Incidence of Cardiac Arrest and Subsequent Survival," *N Eng J Med* 329 (1993): 600-606; M. E. Gornick, P. W. Eggers, T. W. Reilly, R. M. Mentnech, L. K. Fitterman, L. E. Kucken, and B. C. Vladeck, "Effects of Race and Income on Mortality and Use of Services Among Medicare Beneficiaries," *N Eng J Med* 335 (1996): 791-99; H. S. Gordon, D. L. Harper, and G. E. Rosenthal, "Racial Variation in Predicted and Observed In-hospital Death: A Regional Analysis," *JAMA* 276 (1996): 1639-44.

11. Recommendations of the Kerner Commission, *American Journal of Public Health* 58 (1968): 1317.

12. M. M. Heckler, "Report of the Secretary's Task Force on Black and Minority Health," USDHHS 1985: 1 (executive summary).

13. Report to the Board of Trustees, American Medical Association; 50-I-95; Chicago, Ill.

In 1968 the Kerner Commission stated "The residents of the racial ghetto are significantly less healthy than most other Americans. They suffer from higher mortality rates, higher incidence of major diseases, and lower availability and utilization of medical services." Additionally, the commission concluded that disparity in meeting the health care needs of the non-white population was one factor underlying the racial crisis following the assassination of Martin Luther King, Jr.

In 1985 the Heckler-Malone Report contended that there has been a significant difference in death rates between the races ever since accurate federal record-keeping began. There were approximately 59,000 excess deaths (deaths that would not have occurred had the mortality rates been equal for minorities and non-minorities) among blacks each year between 1979 and 1981. Six groups of conditions accounted for approximately 80 percent of this excess mortality (see Table 1).

In 1992, the American Medical Association (AMA) established an Advisory Committee on Minority Physicians (ACOMP) and charged it to improve the health status of minorities, to expand the membership and representation of minority physicians and medical students in the AMA, and to increase the number of minority students and faculty in U.S. medical schools. In its 1994 report, the committee documented major racial disparities in the type, number, and frequency of disease conditions present among minorities along with disparities in disease outcome. In addition, they found differences in delivery sites, availability of care, and access to that care.

The ACOMP Report included a 66-page bibliography of articles published in just two of the major medical journals *(Journal of the American Medical Association* and *New England Journal of Medicine)* from 1984 to 1994 which demonstrated racial health disparities. The Report highlighted four situations (pneumonia, cardiovascular procedures, HIV disease, and kidney disease) in which the patient's race represented a significant determinant of the type and amount of care provided. In 1987 Yergan et al. documented that non-white patients hospitalized with pneumonia received fewer services, fewer consultations, and less intensive care.[14] It was reported in 1993[15] and again in

14. J. Yergan, A. B. Flood, J. P. LoGerfo, and P. Diehr, "Relationship Between Race and the Intensity of Hospital Services," *Medical Care* 25 (1987): 592-603.
15. J. Whittle, J. Congliaarao, C. B. Good, and R. P. Lofgren, "Racial Differences in the Use of Invasive Cardiovascular Procedures in the Department of Veterans Affairs Medical System," *N Eng J Med* 229 (1993): 621-27.

Table 1. Causes of Excess Mortality Among Minorities

cause of death	% excess mortality	approximate number of excess deaths
heart disease and stroke	30.0	17,700
homicide and accidents	18.5	10,900
cancer	13.8	8,150
infant mortality	10.5	6,200
cirrhosis	3.7	2,200
diabetes	3.1	1,800

1994[16] that white patients were more likely than blacks to undergo invasive cardiac procedures (including catheterization, percutaneous transluminal coronary angioplasty and coronary artery bypass grafting) in the Veterans Affairs system. Similar findings have been demonstrated in the private sector.[17] Black patients with HIV disease were significantly less likely than whites to receive anti-retroviral therapy or pneumocystis carinii pneumonia prophylaxis when first referred to an HIV clinic in Moore's 1994 study.[18] Black-white disparities have been documented in the use of both transplantation,[19] and dialysis[20] in patients with end-stage kidney disease.

16. E. D. Peterson, S. M. Wright, J. Daley, and G. E. Thibault, "Racial Variation in Cardiac Procedure Use and Survival Following Acute Myocardial Infarction in the Department of Veterans Affairs," *JAMA* 271 (1994): 1175-80.

17. J. Z. Ayanian, I. S. Udvarhelyi, C. A. Gastonis, C. L. Pashos, and A. M. Epstein, "Racial Differences in the Use of Revascularization Procedures After Coronary Angiography," *JAMA* 169 (1993): 2642-46; E. S. Fore and R. S. Cooper, "Racial/ethnic Difference in Health Care Utilization of Cardiovascular Procedures: A Review of the Evidence," *Health Service Res* 30 (1995): 237-52.

18. R. D. Moore, "Racial Differences in the Use of Drug Therapy for HIV Disease in an Urban Community," *N Eng J Med* 330 (1994): 763-68.

19. B. L. Kasiske, J. F. Neylan, R. R. Riggio, G. M. Danovitch, L. Kahana, S. R. Alexander, and M. G. White, "The Effect of Race on Access and Outcome in Transplantation," *N Eng J Med* 324 (1991): 302-7; R. S. Gaston, I. Ayres, L. G. Dooley, A. G. Diethelm, "Racial Equity in Renal Transplantation: The Disparate Impact of HLA-based Allocation," *JAMA* 270 (1993): 352-56.

20. C. B. Barker-Cummings, W. McCellan, M. Soucie, and J. Krisher, "Ethnic Differences in the Use of Peritoneal Dialysis as Initial Treatment for End-stage Renal Disease," *JAMA* 274 (1995): 1858-62.

Changes in Health Care Delivery

These disparities in illness and treatment are both clear and distressing. They have been worsened, however, by some of the changes that have occurred in the delivery of health care in the past 15 years.

Physician reimbursement by capitation (a fixed payment per patient per month) is a major component of most managed care systems. This departure from traditional fee-for-service payment poses special problems for minority communities and the professionals who provide their care.[21] Since the amount of money received by the physician does not change regardless of the severity of illness or how often the patient must be seen, he or she must, on average, spend more time per dollar of income in caring for minority patients because they are sicker.

The professionals who care for minorities and the medically indigent are more often non-white themselves.[22] Non-white physicians often have difficulty being included in managed care plans.[23] They are often financially penalized when they care for minority patients or practice under a capitation system.[24]

The federal government has encouraged health maintenance organizations (HMOs) to enroll more Medicare patients. This has further eroded the practice base of health care professionals because HMOs are able to offer many perks and benefits to Medicare patients including meals and parties during marketing solicitations, forgiveness of the copayment requirement, pharmacy benefits, and the freedom to disenroll within 30

21. M. E. Stuart and D. M. Steinwachs, "Patient-mix Differences Among Ambulatory Providers and Their Effects on Utilization and Payments for Maryland Medicaid Users," *Medical Care* 31 (1993): 1119-37.

22. B. Rocheleau, "Black Physicians and Ambulatory Care," *Public Health Report* 93 (1978): 278-82; E. May and B. A. Bartman, "Physician Race and Care of Minority and Medically Indigent Patients," *JAMA* 273 (1995): 1515-20; M. Komaromy, K. Grumbach, M. Drake, K. Vranizan, N. Lurie, D. Keane, and A. B. Bindman, "The Role of Black and Hispanic Physicians in Providing Health Care for Underserved Populations," *N Eng J Med* 334 (1996): 1305-10; A. L. Stewart, K. Grumbach, D. H. Osmond, K. Vranizan, M. Komaromy, and A. B. Bindman, "Primary Care and Patient Perceptions of Access to Care," *Journal of Family Practice* 44 (1997): 177-85.

23. D. Grubb, "Medicine's New Face — Minorities Gradually Enter the Mainstream," *California Physician* 12 (4) (1995): 24-32.

24. S. M. Lloyd, D. G. Johnson, and M. Mann, "Survey of Graduates of a Traditionally Black College of Medicine," *Journal of Medical Education* 53 (1978): 640-50; D. G. Johnson, S. M. Lloyd, and R. L. Miller, "A Second Survey of Graduates of a Traditionally Black College of Medicine," *Academic Medicine* 54 (1989): 87-94.

days. Indemnity insurance plans and individual physicians are unable to offer such benefits.

As with Medicare, the federal government has pushed states to use managed care plans to provide health care for poor patients through the federally-funded but state-administered Medicaid programs. Consider, for example, the state of California. To meet the federal mandate, California designed a system to transfer millions of Medi-Cal (California's Medicaid program) enrollees. They set a goal of enrolling 3.2 million beneficiaries in 19 counties by the end of 1997. By August 1, 1997, more than 1.2 million were actually enrolled, but this massive undertaking wrought havoc for both patients and physicians.

For several years, California had been operating successful managed care Medi-Cal plans as pilot projects in five counties. These County Organized Health Systems (COHS) involved all of the major stakeholders in health care and gave them local control and accountability. In response to the federal mandate for the use of more managed care, California abandoned this successful program and began a new experimental Two-Model Plan for each county which was designed to give patients freedom of choice while encouraging competition and efficiency. Under this model, one plan option was to be a local initiative and the other would be a commercial plan such as Blue Cross. The "local" initiative plans had low capitation rates, did not involve local individuals in the planning, and made no provision for the orderly transfer of the massive number of enrollees.

At the same time as the Two-Model Plan was being launched, welfare reform legislation was passed that included provision for immediate implementation. Thus the state found itself trying to start two totally restructured programs simultaneously. The former Aid to Families with Dependent Children program was renamed the Temporary Aid to Needy Families and it was separated from the Medi-Cal program. Thus welfare recipients had to file two sets of complicated forms, and the cover letter explaining this confusing change was printed only in English.

This difficult transition resulted in many Medi-Cal patients failing to select one of the two plans, or failing to select a primary physician as required. The Two-Plan Model included an automatic default assignment policy, and enrollees were defaulting at an alarming rate (85 percent in Alameda County). Tens of thousands of patients were assigned to new physicians resulting in the interruption of ongoing treatment for serious and chronic illness in many cases. Many were assigned to physicians they did not know, often physicians located 40 miles or more away from their homes. Some patients who were able to complete the forms were accidently reassigned to plans or physicians other than those chosen. Quick action by the Alameda-Contra Costa Medical Association pressed the state to allow physicians to enroll patients in the physician's office, and the default rate dramatically declined in that portion of the state to about 10 percent.

There were also significant problems for physicians with this implementation of managed care for indigent patients. Changes in such matters as provider eligibility, referral patterns, and reimbursement rate and structure added to the difficulty of providing continuing care for these patients. In addition, delayed verification of eligibility, low capitation rates, and other problems led to the closure of some public health clinics in Los Angeles County and the threatened closure of the LA County Hospital — averted only by a waiver from the federal government. Of course, the physicians providing care to minorities also felt the impact of managed care common to all physicians such as contract difficulties (treatment authorization requests, gatekeeper issues, hold-harmless clauses, termination-without-cause clauses, gag clauses, one-year lock-in clauses) as well as the increased requirement for prior authorization requests, payment denials, multiple credentialing, and threats of office audits and deselection.

Managed care adds an additional level of complexity in the use of the health care delivery system in minority communities. Added to the injustices of illness and basic access problems are issues of enrollment, limitation of choice of caregivers, default rules, disruption in existing professional relationships, and an increased need for patients to be informed, educated, and knowledgeable about the system. Inadequate and/or inappropriate educational materials and information (e.g., wrong or culturally insensitive language) do not help patients to gain access to needed care. These changes in health care delivery have resulted in disruption of continuity of care, which adversely affects both patients and physicians. In addition, they have led to financial vulnerability for physicians, and a decrease in the number of professional caregivers. These negative results have had a more significant impact on minority physicians and minority patients. This has led to some concerted response by minority physicians.[25]

25. A. Bland, "Minority Physicians Join Forces in Managed Care Market," *California Physician* 12 (4) (1995): 32-33; H. Swan, "Managed Care: Revenge Is the Best Medicine," *Hospitals & Health Networks* (1997).

In summary, differences in illness, disparity in access to care, and disproportionate problems encountered with the transition to a managed care system have resulted in the worsening of the health status of minorities in the United States.

Responses to the Injustice

As Sondra Wheeler has already demonstrated in her chapter earlier in this volume, such injustice should be a priority concern for Christians. It is an affront to God, who has created all people in his image. Accordingly, Christians should not only be developing their own initiatives, such as those described by James Hussey later in this book, but also working with broader coalitions of people at the national, state, and local level.

At the national level, for example, the AMA has taken a number of specific steps including the following:

(a) Project U.S.A. — this initiative, started in 1973 under a government contract, has allowed the AMA to place approximately 7,750 physicians in short-term positions throughout the country, primarily serving minority populations;

(b) the Adolescent Health Initiative — recognizing the unique health care needs of adolescents, the AMA formed a Department of Adolescent Health in 1988 which helps physicians meet the needs of this population;

(c) Federation Outreach — the AMA joined forces with the Robert Wood Johnson Foundation to form "REACH OUT: Physicians' Initiative to Expand Care to Underserved Americans," a major national effort to mobilize physicians to improve care at the local level;

(d) Advisory Committee on Minority Physicians — the AMA formed this committee to formally embody the organization's commitment to take a leading role in improving minority health; and

(e) AMA leadership — in 1995, Lonnie R. Bristow, M.D., became the first African American to assume the presidency of the AMA, and he was instrumental in getting the AMA to adopt the Board of Trustees report 50-I-95 which included recommendations that the AMA should:

210

- maintain a zero tolerance toward racially or culturally based disparities in care;
- consolidate policies regarding health care needs of minorities;
- continue to support physician and patient cultural awareness initiatives;
- develop a series of publications on culturally competent health care;
- consider impact on minorities when testifying in Congress and commenting on regulations;
- develop assessment tools for practices to use to assess racial disparities in care;
- encourage reporting of physicians suspected of racial discrimination;
- strengthen relationships with organizations representing minority physicians such as the National Medical Association;
- communicate its policies on minority health care to pertinent federal agencies; and
- regularly monitor and report progress on racial and ethnic disparities in health care.

The key to these nationwide initiatives of the AMA to improve health care for minorities is that they all seek to influence the delivery of care at the local level.

The California Medical Association (CMA) demonstrates an example of a statewide policy response to racial disparity in health care.[26] The CMA supports a system dedicated to maintaining the physician-patient relationship and continuity of care. They also support guaranteed beneficiary choice of provider and access to traditional providers within the managed care network. They have recommended to the state that all Medi-Cal managed care programs be structured and implemented in a coordinated and integrated fashion. In addition, they support the local administration and control of Medi-Cal plans to allow maximum flexibility, while the state develops minimum standards and provides technical assistance and oversight to ensure quality, beneficiary access, and compliance with federal and state laws.

Another example of response from the professional community occurred when the state's implementation of the new Medi-Cal program caused such disruption in health care services in Alameda and Contra Costa Counties. At that time there was notable cooperation between the

26. Medi-Cal Managed Care. Policy CMA-A-1994; San Francisco; Medi-Cal Managed Care. CMA Board of Trustees Report; July 25, 1997; San Francisco.

state and local chapters of the AMA (e.g., CMA and Alameda-Contra Costa Medical Association) along with the state and local chapters of the National Medical Association (e.g., Golden State Medical Association and Sinkler-Miller Medical Society).

One example of a local response to this increasing problem is the Ethnic Health Institute (EHI) developed in Oakland, California, by Summit Medical Center.[27] This is an outreach program with very specific goals and objectives of enriching the quality of life in ethnically and culturally diverse communities by disease prevention and health promotion. The Summit Medical Center has for a long time served as an example of how communities, academic health programs, and health professionals can work together to promote the health and well-being of all members of the community. The development of the EHI is an extension of this leadership.

Serving as a resource for the entire Bay Area, EHI participates with local health and education agencies to coordinate health education, research, professional training, and community outreach with a special emphasis on underserved and minority populations. It informs these populations about health issues of special concern to them and connects them to resources in the community. It targets all ethnic groups, focusing on those at risk for chronic disease, disability, and death. Trained professionals provide basic health care services, screenings, education, and counseling at a neighborhood level and also make appropriate referrals for treatment. In addition, EHI sponsors community events and develops and distributes health-related materials through traditional and non-traditional media.

EHI operates under the direction and guidance of a local advisory board and Summit's administrative staff. The advisory board, which is racially, ethnically, and professionally diverse, is charged with supporting EHI's goals by helping to develop, organize, and evaluate its projects and services.

Professionals who provide health care services to minority communities have not only had to contend with the issues affecting all physicians in the rush to managed care, but in addition have had to continue to combat the existence of racial disparities and inequities in the health care system. This task has been compounded by the movement toward managed care in the Medicaid and Medicare programs. Christians must be in the

---

27. Ethnic Health Institute. Summit Medical Center, Oakland, Calif.,1997.

forefront of addressing current injustices, including participating in creative initiatives with national, state, and local institutions and agencies to meet these new challenges. God's concern for the marginalized demands no less.

The Impact of Managed Care on Malpractice

Janet E. Michael, R.N., M.S., J.D.

The manner in which physicians, nurses, and others must deliver health care continues to change dramatically. Such change, and the frustrations engendered by it, have caused many health professionals to express a wish to leave health care. Others respond to the change with a sincere desire to meet the challenges effectively so that they can continue to be good advocates for their patients. Regardless of whether they want to leave health care or continue to be patient advocates, almost every health care professional is concerned about the quality of the care that can be given to their patients in today's increasingly managed care environment.

One session at a recent seminar for clinical psychologists was entitled "The Death of Managed Care."[1] It was evident from the questions and comments that most attendees wanted managed care to die a quick death. The speaker, an attorney, spoke of all the opportunities for plaintiff's attorneys to sue health professionals because of bad decisions that were being made as a result of managed care. He implied that eventually such suits would change the behaviors of the managed care companies or eliminate them entirely. One example he discussed with the psychologists was the issue of "single session therapy," the tendency of some managed care organizations to approve only one session of psychological/psychiatric therapy and subsequently to exert major resistance to

1. Brian Welch, "The Death of Managed Care," oral presentation, New Hampshire Psychological Association, Fall, 1996.

214

requests for more sessions. Experience shows that such a policy can cause significant harm in particular cases due to the great variability in the underlying causes of some psychological conditions.

Many plaintiff's attorneys see payment by capitation as the "goose that laid the golden egg," or at least an insurance policy for their retirement. Managed care has created its own new theories of liability, and the attorneys are quick to let people know that they see the opportunities that these new theories bring.

Medical malpractice awards, in general, are on the increase. A study done by Jury Verdict Research showed that the median malpractice award in the U.S. in 1996 reached $568,000, an increase of almost 90 percent from 1988.[2] Other studies done in the past few years also show increases in settlements and awards.

Reasons for Malpractice Claims

Why do people bring medical malpractice suits in the first place? Is there something about managed care that makes people more likely to sue their health professionals and managed care organizations (MCOs) now and in the future? A study done some years ago by the Chicago Risk Pooling Program identified the ten top reasons people file malpractice claims (see Table 1).[3]

The number one reason for claims was anger and frustration. Increasing complaints from patients about MCOs suggest that anger and frustration abound in the current practice environment. It is likely that growing anger and frustration will serve to increase the frequency of malpractice suits in the future. Patients often feel that when an incident occurs which should not have happened, and there is also a bad outcome, the involved health professionals do not respond to the problem. Instead they dig in their heels, thereby creating an adversarial situation — the "we/they syndrome."

Even though consumer fraud was ranked number seven, its presence on the list indicates that patients want compensation when they are expected to pay for (or have already paid for) a service that did not meet

2. William J. McDonough, "Managed Care — Staying Ahead of the Curve: Managing Legal Pitfalls, Risk Management and Liability Shift," presented at the New England Health Care Assembly, March 18-21, 1996.

3. McDonough, "Managed Care."

Table 1. Reasons People Bring Malpractice Suits

(1) anger and frustration

(2) the we/they syndrome

(3) pain and suffering

(4) no response by the health care professional to problems being experienced

(5) desire to recover for financial loss

(6) professional mistakes and incompetence

(7) consumer fraud

(8) professional recommendations to sue

(9) lack of informed consent

(10) lack of willingness by a professional to tell a patient that he/she was involved in an incident

their expectations or a service which was not rendered. This too will be fertile territory for plaintiff's attorneys in the managed care environment.

Although this ranking was compiled several years ago, all of these issues still exist and have only been made worse by managed care. Therefore, we should analyze and address these issues even more diligently today.

Major Managed Care Malpractice Cases

The most famous of the recent managed care legal cases is the *HealthNet* case in California. In that case, a jury awarded an unprecedented $89 million to the plaintiff's estate.[4] HealthNet, an HMO, had refused to pay for a bone marrow transplant for a patient with metastatic breast cancer, claiming that it was experimental and unproven in this situation. After some delay, the patient did have the procedure (paid for with private funds) but she died. The jury found that HealthNet had breached its covenant of good faith and fair dealing and that it had inflicted emotional distress through reckless denial of coverage. The jury award was divided into $12 million in compensatory damages and $77 million in punitive damages. Although this award was reduced substantially on appeal, the ruling stands.

This unusually large award serves as a reminder that juries are made up of people who, although expected to be impartial fact finders, are often

---

4. Fox v. HealthNet, California; Superior Court, Riverside City; December 28, 1993, docket 219692.

216

motivated by their "gut reaction" to what they hear and see in the courtroom. Sometimes jurors sitting on a malpractice case will look at the facts differently if it involves an MCO because they view managed care as big business taking over health care so that profit, not quality of care, is the bottom line. A jury who might have given the benefit of the doubt to the professional in the past will probably not be so gracious if financial considerations were driving the decision of either the individual professional or the MCO.

The case of *Wickline v. State of California* is probably the leading case involving the liability of an MCO for improper use of cost-containment procedures.[5] Mrs. Wickline suffered postoperative complications after bypass surgery for peripheral vascular disease. Her surgeon requested an eight-day extension to her hospital stay for proper monitoring of her condition. Only a four-day extension was granted, and she was discharged home in spite of her protests. She subsequently developed an infection in her leg, which required amputation. The appellate court said that the decision to discharge her was that of her treating physician, and that cost-limitation programs should not be permitted to corrupt medical judgment. The court set forth the following standard:

> The patient who requires treatment and who is harmed when care which should have been provided is not provided should recover for the injuries suffered from all those responsible for the deprivation of such care. . . . Third party payers of health care services can be held legally accountable when medically inappropriate decisions result from defects in the design or implementation of cost-containment mechanisms. . . . However, the physician who complies without protest with the limitations imposed by a third party payer, when medical judgment dictates otherwise, cannot avoid his ultimate responsibility for his patient's care.

A third type of case arising in the context of managed care involves improper triage of patients. A patient in Massachusetts sued her HMO because they had negligently failed to provide the appropriate intervention for a lump that had appeared in the area of her navel.[6] Although she had been assigned a primary care physician, she was generally seen by nurse practitioners or physician assistants. She was eventually seen by a phy-

5. Wickline v. State of California, 239 Cal. Rptr. 810 (Cal App. 2d Dist. 1986), review dismissed, 741 P.2d 613 (Cal. 1987).

6. Larry Tye, "Cancer Victims Can Win Malpractice Suit," *Boston Globe,* June 26, 1997.

sician from another HMO who diagnosed metastatic ovarian cancer, for which she had numerous surgical procedures. The case was settled for $1.5 million six weeks before it was scheduled to go to trial. Commentators on this case point out that the almost total delegation of the patient's care to non-physicians may have caused the problem.

Perhaps even greater than the improper delegation in this case was the lack of continuity of care. The patient was seen by a variety of professionals and did not receive the in-depth examination that she needed to determine her problem until it was too late. She did see her primary physician for one 15-minute visit during this period. However, quite often a patient's problem cannot be addressed adequately in a 15-minute visit; that is simply not long enough to take a thorough history, perform an appropriate exam, and order tests and/or discuss treatment options. Recently some HMOs have insisted that primary physicians spend no more than 15 minutes with a patient. In such situations the patient receives less than optimal care and professionals open themselves up to allegations of malpractice.

Another type of triage problem may arise from the use of a triage nurse. In the case of *Adams v. Kaiser Foundation Health Plan of Georgia*,[7] an ill six-month-old baby became worse after being seen by a Kaiser physician who had minimized the seriousness of the baby's condition. When the baby's condition worsened, the triage nurse was called. The triage nurse requested only limited information from the family and then called a pediatrician who did not become concerned due to the limited information he was given. The nurse directed the family to take the baby to an emergency room (ER) which was 42 miles away because it was the closest approved ER under the managed care plan. Thirty miles into the trip, the baby had a cardiac arrest. His parents took him to the nearest ER where he was resuscitated. Unfortunately, the circulation did not return to his extremities and he subsequently required a quadruple amputation of his hands and feet. The jury returned a guilty verdict and awarded $45 million in the case.

Dearmas v. Av-Med, Inc. is another case involving a patient who was routed to an ER at a hospital that participated in her managed care plan.[8] In this case, a five-month pregnant woman was taken by ambulance to a local hospital after having been involved in an auto accident. The local hospital did not treat her because it did not participate in her managed care plan. The patient was sequentially transferred to several other hospitals

---

7. Adams v. Kaiser Foundation Health Plan of Georgia, Inc., No. 93-VS-7985-E (State Ct. Fulton County, Ga., decided Feb. 2, 1995).

8. Dearmas v. Av-Med Inc., 814 F. Supp. 1103 (S.D. Fla. 1993).

before she was finally treated at a participating hospital. She had a back fracture which she claimed was unstable. She eventually underwent surgery, but was left with significant disability. The patient sued her HMO for compensatory and punitive damages claiming in part that they had violated the federal Emergency Medical Treatment and Labor Act's (EMTALA) anti-dumping provisions. The court dismissed both the patient's malpractice claim against the HMO (state law) and the EMTALA claim (federal law). The federal claim was dismissed because EMTALA applies only to hospitals who fail to treat ER patients in a timely and appropriate manner, and the claim was brought against her HMO rather than against a hospital. The state claim of malpractice against the HMO was dismissed because the court ruled there was an ERISA preemption. ERISA is the Employment Retirement Income Security Act,[9] which has provisions that work in favor of managed care plans in many instances. Preemption is a legal principle which allows federal laws to take precedence over state laws. The federal ERISA preempts all state laws that relate to any employee benefit plan except those that regulate insurance, banking, and securities.

Another example of ERISA preemption is *Corcoran v. United Healthcare.*[10] In this case, a physician sought pre-certification for hospitalization of his patient for the third trimester of her pregnancy. The MCO denied the request for hospitalization, but instead authorized ten hours per day of home health nursing care. Fetal distress occurred at 32 weeks gestation while there was no nursing supervision, and the baby died. The patient and her husband sued for wrongful death. The MCO argued that ERISA preemption applied because the MCO had not made a medical decision, but had merely determined whether or not the patient was eligible for benefits under the plan. The plaintiff argued that ERISA preemption should not apply because this was a malpractice case against the MCO. The court ruled that the MCO had made a medical decision, but it was made in the context of determining benefits. Therefore, the court said, the stated cause of action for wrongful death was preempted by ERISA. Since the Corcoran decision, there have been numerous cases in various jurisdictions that have held that ERISA does not preempt claims for medical malpractice against HMOs when (a) the state law claims do not rest on the terms of the managed care plan,[11] (b) it is alleged that the HMO is vicariously liable for the alleged

9. Employment Retirement Income Security Act. 29 U.S.C. sections 1001-1461.
10. Corcoran v. United Healthcare. 935 F.2nd 1321 (5th Cir. 1992), cert. denied, 113 S.Ct. 812 (1992).
11. Rice v. Panchal, 65 F.3d 637 (7th Cir. 1995).

malpractice of one of its physicians,[12] or (c) claims for medical malpractice against HMOs involve the quality of medical care provided by their physicians, as opposed to claims that the HMO plan erroneously withheld benefits.

Professional Liability Issues

In addition to the cases discussed which involved denying experimental treatment, inappropriate cost-containment procedures, inadequate triage, and ERISA preemption, other managed care malpractice cases have been brought based on both old and new claims of professional liability. Theories of health care liability have expanded due to the layers of health care decision-making and constraints on health care decision-making created by managed care. Some of these theories are listed in Table 2. The managed care setting is indeed fruitful territory for malpractice claims, settlements, and awards.

There are special liability issues regarding the gatekeeper position. When health professionals become gatekeepers for MCOs, they often find themselves filling a role they really had not analyzed prior to accepting. Whether gatekeeping for established patients or for a panel of unfamiliar patients, there are numerous challenges from both an administrative and a clinical perspective. Since gatekeepers must often discharge patients sooner under managed care, they need to pay special attention to the way they terminate the physician-patient relationship, whether it be a hospital discharge situation or the end of a course of outpatient treatment. Moreover, the gatekeeper will likely be called upon to approve or deny care for individuals within the patient population even when the professional does not have access to the specialized knowledge about the individual that is required to make appropriate decisions. In emergency situations, this decision-making process becomes especially difficult, and mistakes in decision-making may lead to allegations of malpractice.

Physicians need to be careful to learn the rules before they accept the responsibility of being a gatekeeper. Also, it is important to understand the parameters of the practice expectations of the MCO. For example, primary care physicians may be asked routinely to do procedures that were previously only done by specialists. If primary physicians undertake to do such procedures, they will be held to the same standard of care that

12. Pacificare of Oklahoma, Inc. v. Burrage, 59 F.3d 151 (10th Cir. 1995).

Table 2. Various Theories of Liability

- negligent choice of specialist
- negligent failure to refer to a specialist
- premature discharge
- failure to provide treatment
- negligent credentialing
- inadequate peer review
- decision-making by non-physicians
- breach of contract to provide care
- refusal to admit to a hospital
- limitations of benefits
- non-disclosure of research interests
- non-disclosure of financial incentives
- inadequate enforcement of practice guidelines
- defective equipment or facilities
- gatekeeping
- advertising
- lack of informed consent due to prohibitions against discussing treatment options ("gag clauses")
- lack of communication (unavailability of records or test results; lack of continuity of care)

would be applied to a specialist. They can be successfully sued for malpractice for a failure to have the requisite training and skill necessary to perform a given procedure. In addition, the MCO itself may incur liability for employing gatekeepers who do not have the appropriate credentials to perform their duties. For this reason, the issue of credentialing is becoming increasingly important for MCOs and for individual professionals.

Impact of Managed Care on Health Care Standards

Will the increasing influence of managed care erode the standard of care for physicians, nurses, and other health care professionals? Many MCOs are developing guidelines for patient care. In addition, many professional associations are developing clinical pathways and practice parameters. MCO guidelines are sometimes in conflict with these professional practice parameters or with the actual practice patterns within a given specialty.

For example, the short hospital stays authorized as standard by many MCOs after surgery ("drive-through mastectomies") or obstetrical delivery ("drive-through deliveries") are considered to be inappropriate by many practicing physicians and some professional groups.

One difficulty in trying to resolve this discrepancy is that we have little data that can support the actual practice standards versus those chosen by the MCOs. Everyone hears the horror stories when MCO standards prove to be disastrously inappropriate, but these stories do not constitute adequate data.

The State of Maine has a Medical Liability Demonstration Project until the year 2000. As part of that project, there have been practice parameters developed for four areas of practice: Emergency Medicine, Radiology, Anesthesiology, and OB-GYN. If a physician participating in the practice parameters project is sued for malpractice, the fact that he or she followed the set of parameters can be used as an affirmative defense. This is a good idea in theory, but there is insufficient data thus far to know if the practice parameters are valid.

Legislative Attempts to Deal with Managed Care Liability Issues

In 1996, 40 states passed laws about HMO consumer protection. Moreover, many states are in the process of drafting additional laws dealing with issues that have arisen from managed care, particularly the widely known practices such as the so-called "drive-through deliveries" and "drive-through mastectomies." For example, a Texas law allows HMOs and other managed care entities to be sued for medical malpractice when a treatment decision adversely affects a patient's health. However, Aetna Health Plans of Texas, Inc. has sued the state of Texas in federal court in an attempt to block this law.

Many other bills have been introduced in state legislatures and in Congress to address the liability and other problems raised by managed care, and it is anticipated that this trend will continue. In addition, it is likely that more suits will be brought against MCOs for health care decisions they make until such time as we see a correction in the direction that managed care is taking.

Special Challenges for the Physician

In the meantime, physicians will continue to face some challenging questions. For example, what should a physician do when he or she determines that a patient needs treatment which the managed care plan will not pay for? It is imperative to know the current standard of care for the patient's problem. If the best course of action is one that the MCO will not pay for, the physician should still recommend the most appropriate treatment to the patient and explain why a lesser treatment might not be effective. In reality, the physician's responsibility to provide the patient with information that will allow the patient to make an informed decision actually increases under managed care.

It may also be important to explain to the patient how much the recommended course of treatment would cost versus other potential treatments. The physician can also advocate on the patient's behalf with the MCO for an exception to be made in this individual case, or for a general change to be made in the policy benefits. When acting as advocate for a patient, it is best to climb the chain of command within the MCO and to send follow-up letters regarding conversations one has had with all parties involved, including the patient.

A second recurrent challenging question is whether a physician may discontinue treatment for a non-compliant or difficult managed care patient, as with other patients in the past, or whether the physician must handle such patients differently if they are covered by an MCO. Treatment may be discontinued, but doing so may be more difficult in that the physician may have a limited number of options regarding to whom the patient can be transferred. The patient will have to be transferred to another physician within the MCO panel, and continuity of care must be assured. In addition, as with indemnity insurance, the professional relationship cannot be terminated during an acute illness. It is best to involve the patient from the beginning in the transfer process, and to give him or her several choices of other physicians who are able to give appropriate care.

Another important question for physicians today is what process they should use when referring a patient to a specialist on an MCO panel about whom nothing is known. The referring physician must personally ensure that the specialist to whom he or she is referring is an appropriate choice. A patient can always allege that the physician made a negligent referral if he or she has not adequately checked on the specialist and a bad result ensues. Credentialing information should be made available

223

by the MCO, but the referring physician should make additional checks with other physicians about the specialist's reputation. It is important to determine if any significant complaints have been made about the specialist.

Health care professionals today have the power to make decisions, lobby in a political sense, and act as advocates for patients. What each health care professional does with that power, and what he or she does to avoid professional liability, is an individual choice. May God grant each clinician the wisdom needed to meet the clinical, ethical, and legal challenges that will continue with the growth of managed care.

ASSESSING ALTERNATIVES

Meeting the Needs of Poor Persons under Managed Care

James M. Hussey, M.B.A.

The United States currently views health care as a poor value. Coupled with deep concern about quality, a convergence of factors is creating great distress among patients, providers,[1] employers, and the government. The public especially worries about the "affordability/quality" gap in the current health care system. Poor persons find themselves especially vulnerable to this problem. As the cost of health care increases, the number of uninsured patients and those on public assistance will likely increase.

The current approach to cost control revolves around managed care. This form of health care delivery has been extremely effective in reducing the increases in health care costs. Unfortunately, patients have viewed some cost cutting initiatives in managed care as "poor quality." In managed care, providers are either reimbursed under a reduced fee-for-service or they work under a capitation program. In either system, abuses can occur. Under fee-for-service, there is great incentive to order unnecessary tests and procedures to increase provider revenue. Under capitation (prepayment), the opposite tends to occur. Patients are denied needed health care treatment and de facto rationing occurs. The Health Care Financing Administration and Federal Bureau of Investigation are currently investigating fraud and abuse in the health care system. The results are not encouraging. Several health care executives and physicians have been

---

1. The term "provider" will be used here as a convenient umbrella term for everyone working in the health care arena. Its use is not intended to "commodify" the work of physicians or other health care professionals.

indicted for health care fraud and excessive billing. At the same time, the stories of care being withheld under capitated payments systems are legion and have prompted legislation regarding maternity stays and other procedures.

Both uninsured and Medicaid patients are caught in this debate over the optimal system to control costs and improve quality. Health care costs are rising again after several years of moderation or retreat. Even under a reasonably good economy and low unemployment, the rising cost of health care will push many poor patients to drop coverage or go back onto Medicaid rolls. Among Christian health care providers, there is a growing sense of angst, especially about our approach to poor persons in our community. However, this sense of despair about the system comes from not understanding the business side of health care, and the need for appropriate strategies to confront the changes. These strategies should rely on both biblical principles ("God is Sovereign") and business principles ("How to Increase Revenues and Efficiency in the Clinic"). First, the Christian health care provider must understand the problem.

The Patient's Predicament

In January 1997, the National Coalition on Health Care published a study of over 1,000 patients on their perceptions of and experiences in the health care system.[2] The study was remarkable in the depth of concern expressed from an economically diverse range of patients, 40 percent of whom could not afford health insurance. Broadly, study participants reported a lack of trust in a health care system they viewed as inefficient, uncaring, and expensive. They view the vices of the system as legion. Results of the study include the following:

87% of patients believe the quality of medical care must be improved.
79% believe there is something seriously wrong with our health system.
80% believe hospitals have "cut corners" to save money.
74% believe quality care is often compromised by insurance companies to save money.

2. "The National Coalition on Health Care Consumer Attitudes Survey," available from the National Coalition on Health Care, 555 13th Street NW, Suite 1300 East, Washington, DC 20004.

In other words, nearly nine of ten patients believe the quality of medical care must be improved. About four of five believe there is something seriously wrong with the current health system. The vast majority of patients believe providers, insurers, and others do not operate in the best interest of patients.

64% believe medical care costs have increased but quality has gone down.

79% believe quality health care is almost unaffordable for the average person.

74% believe the high cost of medical care is due in part to the greed of the insurance companies.

82% believe medical care has become big business that puts profits ahead of people.

24% believe health insurance companies put the needs of customers ahead of profits.

53% believe there is not much "care" left in health care these days.

32% believe health insurance companies really care about their customers.

44% do not have much confidence in the health care system to take care of them.

Again, this second set of figures reveals a remarkable lack of trust by patients in the health care system. About two-thirds of patients believe medical care costs have increased while quality has gone down. About 80 percent believe quality health care is almost unaffordable for the average person. Patients believe the health care system has become "big business" and has lost its focus on the patient. Well over 40 percent no longer believe that they can rely on the health care system to be there when they need it.

The study reveals that patients have other concerns as well. For example, over half of patients worry about their decreasing health care coverage. Over one-third of patients feel they do not have much choice of physicians with their current medical plan. Less than half believe they can trust their insurance company to do the right thing for them by providing the proper oversight and care.

The most dramatic change in patient attitudes concerns how patients view the government's role in health care. Just a few years ago, the public overwhelmingly rejected a government proposal to revamp the health care system. Now, the vast majority of the public perceives a major role for the government in health care. Patients are looking for government oversight of health care in order to restore trust, improve quality, and reduce price. The figures are as follows:

72% believe the federal government can play an important role in making health care more affordable.

69% believe the federal government can play an important role in making health care better.

Only 40% now believe the government should stay out of health care altogether.

86% of patients believe the government should set standards for quality of care.

84% believe the government should intervene when providers do not meet standards.

Christian health care providers face increasingly hostile and distrustful patients, an expanded role for government, and an affordability gap for patients and payers that will likely accelerate cost-reduction programs including managed care. Poor persons will increasingly be placed into managed care programs as health care costs increase. Providers face large corporate entities they do not understand and do not trust. This has led to tremendous frustration and anger among providers, including Christian providers.

For poor patients, the problem is more acute. Working poor and Medicaid patients rely heavily on the charity and social mission of the Christian community for health care. Government programs generally either provide insufficient coverage (working poor) or are poorly staffed (Medicaid). In Illinois, there are only 240 physicians willing to see the over 1,000,000 patients on Medicaid. This has led to patients seeking primary care services at the local hospital emergency room. This is an extremely expensive and inefficient option for Medicaid patients and provides little long-term care or follow up. It does, however, provide patients acute care they need in a timely manner.

Physicians Quality Care:
One Successful Approach to Poor Patients

Physicians Quality Care is a physician-owned equity model in Chicago.[3] The company provides services to over 150,000 patients in a variety of

3. Physicians Quality Care, 1415 W. 22nd St., Suite 625, Oak Brook, IL 60521.

managed care settings. This includes over 5,000 Medicaid patients. The company is actively involved in establishing church-based health clinics through the Jericho Road Foundation, discussed below. For example, the company provides management services to the Roseland Christian Health Care center in an underserved area of Chicago for Medicaid patients in managed care. Our company philosophy is twofold. First, we hold to our biblical principles in business. For example, we do not accept or provide abortion services for patients. We also sponsor health care fairs for the community and provide hundreds of school physicals and immunizations for children in the neighborhood. Second, we have established good working relationships with the local hospitals, health plans, and other agencies involved in care. We have an opportunity to share the gospel of Jesus Christ with key persons and to provide excellent health care to patients in need.

We have invested in excellence in operations and personnel to administer managed care. Our information systems are "state of the art" and our employees are carefully trained and well compensated in line with biblical principles. We have grown from a beginning in December, 1994 to over 150,000 patients in less than three years. God has richly blessed us, we believe, for seeking out those persons and companies in the health care system who historically have been the target of provider anger and frustration. We now count them as friends and potential believers in Christ. We are confident that our "open door" philosophy of endeavoring to treat all patients regardless of ability to pay is pleasing to God as a matter of biblical justice.[4]

In health care, *"no man is an island."* The health care system has myriad participants with competing interests. Christians are torn between a desire to remain free of the world and a commitment not to abandon the world. Several basic principles provide helpful guidance for Christians in health care who would establish or operate facilities to treat the poor:

> *Understand the changes in the health care system.* Christian health care providers, especially those treating the poor, must adapt to changes in the marketplace. Managed care or other cost-driven health care models may feel uncomfortable to Christians. However, it is unreasonable to assume rising health care costs are not going to bankrupt the country at some point in the future if they are not somehow significantly constrained.

4. See the earlier chapter on justice in this volume by Sondra Wheeler.

Develop core competencies in managed care. Many Christian health care providers consider managed care evil. Conversely, managed care companies suffer from the lack of committed Christians actively participating inside these organizations. Christians should become actively involved in managed care committees, companies, and organizations to share a Christian perspective. Many Christians have simply abandoned managed care organizations and speak of them with hostility. We need to develop core competencies and understand how managed care affects all aspects of health care.

Commit to treating both paying (Medicaid) and nonpaying (uninsured) poor persons. Christians need to develop a Christian policy toward accepting patients. Many Christian providers complain about losing "paying" poor patients and gaining "nonpaying" poor patients. Such a situation must be reevaluated based on our Christian mission. Would Christ want a "wallet biopsy" at the door? Christians should consider community outreach or other fund-raising to help defray the cost of treating uninsured poor persons. Documenting the number of uninsured poor patients the clinic treats would help greatly in community fund-raising.

Build the effort around the church, but engage the entire community. The church should be the bedrock of our efforts with poor persons. Many diseases afflicting impoverished people stem from destructive behavior. Christ changes behavior through the Holy Spirit after conversion. Involve as many churches as possible in the clinic. Clinics should involve as many churches as possible in their work. They should also involve local charities and health plans. Health plans are often willing to make a large donation to build clinics to assist poor persons. Hospitals also help with funding the local operations of free clinics. Partnering with such groups need not be a problem for Christians unless the involvement of churches is somehow weakened in the process. We must remember that even in the areas of the city where crime, drug abuse, and poverty are the worst and Satan seems to have a firm stronghold, the church is still there. According to Christ, "the gates of hell will not overcome it" (Matt. 16:18).

Recognizing the importance of involving the church, and accomplishing this involvement, are two different matters. Another model may prove helpful at this point.

The Jericho Road Foundation

The Jericho Road Foundation[5] is a not-for-profit Christian health care organization providing advice and selected support services to organizations interested in clinic initiatives. The Foundation has a national network of support services to assist churches in starting a church-based clinic. Starting a medical clinic requires a very different set of skills than is commonly present in the church. The clinic must deliver high-quality medical care in order to be successful. Churches need to understand the quality aspects of delivering health care in their communities.

Starting a church-based clinic typically involves a few fundamentals. The clinic needs to be supported by several churches in the area sharing a similar theology and desire to work together. The committee should meet in prayer for several weeks to seek guidance from the Lord before proceeding. Starting a church-based clinic is a major undertaking and commitment. If the group is led of the Lord, then it should proceed to the next step. The clinic needs to raise funds to begin a feasibility study and assessment. The clinic committee needs to raise about $10,000 for this initial phase. These funds will enable the group to gather the information required to assess the feasibility of the project. If the church-based project looks feasible, the committee will need to identify people with the necessary skills and information to begin building and staffing the clinic. Counsel on building the clinic and retaining professional staff is available from the Jericho Road Foundation. It is very important to garner the needed expertise prior to beginning to raise funds for the clinic.

The clinic will need about $250,000 to start operations. Depending on the mix of patients seen at the clinic, it may break even within a few years. It is important for the church clinic to become a Federal Qualified Health Center and offer services to patients with or without insurance. It is also important that all patients pay something for their services, even a nominal amount. The clinic also should offer Christian counseling services and other church-sponsored outreach programs. The clinic should provide services to all members of the church, including those without insurance or the ability to pay. Over time, the church will find that the health clinic, if done well, serves as a vehicle to bring more people into the congregation.

5. Jericho Road Foundation, 10838 S. Wallace, Chicago, IL 60628. Telephone: 301-990-4311.

If Christians in the health care arena can set aside their anger and frustration, they can respond to current changes in the marketplace. Jesus commands us to "Go forth and make disciples of all." He also commands us to care for the poor and sick among us. Christians in health care must reach out to the persons and institutions controlling health care. They must also be good stewards of what they are given. Good business principles require meeting the needs of patients in an increasingly competitive marketplace. We are reaping the harvest of our bitterness toward certain entities in the health system. Christians in health care need to set aside anger and bitterness and move toward establishing good working relationships with hospitals, health plans, and governments to develop a biblically solid and financially sound approach to health care problems. In the end, we will care for more patients, and win more to Christ, by engaging the health care system than by wringing our hands in frustration and worry.

Funding Health Care through the Church

Alieta Eck, M.D.

Soon after beginning our joint medical practice in the United States, my husband and I decided that we would not participate in Medicaid, the government health insurance program for the poor. Instead, we would care for the poor, either without charging a fee, or at a very reduced rate. Although we have taken some Medicaid patients on a case-by-case basis, we do not trust the government to screen these people carefully. Some of our Medicaid patients have taken trips to visit their families in the Philippines. One just left for a three-week vacation trip to Italy. It does not seem right for hard-working taxpayers, paying for their own health care, to be forced to pay for the health care of people who can take such trips. Also, since the government Medicaid reimbursement is so low, taking on too many Medicaid patients would jeopardize our survival. If our practice went under, we would not be able to help *anyone*, rich or poor. Something seems disingenuous in the government promising *they* will provide free health care for the poor, then expecting *us* to actually provide it practically for free.

Furthermore, our experience with health insurance in the state of New Jersey has convinced us that the whole system is expensive and unwieldy. The government has burdened the insurance industry with so many costly mandates. Hospitals and doctors have been known to double-bill and inflate their prices, and patients are quick to overuse and abuse the system that is designed to help them. Fraud and abuse abound, so that an increasing number of watchdogs have been hired to minimize misuse. Premiums have sky-rocketed out of control. Since 1993, New

Jersey residents want to purchase health insurance, they must purchase one of the five plans designed by the state. No other health insurance is legal, and the premiums are not tax deductible. In the state-approved plans the insurance companies must fulfill two mandates. One is *guaranteed issue*, where anyone willing to pay the standard premium, regardless of prior or existing illness, cannot be turned away. The second mandate is the *community rating*, for which everyone pays the same premium, regardless of age. Our family policy jumped from $385 per month to $585 per month in one year. It is slated to go over $1000 per month shortly. Something is drastically wrong. A cost crisis is looming.

We first learned about Medical Savings Accounts (MSAs) in 1988, and have been avid supporters ever since. MSAs give patients more control by requiring them to pay for most of their own health care. They also eliminate much of the paperwork associated with low-deductible policies. Coupled with high-deductible insurance policies, they could provide complete health security.[1] Legislation to make them tax-deductible is desirable, but more is needed than the highly restrictive trial of MSAs authorized by Congress in the 1996 Kassebaum-Kennedy legislation. It almost appears that they were designed to fail. Indeed, they are not catching on, and detractors of MSAs have taken this as evidence that people don't want them. The insurance lobby and government bureaucrats have so dominated the discussion that, unless everyone takes a crash course in the intricacies of health insurance, deception will likely prevail. Thus far, at least in our state, the insurance industry has been unwilling to support the MSA concept with a reasonably priced high-deductible policy, so the concept is unworkable with traditional insurance.

We agonized, prayed, lobbied, contacted our legislators, networked with experts from across the country, and left no stone unturned. Finally, we gave up in disgust. However, when we began to discover the concept of true security clearly addressed in the Scriptures — in matters of health and otherwise — we began to see light at the end of the tunnel.

The Bible says, "Bear ye one another's burdens, and thus fulfill the law of Christ" (Gal. 6:2). What does this mean? What are the burdens we are to share? Are they spiritual shortcomings? Or could they mean financial and physical calamities that can befall any of us? People in modern United States Christendom have been misled by an overemphasis on the American notion of rugged individualism. A general attitude

---

1. John C. Goodman and Gerald L. Musgrave, *Patient Power* (Washington, D.C.: Cato Institute, 1994), pp. 92-96.

prevails that health care expenditures are one's own business — and if people get into big trouble, hopefully they were smart enough to have insurance. If not, they should look to the state, or simply bank on the fact that hospitals, by law, cannot turn people away if they are sick enough.

The U.S. has erected a system of employer-based insurance that is incredibly illogical. Imagine — a man and his family are "covered" as long as he, the breadwinner, is healthy. What happens when he gets too sick to work? He goes on short-term, then long-term, disability. His paycheck becomes a fraction of its original amount. His employer might pay his health care premiums for a few months, but a cost-effective business cannot keep that up for long. They will need to hire a replacement and soon will be paying for the new employee's health insurance. The government has seen his plight, so has initiated a system called COBRA (Comprehensive Omnibus Benefits Reconciliation Act). It allows him to continue to pay, at his own expense, the premiums his employer was paying for his health insurance. This can continue for the 18 months after he has stopped working due to illness. Presumably the rate for the continued employer-based insurance is lower than that which he could obtain on the open market. But he is on disability, a lowered salary. Where does this extra money for health insurance come from? And what happens after the 18 months are up?

How does the church look at this? If a woman gets very sick, she makes them very uncomfortable. They wish her problem would just go away. The benevolence fund is rather scanty and they have so many other programs to fund. How can they help her? The ladies are kind to bring over some meals — but what about her prescriptions? What if the church is small? Her problem threatens to overwhelm them.

A man in our practice had this very thing happen to him. He happened to be in an accident that caused him severe, unrelenting back pain. His job required physical strength, and it was clear that he could no longer perform the tasks. His wife was already working, so she could not bring in more funds. His bills are piling up and the bank may soon foreclose on their house. He scrapes together money to continue his COBRA payments, but the 18 months will run out soon, after which he will have no more health insurance, no reserve, and no end in sight. His wife is depressed and does not feel she can continue much longer. Where is the church in this? They are very kind. They smile at the family. They assure them that they are praying for them — that somehow their problems will be relieved — that God will intervene. Are they bearing the burdens of this family?

The apostle James asks: What good is it, if a man claims to have faith but has no deeds? Can such faith save him? Suppose a woman is without clothes and daily food. If someone says to her, "Go, I wish you well, keep warm and well fed," but does nothing about her spiritual needs, what good is it? In the same way, faith by itself, if it is not accompanied by action, is dead (James 2:14-16).

The church has become complacent in this country because the government has usurped its role. Why does the church have to worry when the local welfare office is there to help victims who have fallen into hard times? And we have Medicaid for people who are too poor to purchase health care coverage. Let the government worry about these people.

Government health care programs are often top-heavy, poorly responsive to real needs, easily abused, and wasteful — and the taxpayers are paying dearly for the fact that the church has given away its job. The patient described above would have to uproot his family, sell his house, and be homeless to get the help he needs from the government. When the help comes, it will be inadequate. What will happen to the children? They will feel uprooted, insecure, and bitter. Is there no one to come along side and help?

A fundamental problem here is that Christians have been financing health care in the wrong way. We have been sending our money off to "Egypt" and have expected them to treat us well. As believers, we have reached the Promised Land of God's love and protection, but have murmured that we do not really believe God can meet our needs. We know in our heads that God is our provider, protector, and husband, but we want a king like the other nations. Can we trust God and his people to help us pay our bills when we get sick?

Health care used to be a church enterprise. The names of many of our hospitals tell the tale of their beginnings. St. Mary's, St. Peter's, St. Luke's, Deaconess, Presbyterian, Methodist, Lutheran General, Baptist Hospital Systems, and the like. These places were built to meet a need. They were not fancy and elaborate, and technology was sparse. Nevertheless, compassion abounded. Volunteers gave freely of their time in caregiving and fundraising. The job got done.

After WW II, during the time of price and wage controls, the U.S. Congress decided to allow employers to give health insurance as a benefit, and not call it taxable income. This seemingly small, well-meaning decision totally revolutionized the funding of health care. It led to a system of prepaid health care where essentially the first dollar of care was covered. From this time forward, the consumer no longer paid directly for health care services, and health care inflation began to rise precipitously.[2] In 1960, a normal delivery cost about $500 — and the mother and child were welcome to spend a week in the hospital getting to know each other. Contrast this with eight-hour hospital stays for a cost reaching up to $10,000. In 1965, with the inception of the two huge government entitlement programs — Medicare (government-financed health care for the elderly and disabled) and Medicaid (government-financed health care for the poor) — third party payment of health care bills became the norm. This is where the "monetarization" of health care began and the emphasis on human touch began its inexorable decline. When government money flowed, the money-changers arrived on the scene.

We have reached the point where health care premiums are approaching the level of a home mortgage, and people live in fear of not being "covered." Three-day intensive-care stays can command a price tag of $30,000 and people feel completely vulnerable to bankruptcy due to illness. This ought not be.

Our policies are now mandated in New Jersey to cover abortions in all three trimesters. They are toying with the idea of physician-assisted suicide, and young doctors are trained to obtain advance directives from every patient that gets admitted to the hospital. I envision the day when an insurance application will be accompanied by a vial of serum so that companies can do genetic mapping and thus decide whether we are worthy of being covered.

Where is the caring? We have abandoned every tenet of the Hippocratic Oath, from proscription of abortion to the principle of doctor/patient confidentiality, to the shunning of physician-assisted suicide. Are we physicians or *providers?* Do we work on behalf of our patients, or of the insurance industry and the State?

In some ways, people have not changed. Back in the time of Samuel, the people clamored for a king. They said, "We want a king to lead us and fight our battles" (1 Sam. 8:20). Samuel was disturbed that the people were calling for big government, and turned to the Lord for guidance. God said something surprising. He replied, "Listen to all that the people are saying to you; it is not you they have rejected, but they have rejected me as their king" (1 Sam. 8:7). This scene resembles our present time, when we are clamoring for the government to solve our social and economic problems. But Samuel had it right when he warned them that the king, or big government, would impoverish them. He told them that the king

---

2. *Patient Power,* pp. 19ff.

would take their sons and turn them into servants; he would take their daughters and make them work. A king would take the best of their workmanship and give it to his bureaucrats. And he warned, "When that day comes, you will cry out for relief from the king you have chosen, and the Lord will not answer you in that day" (1 Sam. 8:18). If they did things their way, goods would cost more and events would not go well — and the Lord would seem absent.

In the Old Testament, the tithe did not only go toward paying for worship centers and priests' salaries, but it actually ran the entire civil government as well. You might say that ten percent would never be enough to do all that, but it was. Deuteronomy 14:22-29 explains that God intended the tithe to teach his people to rely on him for all things, and to revere the name of the Lord always. It was to be gathered on a regular basis and brought to a pre-determined storage location. It was used to pay for the priests and Levites, because otherwise they would have no source of income; but it was also used to provide for the aliens, orphans, and widows. It was intended to meet the social and physical needs of the people. Furthermore, it came with a promise. If God's people obeyed, the Lord would bless them in all the work of their hands.

Malachi records that God was very angry because the people were not bringing their tithes into the storehouse as he had commanded. God gave a great promise that would accompany their obedience when he said, "Test me in this, and see if I will not throw open the floodgates of heaven and pour out so much blessing that you will not have enough room for it. I will prevent pests from devouring your crops. . . . Then all the nations will call you blessed, for yours will be a delightful land" (Mal. 6:10-12).

When God spoke through Ezekiel the prophet, he expressed anger and likened his people to prostitutes. He said, "You adulterous wife! You prefer strangers to your own husband" — me! (Ezek. 16:32). They were turning to strangers for comfort and security. And to make matters worse, instead of them paying God's people to be prostitutes, God's people were giving *them* money — "You give payment, and none is given to you!" (Ezek. 16:34). God wants to be our source of supply. God wants us to turn to *him* when we are in trouble. Why do we run to an insurance company or the government when we are in financial and health-related difficulties? They do not love us. They will take our hard-earned money and meet their own needs before they ever dispense to us some of what is left over. No, we ought to be turning to God and his Church.

On June 1, 1997, our family dropped our health insurance completely. One of the large central New Jersey newspapers did an article about us, complete with a picture of our five "uninsured children." Two physicians dropping their health insurance by their own choice was considered that radical. We decided that we could no longer work within the system, and that reforming it was very unlikely in the near future. We have chosen to get our health security from the place where we believe God intended — the churches and God's people. We are willing to bear the burdens of other believers and they have promised to bear ours if a major medical event occurs in our family. The vehicle that facilitates this burden-sharing is the Christian Brotherhood Newsletter (CBN). This organization was founded by a poor pastor, the Rev. Bruce Hawthorn, 15 years ago under the tragic circumstance of the accidental death of his wife and four-year-old daughter. He had been working in a home for alcoholics and had a mailing list through which he informed other believers of his tragedy. He was astounded when money poured in from all over the country to defray the $54,000 in hospital bills of his two other children, also injured in the accident. The warmth and caring he felt was such a comfort, and he determined that this was the way Christians ought to be "bearing one another's burdens, thus fulfilling the law of Christ." Since then, the Newsletter has grown from about 200 subscribers to an amazing 100,000, and they share in the paying of $4.3 million in health care bills per month.[3]

We have dropped our family's health insurance and now will be sending one family somewhere across the country $150 per month. Each month, the Christian Brotherhood Newsletter will tell us where to send our money. And, if someone in our family has a health care event that goes over a thousand dollars, subscribers will send us the money. This is the true insurance principle. There are several other Christian organizations patterned after the Christian Brotherhood, and all are worthy of consideration.

In keeping with Galatians 6:5, and "carrying our own loads," we are planning to put away $300-$400 per month into our own family's Medical Savings Account. We will not worry about it being tax deductible, since there is no way we can meet the stringent requirements set out by the government. Correspondingly, we will not be responsible to the government for how we spend the money. In an age when doctors are increasingly vulnerable to prosecution for "providing unnecessary care," governmental control is increasing. Who knows best what is unnecessary? Why not allow the families to make that determination? If our account

---

3. Christian Brotherhood Newsletter, P.O. Box 3948, Akron, OH 44314 USA.

had been started when we were 20 years old and newlyweds, and we had used it for all the routine health care that we have needed thus far, it would have reached half a million dollars by the time we reached retirement. Since we cannot count on Medicare being solvent by then, I would recommend every young Christian do the same.

Interestingly, while the Christian Brotherhood Newsletter's only statement of faith is a belief in Jesus Christ and a confession of inclusion in the Body of Christ, it has some rather strict health requirements: *no* alcohol, *no* smoking, *no* homosexual lifestyle, and one must go to church 3 out of 4 Sundays per month. These requirements are one reason the rates are kept so low. The $150 we send to a Newsletter family is equivalent to the $585 insurance policy that we once had. An individual can have the same health security by simply donating $50 per month to someone out there who needs it. This is decidedly better than insurance. It covers 100 percent over $1000, while our more expensive health insurance policy covered only 80 percent. The Christian Brotherhood is *not* insurance, but a commitment to share. All legitimate health care bills have been paid to date. It is biblically sound to escape from the world's health care financing system and get into one of these networks.

The Rev. Robert Sirico is a communist turned capitalist, turned Christian, and finally, a Catholic priest.[4] He clearly articulates the virtues of the free market as the most just form of economy. He speaks of the subsidiarity principle — a principle that one needs to understand to comprehend fully the logic behind Medical Savings Accounts and the Christian Brotherhood Newsletter. The greatest funding and the greatest responsibility should be located at the point where the people are closest to the problem. This is why people need to be more accustomed to paying their own routine health care bills. They will be careful consumers of their health care dollars and they will eliminate much fraud and abuse. When one family experiences a greater health care need (over $1000) the Christian Brotherhood Newsletter is there to subsidize its needs. We first carry our own loads (the smaller medical expenses) but then we bear each other's burdens (the bigger and more overwhelming medical expenses). In contrast to insurance, we can thus minimize fraud and abuse, the padding of bills, and the siphoning off of premium money for questionable administrative costs.

We need to disavow the ideas that we are each on our own, and

4. Father Robert Sirico, Acton Institute, 161 Ottawa St. N.W., Suite 301, Grand Rapids, MI 49503 USA.

must turn to the government to meet our collective health care needs. The 60-year-old Christian widow, while she is unable to afford health insurance, can probably come up with the $50 per month it will cost her to enroll in the Christian Brotherhood. If the local churches join forces, they could even see to it that the Christian Brotherhood Newsletter subscription is paid even when the primary wage earner becomes too sick to work or people are otherwise too poor to cover the monthly cost. We could work together as the corporate Body of Christ and bear each other's greater needs such as child care, meals brought to the house, and the like. We could develop a Christian, church-based visiting nurse network and a health care chaplain to meet families in their need. Chaplains have traditionally been a hospital-based enterprise — but why not have chaplains work, church-supported, on a home-visit basis as well? This is our vision for the newly forming Family Health Fund.[5]

We dream of harnessing the health care dollar in such a way that the church will explode in its influence. If the entire civil government could be funded with the tithe in the Old Testament, how much could God's people do with the tremendous health care dollars we are currently squandering in insurance companies and top-heavy government programs? Opportunities to share the gospel will abound, and the world will say, "See how they love one another." Why not? Why should we allow the ways of Egypt to influence our health care delivery system? They would pound us into slavery and make us gather the straw, as well as make the bricks. They would look at us as units of productivity rather than kind, caring professionals. They would degrade us into being just health care providers and would "de-select" us if we took too much time explaining the way of salvation to a frightened patient with a grim prognosis.

God has blessed our practice. We are now four doctors strong and able to display a clear Christian witness in our waiting and examining rooms. Christian evangelistic literature from *Focus on the Family*[6] is freely distributed, and the gospel goes out daily. People find a warm, caring environment and many have come to find Jesus. We are not affiliated with any capitated HMOs (where doctors are compensated with a fixed sum per patient per month) and do not have any strings attached —

5. Family Health Fund, c/o Affordable Health, Inc., 1056 Stelton Rd., Piscataway, NJ 08854 USA.

6. Dr. James Dobson, Ph.D., Focus on the Family, P.O. Box 35500, Colorado Springs, CO 80935-3550 USA.

strings that would force us to compromise our witness to a dying and disheartened world. By dropping our health insurance, for example, we have escaped from the funding of abortion. Medical Savings Accounts allow for complete doctor/patient confidentiality, as there are no claim forms going to an indifferent, and even hostile, insurance company. There are no profiteers looting the system with our plan. There is no reason why this concept cannot be multiplied across the country, in each state. And there is no reason why we cannot all live in the Promised Land of kind and compassionate Hippocratic medicine.

George is a 61-year-old patient who was referred to us by a small church. He had lost his job and was doing odd jobs to pay his bills. He had no insurance. When my husband saw him in the office, he diagnosed his abdominal pain as being due to a large hernia. He referred him to the clinic of the medical school, assuming that they had some mechanism of caring for the indigent. They told him that since he owned a house, they would put a lien on it — $7000 for the hospital stay, $2000 for the surgeon, $2000 for the anesthesiologist, plus probably more. George came back to John, dejected and worried that he would be left with such a big bill. John began to talk about some missionary hospitals, and, to make a long story short, George is going to a missionary hospital in Quito, Ecuador. The cost will be under $1000, and American Airlines will fly him there for $550. He will stay a week or so to recuperate beside a nice hotel pool following his surgery. George is signing up to join the Christian Brotherhood Newsletter — this will take care of any future medical needs. But for now his crisis is over, thanks to a wonderful Christian network.

Insurance actually was God's idea. As the apostle Paul writes in 2 Corinthians 8:13-14a: "Our desire is not that others may be relieved while you are hard pressed, but that there might be equality. At the present time, your plenty will supply what they need, so that in turn their plenty will supply what you need." Paul knew what we have learned afresh in the contemporary health care arena — that "Like a bad tooth or a lame foot, is reliance on the unfaithful in times of trouble" (Prov. 25:19). James adds to Paul's counsel the reminder that "Religion that God our Father accepts as pure and faultless is this: to look after orphans and widows in their distress and to keep oneself from being polluted by the world" (James 1:27).

Let us carry our own loads and bear one another's burdens — thus fulfilling the law of Christ.

Physician Unions:
Guardians of the Covenant
or Keepers of the Contract?

Mary B. Adam, M.D.

Physicians have long received money for their services in order to cover their costs and generate an income. The tension between patient care and the business aspects of medicine is far from new. However, it has escalated in today's world where physicians and nurses have become providers, patients are now called consumers, and medical care is now a product. Physicians are struggling as never before to understand how to function ethically both in the marketplace and at the bedside. It is against this backdrop that physician unions have entered the picture.

In order to examine the ethical implications of this tension in the context of physician unions, the history of the physician-patient relationship and the commercialization of medicine will be explored. Next, specific examples of the impact of physician unionization will be considered. Finally, a group of ethical diagnostic questions will be presented to help physicians build a framework for evaluating physician unions.

Competing Views of the Physician-Patient Relationship

Professionalism in medicine has been a topic of debate for centuries. Hippocratic medicine was at odds with the prevailing medicine of its time when introduced 2500 years ago. Yet, over a period of several centuries the Hippocratic Oath became a standard for ethical practice in Western medicine. The Oath clarifies that the relationship between the patient and the physician is based on the expectation that the physician will put the needs of the patient first, over and above his own needs, his financial welfare, or the needs of any other party. A physician who swears this Oath puts himself in a covenant relationship to his teacher, his patient, and his god. For the physician, a covenant relationship is a beneficent promise to put the interests and needs of the patient first. Therefore, the practice of medicine becomes a moral commitment.

Alternatively, the physician-patient relationship can be understood in contractual terms. Contracts are negotiated between two parties, each concerned for his or her own welfare. A patient contracts for the care of a physician because of his or her specialized knowledge and skills. It has been stated that physicians have a "monopoly of information" because of "the technical nature of the basic biomedical sciences and the need for prolonged direct experience in order to master clinical medicine."[1] Negotiation is viewed as an important way to define the dimensions of the physician-patient relationship. An article in the *American Medical News* observed, "As our patients become more-educated consumers, negotiation becomes a natural framework for guiding our physician-patient relationship."[2]

In the medical marketplace, patients are referred to as "consumers," "covered lives," "clients," or "members per month," all of which are terms of business. Physicians — along with nurses, respiratory technicians, and a host of others — are called health care providers. Relationships with physicians are defined by contracts to provide care, which can be changed when a less expensive contract is negotiated. The impact of contractual relationships is especially vivid in managed care models where employers can, on a given date, change health maintenance organization (HMO) providers, leaving thousands of patients to find a new set of "providers."

Indeed, many share the view Grace Budrys states in her book, *When Doctors Join Unions:* "The meaning of professionalism [has] evolved over the past two centuries from sacred vocation to secular occupational identity."[3] Professionalism was previously defined by the Hippocratic tradi-

---

1. D. M. Mirvis, "Physicians' Autonomy: The Relation Between Public and Professional Expectations," *New England Journal of Medicine* 328 (1993): 1346-49.

2. L. J. Marcus and B. C. Dorn, "Negotiating an Effective Physician-Patient Relationship," *American Medical News* (July 7, 1997): 23.

3. G. Budrys, *When Doctors Join Unions* (Ithaca, N.Y.: Cornell University Press, 1997), p. 33.

tion, in which the needs of the patient were placed above the needs of the physician. In contrast, the current understanding of professionalism is defined by the physician's level of technical expertise.

These competing views of the physician-patient relationship are evident in medical school training and in professional societies. For years, physicians have taken the Hippocratic Oath or some form of oath at graduation. Currently, many schools participate in "White Coat Ceremonies" for incoming students, in which they hear an inspiring address by a physician role model, are cloaked with their first white coat, and swear the Hippocratic Oath. The goal is to impress upon students early in their training the primacy of the doctor-patient relationship, and to call them to pursue excellence in science, to demonstrate compassion, and to lead moral and upright lives.[4] Students spend most of their training gaining technical skills and expertise. They are schooled in issues of medicine and business. Daily there are discussions of cost-containment and risk-benefit and expense-benefit ratios. The constant challenge for medical professors is to teach which medications or treatment options are efficacious while also teaching students to discern efficiently which valid treatment option is covered by the patient's insurance plan. For example, questions such as whether or not a patient is ready for intravenous therapy at home (a less expensive environment) may be presented by the case manager on the second day of hospitalization.

Professional societies like the American Medical Association (AMA) also experience the tension produced by the competing contract versus covenant views of the physician-patient relationship. The AMA Code of Ethics, first adopted in 1847 and subsequently revised,[5] has also profoundly influenced the profession. The Code voices a clear call to ethical conduct by outlining a virtuous and high moral standard for the physician-patient relationship. In this code of ethics, a discussion of the "rights and responsibilities" of the physician is followed by a discussion of the "rights and responsibilities" of the patient. Baker et al. summarize it well:

> The AMA's Code of Ethics was unlike any ethics subscribed to by any earlier group of medical practitioners. No national assemblage had ever proposed to bind all of its members by a uniform code of ethics, and no previous code of ethics had ever been formulated as an explicit social contract between the profession, its patients, and the public. In the

4. The ceremonies have been encouraged and funded by The Arnold P. Gold Foundation (260 Lincoln St., Englewood, NJ 07631).

5. *Code of Medical Ethics* (Chicago: American Medical Association, 1997).

Code of Ethics, each of the contracting parties is envisioned as having correlative rights and responsibilities.[6]

This code is essentially a social contract rather than an oath — any reference to a higher power is removed. Unfortunately, it is rarely invoked at stockholder meetings or in the boardrooms of today's mega health care corporations, where physicians are valued more for their ability to generate profit than their compassion for patients. At best, they are evaluated on the basis of their technical competency by hospitals and health plans. More ominously, they are now regularly evaluated by their respective employers or insurance groups to determine if they are cost-efficient. It is presently rare for physicians to be evaluated on the basis of their values or professionalism.

Patients are also caught in the conflict between the covenant and contractual views of the physician-patient relationship. On the one hand, patients are instructed to be educated consumers of their health care. Patients and employers treat the physician-patient relationship like a commodity or service that can be bought or sold for the best price. Some patients will change their physician for as little as a $2 difference in co-payment. They may demand services or convenience care with a self-righteous, "I've paid for this and I want it now" attitude.

On the other hand, patients state that they want a physician who can be trusted to care for them regardless of circumstances. They want someone who will not withhold care because of financial pressures and they will often ask the physician, "Are you omitting this test because of its expense?"

Nigel Cameron, author of *The New Medicine*, phrases the tension between the two views as follows: "Is medicine essentially a matter of medical technique? Or is it rather, a matter of values, of moral commitments in the exercise of clinical skills?"[7] The answer to this question is currently being debated throughout the medical and business communities. It has profound implications for medicine as a profession, the business aspect of medicine, and for society.

6. R. Baker, A. Caplan, L. L. Emanuel, and S. R. Latham, "Crisis, Ethics, and the American Medical Association: 1947 and 1997," *Journal of the American Medical Association* 278 (1997): 163-64.

7. N. M. de S. Cameron, *The New Medicine: Life and Death after Hippocrates* (Wheaton, Ill.: Crossway Books, 1991), p. 23

The Commercialization of Medicine

Business has provided the impetus for many of the changes in today's practice of medicine. Managed care and corporate mergers have nearly eliminated solo practitioners and small groups of physicians. In the early twentieth century, medical care was strictly a service provided to a sick patient, and financial arrangements were made between the physician and the patient. Physicians were able to give as much or as little charity care as they wished. The church also played a vital role in caring for the sick and many hospitals were developed with charitable care for the poor as an essential part of their mission.

However, the advent and expansion of third party payers and Medicare coupled with the growth in medical technology resulted in dramatic increases in health care costs. Health care spending was $27 billion in 1960, $75 billion in 1970, and $1 trillion in 1994. Managed care grew in large measure as a response to pressure from private and public purchasers to slow the rising costs of health care. Budrys states it well: ". . . one of the arguments for introducing market mechanisms during the 1980s was the claim that the professional dominance of doctors permitted them to ignore market controls; this dominance was targeted as a major reason for rising costs. Accordingly, policy makers passed laws aimed at imposing greater control over doctors' treatment decisions and the charges accompanying those decisions."[8] The growing financial base of health care has not escaped Wall Street, where many of the major health care organizations are now traded on the New York Stock Exchange.

Physicians are now much more likely to be employed, and their paycheck is more likely to depend on their success in cutting costs than on the quality of their medical care. In his article, "Managed Care and Merger Mania," Victor Fuchs writes: "Of special importance to physicians is the deleterious effect of managed care on professional norms. At its best, the patient-physician relationship was an integrative system characterized by reciprocal rights and responsibilities. Managed care tends to transform this into an exchange system characterized by market mentality similar to that found in the market for most commodities."[9] Physicians are no longer free agents able to act out of their knowledge and expertise, in the interests of the patients.

Physicians in this commodity system are interchangeable workers,

8. Budrys, p. 67.
9. V. R. Fuchs, "Managed Care and Merger Mania," *JAMA* 277 (1997): 920-21.

accountable only for their financial performance. Many hospitals and physician practices have been bought by for-profit entities like Columbia HCA with a drastic alteration in their staffing and patient services, usually resulting in an improvement in their balance sheet. However, this "improvement" comes at a cost. Patients also are viewed as a commodity, charitable care is diminished, teaching and research are compromised, and money-losing services may be eliminated regardless of need.[10] The financial considerations of the business now seem to override the ethical concerns of the physician and patient. McArthur and Moore state in their article, "The Two Cultures and the Health Care Revolution: Commerce and Professionalism in Medical Care": "When a corporation employing physicians seeks profit by selling their services, the physician-employees cease to act as free agents. Professional commitment to patient care is subordinated to new rules of practice that assure the profitability of the corporation."[11]

Medicine and business have two different cultural traditions. Threats to the quality of medical care arise when the commercial ethic overtakes the medical ethic. Indeed, a business actually has a fiduciary responsibility to its shareholders to make a profit. McArthur and Moore state it this way: "The fundamental objective of commerce in providing medical care is achieving an excess of revenue over costs while caring for the sick, ensuring profit for corporate providers, investors, or insurers. A central feature in enhancing net of income over expenses in a competitive market is a reduction in volume or quality of services so as to reduce costs, while maintaining prices to the purchaser."[12] This phenomenon is seen in both "for-profit" and "not-for-profit" hospitals, but is of greater concern in the former type of institution, where the profit goes to the shareholders instead of into teaching, research, and charitable care. In a commercial model, physicians and insurers (including both indemnity plans and HMOs) have compelling reasons to shun sick patients in favor of healthier, more profitable patients. In fact, it is quite difficult if not impossible to find an HMO model that emphasizes care to special needs children or adults because of the increased cost of their care. Physicians who care for patients with complex medical problems have legitimate

---

10. R. Kuttner, "Columbia/HCA and the Resurgence of the For-Profit Hospital Business," *N Eng J Med* 335 (1996): 362-67 (Part 1) and 446-51 (Part 2).

11. J. H. McArthur and F. D. Moore, "The Two Cultures and the Health Care Revolution: Commerce and Professionalism in Medical Care," *JAMA* 277 (1997): 985-89.

12. McArthur and Moore.

fears about being "deselected" (having their contract terminated) from an HMO because their utilization of services is too high, putting them at risk for serious financial loss. Physician James Li asserts: "In the commercial model of medicine the patient is at best a consumer; at worst, the patient is a revenue stream when well and a source of medical (financial) loss when sick."[13]

It is in this context that doctors have experienced a sense of loss. They have lost autonomy over patient decisions. They have lost status in their communities. And they have lost income. These losses have caused a sense of powerlessness. Physician unions are a response to this powerlessness felt by so many physicians.

Labor Unions and Professional Societies

The labor union movement in America was formed in response to industrialization in order to empower workers who wanted a bigger piece of the industrial pie. Their primary focus was wages, work conditions, and benefits. Labor law, which evolved during this industrial period, has restricted unions to dealing with these same issues, yet today's white collar workers, and especially physicians, have issues outside these boundaries.

Physician unions first emerged in America in the early 1970s. Twenty-six different physician unions were formed during the 1970s, of which one is still in existence.[14] They arose as a response to changes in reimbursement patterns and growing Medicare regulations. Doctors were frustrated with their loss of control. Nonmedical people were giving them orders (e.g., pre-approval was required from an insurance company clerk). Many health care decisions were being made by third parties, removing personal responsibility for the patients from the physicians. Comments like those of Dr. George Lagorio who organized the Illinois Physician Union in 1973 sound surprisingly contemporary: "Professional freedom is rapidly disappearing. Dignity, prestige and respect which are the symbols of medical professionalism have been eroded by insurance carriers and governmental agencies desiring to gain control of medical practice, as well as the biased anti-physician diatribe of the press. . . . the physician

---

13. J. T. Li, "The Patient-Physician Relationship: Covenant or Contract?" *Mayo Clinic Proceedings* 71 (1996): 917-18.

14. Budrys, p. 16.

who has joined organized labor has merely joined with his patient who is already a part of that movement, so as to achieve the ultimate goal of good medical care."[15] Similar sentiments were echoed in the preamble to the organizational charter of the Union of American Physicians and Dentists (UAPD) which was also established in 1973.[16]

Doctors who were in the habit of reaching agreements primarily with individuals on the basis of trust were now having to negotiate with large organizations while battling for their own financial survival. The goals and functions of these unions were to bring doctors together to negotiate with large corporate or government agencies. Unions have used a traditional bargaining approach to improve wages and benefits, but have also addressed specific contract issues such as medical staff privileges, peer review, and the handling of malpractice suits. Unions have defended the due process rights of doctors, and in so doing, often assisted doctors in private practice by helping them obtain reimbursement when denied by third party payers.

Unions have used various methods in order to accomplish these goals. Expertise in negotiation and labor law has been central to progress on union issues. Use of the media and other forms of information disbursement (i.e. informational picketing) has allowed them to gain broader public support for their causes. Strikes and other forms of work stoppage have also been employed.[17] Germany had a militant physician union as early as 1898 and in the early years struck 200 times because of what they considered arbitrary reimbursement from sickness funds. Canadian physicians in Ontario staged a visible and successful strike for 25 days in 1986 over the issue of "balance-billing." However, many physicians actually saw patients even though they spent some of their time on a picket line. In 1972, Nevada physicians were angered when some Las Vegas hospitals required physicians to spend one afternoon a week doing chart review to fulfill Medicare requirements, so the union organized a "white-in." Doctors provided complete care for all patients who came to the ER and invited every patient to have a bed in the hospital, then intentionally neglected to complete the necessary paperwork. After one and a half days, hospital administrators agreed to the union demand to pay physicians $50 per hour for their chart review services. The issue of strikes has been a key differentiating feature between professional societies and physician unions.

15. Budrys, p. 12.
16. Budrys, p. 9.
17. Budrys, pp. 11-31.

Organized medicine has a long history in the United States. The AMA and other professional organizations like the American Academy of Pediatrics and the American Board of Internal Medicine have done much to make the profession of medicine a true asset to the public, a profession with high standards that is worthy of trust. Since its inception, the AMA has functioned as a collective voice on issues ranging from quackery to reimbursement from Medicare. Indeed, there was much dialogue in the early 1970s between the AMA and unions about how best to be the voice of physicians. Union leaders like Dr. Stanley Peterson, then president of the newly formed Federation of Physicians and Dentists, made a formal proposal as delegate to the 1973 AMA convention that the AMA establish guidelines for collective bargaining. The AMA's response was clear: negotiation without unionization.[18] Seeking a collegial solution of grievances was deemed more "professional" and less "industrial" than an adversarial approach.[19] Currently the AMA is actively promoting collective bargaining in an effort to respond to doctors who increasingly believe insurers have gained control over medical decision making. Nevertheless, the AMA has also consistently opposed the idea of physician strikes. As Julie Johnsson observed in an article on collective bargaining in the July 1997 *American Medical News:* "Many doctors are drawn by the union's potential might, but are disturbed that this power traditionally has been exercised through work stoppages."[20]

The Union Movement at Thomas Davis Medical Centers

The story of the union movement at Thomas Davis Medical Centers (TDMC) has been chronicled in *Medical Economics,*[21] *The New York Times,*[22] and *JAMA.*[23] Thomas Davis Medical Centers is a large multispecialty clinic which began about eighty years ago and developed its own

18. Budrys, p. 88.

19. Budrys, pp. 87-96.

20. J. Johnsson, "Physicians Want to Collectively Bargain; AMA to Further the Quest," *American Medical News* (July 7, 1997): 33.

21. D. Azevedo, "Taking Back Health Care: New Owners Drive This Group to Unionize," *Medical Economics* (March 24, 1997): 194-207.

22. A. Adelson, "Physician, Unionize Thyself: Doctors Adapt to Life as H.M.O. Employees," *The New York Times,* 5 April 1997, p. 21.

23. U. E. Reinhardt, "Economics: Hippocrates and the 'Secularization' of Patients," *JAMA* 277 (1997): 1850-51.

HMO in the early 1980s. The TDMC physicians sold their profitable HMO and their unprofitable physician group practice to Foundation Health (FH), a California health plan. By selling their assets, the individual physicians who were shareholders became wealthy. The sale changed TDMC from a physician-owned-and-operated clinic to a business with a fiduciary responsibility to shareholders.

Following the sale, a broad range of cost-cutting measures were instituted. These changes in business practices were perceived by the physicians as subordinating patient care to the financial profitability of the corporation. For example, physicians were denied the opportunity to continue their volunteer service at a clinic for the indigent during work time, but were told to do it during their free hours. Physicians were told they should see more patients, work longer hours, and send fewer patients to Urgent Care or face salary cuts. In August of 1996, FH outlined a plan to cut another 2 million dollars from the budget because of continued financial losses, and they sold the money-losing physician practice to FPA Medical Management (FPA), retaining the more lucrative outpatient surgical center and the pharmacy.

The physicians were incensed and feared they might lose their jobs. Many believed the financial losses were accounting ploys by FH to make TDMC appear unprofitable, although in reality, the group had been subsidized by its profitable HMO for years. Increasing loss of autonomy and paperwork for referrals continued to irritate the physicians. Thinking they had nothing to lose, the doctors of the Tucson branch of TDMC voted to unionize by a 93 to 32 margin. The TDMC Administration and the new owners (FPA) attempted to block unionization by saying that the union was invalid because the physicians were supervisors not employees, a claim which has so far been rejected by the National Labor Relations Board. The union publicly announced the doctors' concern that patients could not obtain good care at TDMC because corporate concern for profit kept them from taking care of patients adequately. The message of the union to the press was, "this isn't about money, it's about being a good doctor." Media coverage grew from local newspaper reports to national network television.

Hostility between physicians and administration grew and resignations began. All department chairmen resigned their leadership positions on the same day. Patients asked their individual physicians whether they could still get good care at the clinic after their confidence was eroded by a work stoppage in early January 1997. While not formally supported by the union, a chief union organizer had called each department, urging physicians to stop seeing patients because the new malpractice policy provided inadequate coverage. The work stoppage lasted about three hours, during which time the malpractice crisis was resolved. However, many of the TDMC physicians continued working. Many who believed the work stoppage was unethical, including some who were active in the union, circulated a letter to their colleagues denouncing the action.

Further unrest was precipitated by the implementation of a new physician compensation system which resulted in salary cuts of 25 to 35 percent for most primary care physicians. At the time of this writing, the National Labor Relations Board is suing TDMC for its refusal to negotiate with the union, patients are unhappy, doctors are angry, and the nurses are terrified. Uncertainty prevails.

Ethical Questions for Physicians

In this time of uncertainty, it is important for physicians to ask and answer pertinent ethical questions, the most important of which concerns the definition of the physician-patient relationship. Are the parameters of that relationship primarily determined by contracts or covenant? Dr. Li, in his analysis of the patient-physician relationship, outlines three provocative self-diagnostic questions which are presented for individual self-examination: (1) Am I a caregiver or a gatekeeper? (2) Which principle governs my relationship with my patients: morality or the marketplace? (3) What is my relationship with my patients: a covenant or a contract?[24]

For physicians who adhere to the Hippocratic tradition, and especially for Christian physicians, the compassion shown by Jesus to those with leprosy is to be our example. Christian physicians must touch the untouchable, care for the outcast, and offer healing techniques to the best of their abilities, regardless of a patient's ability to pay. Jesus gave the story of the Good Samaritan to non-medical people. Is not the call to physicians even greater?

Christian physicians must, fundamentally, be caregivers governed by morality, not gatekeepers ruled by the marketplace. Christian physicians need to have a covenant relationship with their patients, recognizing them as people made in the image of almighty God. The faithful covenant

24. Li.

255

relationship offered by God to humanity provides an example for our physician-patient relationships.

Other ethical questions are important as well. In relation to physician unions, we must first ask: Whom does the union serve? Much union rhetoric blurs the obvious answer. A union serves or cares for physicians and is concerned about their wages, benefits, and work conditions. A union does not care for patients. Physicians care for patients. Unions are external to the physician-patient relationship and therefore occupy a sphere of influence shared with employers or third party payers, including government. Physicians are the last defense in advocating for patients. This distinction is important because it reminds one that while the doctor-patient relationship can be described by either a contract or covenant, the doctor-union relationship is always contractually driven. Since unions occupy the same sphere of influence as other business entities, important ethical questions for evaluating unions are similar to questions that could be used in evaluating the business aspect of medicine. However, we will here address these diagnostic questions with respect to physician unions:

1. Does the union assist me in putting the needs of the patient first? If so, how? Any group of physicians could come together and encourage each other to put the needs of the patient first. Unions, like professional organizations, certainly could be a vehicle for patient advocacy but this has not been a priority for either. Nevertheless, unions have impacted the physician-patient relationship for good by addressing dangerous work standards.[25]

2. Does the union propose any action that would violate my role with patients? Strikes are a difficult issue for physician groups because work stoppage by any name does affect patient care.[26]

3. Does the union assist physicians in making the profession a public asset worthy of the trust of government and citizens? Is the profession encouraged to fulfill its role to the indigent and uninsured, to teaching and research? Unions, by virtue of being a group of physicians, could potentially advocate high standards for the profession as a whole. However, this is an advocacy role already taken by professional societies, not by unions.

4. Do the lives of union leaders and the language that they use give

25. Budrys.
26. Budrys, ch. 3. See also Azevedo.

256

me confidence in their moral character? Personal moral character assessments are necessary and prudent in assessing any type of professional alliance.

5. Can the contracts negotiated by the union improve my business position without adversely affecting those with whom I work, such as nurses and staff? Addressing how other workers will be affected by contracts may be difficult but it is essential to attempt to do so if one is to behave in an ethical fashion.

The physician/union interface is about what the physician gets in terms of wages and benefits, while the physician/patient interface is about what the physician gives in terms of care and concern in the exercising of clinical skills. While unions are legal and valid tools for negotiating contract issues, they have seldom helped physicians protect the physician-patient relationship.

Unions can certainly exert an impact on the physician-patient relationship, but in the covenant model the impact of unions is on the same level as other external forces such as society and business. All these influences are subordinate to the covenant relationship that starts with God and is extended to the physician and the patient.

A Christian physician could ethically and morally join a union as long as he or she maintains a covenant view of the physician-patient relationship. However, this would entail not participating in strikes or work stoppages, the union's most powerful weapon. Once unions are reduced to negotiation alone, they are in no better position to affect business than "organized medicine," like the AMA. Unions, without a call to moral action like the AMA Code of Ethics, are at a disadvantage.

Christian physicians are uniquely positioned to influence their colleagues by calling them to a covenant relationship with their patients. It is essential for our generation of physicians to adhere to the Hippocratic tradition if we are to combat the incredible forces of market pressure and cost containment as they are increasingly applied to practice guidelines, end-of-life care, and quality-of-life decisions. An understanding of the ministry of Christ Jesus, the Great Physician, can empower Christian physicians to do the work to which he has called them.

Emerging Alternative Therapies

Dónal P. O'Mathúna, Ph.D.

The face of health care is changing dramatically in the area of alternative medicine. It has become a regular feature of cover stories and TV news programs, especially when a major medical center or academic institution joins those offering alternative therapies. Huge numbers of books on alternative medicine are being sold. Physicians like Andrew Weil, Deepak Chopra, Herbert Benson, Larry Dossey, and Bernie Siegel have become celebrities with best-selling books on alternative medicine.

In America, increasing amounts of money are being spent on alternative medicine: $13.7 billion dollars in 1990, for example — three quarters of which was paid out-of-pocket.[1] In Europe in 1991 herbal medicine sales were estimated at more than $2 billion, and the same amount was spent in the U.S. in 1995.[2] Americans spend $6 billion annually on all sorts of nutritional supplements, and the market is growing by 20 percent every year.[3]

The British National Health Service is under pressure to make alternative therapies available, while health insurance companies are starting to provide coverage for them. The pressure is coming from patient

1. David M. Eisenberg, Ronald C. Kessler, Cindy Foster, Frances E. Norlock, David R. Calkins, and Thomas L. Delbanco, "Unconventional Medicine in the United States: Prevalence, Costs, and Patterns of Use," *New England Journal of Medicine* 328 (Jan. 1993): 246-52.

2. Peter Fisher and Adam Ward, "Complementary Medicine in Europe," *BMJ* 309 (July 1994): 107-10; Joseph Weber and Sandra Dallas, "Cure? Well . . . Profit? Sure," *Business Week*, 23 Oct. 1995, pp. 58-59.

3. Geoffrey Cowley, "Herbal Warning: Health-Food Stores Have Built a New Natural-Drug Culture. How Safe Are Their Wares?" *Newsweek*, 6 May 1996, pp. 60-68.

demand and the need to cut costs. In April 1997, the U.S. National Managed Health Care Conference included a half-day symposium on how to integrate alternative medicine into managed care plans. The manager of Oxford Health Plans, which already covers alternative medicine (for an extra charge), claimed: "I believe that if the competitors don't listen to what their customers are saying and enter this [alternative medicine] market they are going to lose a lot of business, and I'm going to take it from them."[4]

In more academic settings, over 40 U.S. medical schools teach courses in alternative medicine, with one or two of them making this a requirement.[5] Therapeutic touch, one type of alternative therapy, has been taught in over 80 U.S. nursing schools and in 68 other countries.[6] Harvard Medical School hosts an annual academic conference on alternative medicine. The journal *American Family Physician* put alternative medicine on its November 1996 cover and included articles calling for its acceptance.[7] The U.S. National Institutes for Health has established an Office of Alternative Medicine to investigate its scientific claims. Although fraught with controversy over its precise role, the very existence of this office is frequently used to justify interest in and funding of alternative medicine.

Numerous studies have tried to quantify the level of interest in alternative therapies. In Europe, 20-50 percent of the populations of various countries use alternative therapies. Some studies have documented large increases in their use. For example, in 1981, 6.4 percent of the Dutch population visited an alternative medicine provider. This figure had increased to 9.1 percent by 1985 and to 15.7 percent by 1990.[8]

The most highly publicized and frequently cited U.S. study was conducted by David Eisenberg and published in the *New England Journal*

4. Hasaan Rifaat, M.D., "Integrating Alternative Medicine & Managed Care," Pre-Conference Symposium at the National Managed Health Care Conference (INFOCUS: 4 April 1997), audiocassette #320-S3B.

5. "Integrating Alternative Medicine & Managed Care," Pre-Conference Symposium at the National Managed Health Care Conference (INFOCUS: 4 April 1997), audiocassette #320-S3C.

6. Dolores Krieger, *Accepting Your Power to Heal: The Personal Practice of Therapeutic Touch* (Santa Fe, N.M.: Bear & Co., 1993), p. 5.

7. M. Kyu Chung, "Why Alternative Medicine?" *American Family Physician* 54 (Nov. 1996): 2184-85; James S. Gordon, "Alternative Medicine and the Family Physician," *American Family Physician* 54 (Nov. 1996): 2205-12; and a patient information handout.

8. P. Van Dijk, *Geneewijzen in Nederland* (Deventer: Ankh-Hermes, 1993); cited in Fisher, p. 107.

of Medicine. His study found that one out of every three Americans had tried some form of alternative therapy in 1990.[9] Alarmingly, 70 percent of these people did not inform their medical doctors that they were pursuing such alternatives.

Defining Alternative Medicine

Eisenberg's article leads us to the first major difficulty in understanding, evaluating, and thinking theologically about alternative medicine. Discussions about it are plagued by problems of terminology. This movement, or group of therapies, goes by many different names, such as alternative, complementary, unorthodox, unconventional, unproven, holistic, fringe, integrative, natural, or New Age medicine. "Alternative medicine" will be used here because it remains the most popular term. This type of medicine is an alternative to the medicine associated with physicians and hospitals, also known by many names, including conventional, modern, scientific, orthodox, allopathic, reductionistic, biochemical, or physicalistic medicine. "Conventional medicine" will be used here.

To understand and evaluate alternative medicine, the practices and principles it encompasses must be examined. Eisenberg's study defines alternative therapies "as medical interventions not taught widely at U.S. medical schools or generally available at U.S. hospitals."[10] His broad definition includes a very diverse group of practices. For example, the most common alternative therapies included are relaxation techniques (used by 13 percent of respondents), chiropractic (10 percent), and massage (7 percent). Of intermediate popularity are therapies like commercial weight-loss programs (4 percent), lifestyle diets (4 percent), and self-help groups (2 percent). Many of these practices would be regarded by most people as part of a common-sense approach to healthy living. Yet their inclusion as alternative therapies helps to bolster the overall numbers of people pursuing alternative medicine. Eisenberg's study reveals that therapies that are very different from conventional medicine have been used to a very small degree, for example: energy medicine (used by 1 percent of respondents), homeopathy (1 percent), and acupuncture (less than 1 percent).

Eisenberg's pilot study also includes exercise (used for medical pur-

9. Eisenberg, pp. 246-52.
10. Eisenberg, p. 246.

poses by 26 percent of the respondents) and prayer (used by 25 percent). The researchers excluded these practices from their main study, however, citing methodological difficulties. Yet these practices fit Eisenberg's definition of alternative medicine. It seems arbitrary to exclude these, especially since his data show that people have engaged in these practices twice as frequently as in the next-most-popular therapy. Inclusion of prayer and exercise, though, would have led to the conclusion that an extremely high percentage of people use alternative medicine, thereby undermining the usefulness of the term.

Other authors use even broader definitions. One study reports that physical therapy, counseling, nutrition, and massage are the alternative health therapies most frequently used by people with multiple sclerosis.[11] Another includes active listening and patient advocacy as "natural therapies"![12] Factors such as diet, exercise, stress reduction, and patient advocacy are indeed important in promoting and maintaining health. However, inclusion of these factors within alternative medicine suggests that conventional medicine does not consider them important, when in fact it does.

An overly broad definition portrays alternative medicine as more popular than would a narrower definition that more accurately captures the concept. Dubious and questionable therapies, some of which will be examined later, gain credibility and acceptance on the coat-tails of obviously important factors like nutrition, exercise, and relaxation. Grouping energy medicine along with diet and exercise makes it difficult to provide a reasonable analysis. Those concerned about fringe therapies are viewed as questioning the importance of nutrition and mental attitude for good health. Before proposing a set of categories to help clarify these discussions it will be helpful to suggest some reasons why alternative medicine has become more popular.

Understanding the Popularity

Part of the popularity of alternative medicine can be explained in the way that it is commonly distinguished from conventional medicine. Dichot-

11. Jacqueline Fawcett, Joan S. Sidney, Mary Jane S. Hanson, and Kathleen Riley-Lawless, "Use of Alternative Health Therapies by People with Multiple Sclerosis," *Holistic Nurse Practice* 8 (1994): 36-42.

12. Gareth J. Daniels and Pauline McCabe, "Nursing Diagnosis and Natural Therapies: A Symbiotic Relationship," *Journal of Holistic Nursing* 12 (June 1994): 184-92.

omized terms are often employed to present alternative medicine in the best possible light. For example, conventional medicine is said to take an aggressive, invasive approach, while alternative medicine adopts a gentler, more natural approach. Conventional medicine is reductionistic and focused on diseases, while alternatives are holistic and attentive to body, mind, and spirit. Conventional medicine has a negative focus on eliminating disease, while alternatives are positive, focused on optimizing health. Conventional medicine has a magic bullet or technofix approach, while alternatives address broader lifestyle issues. Conventional medicine is paternalistic, while alternative medicine promotes partnership and encourages responsibility and self-care. Even the different terminology used for the two groups is noted. Conventional medicine seeks to cut, cure, and kill, while alternative medicine encourages relaxation, balance, and empowering.

These descriptions portray alternative medicine as the small, gentle guy pushed aside by the big, bad medical and pharmaceutical establishment. This image fits a general reaction against a medical system that focuses too much on a purely physical approach to health and healing. Conventional medicine has at times neglected the importance of lifestyle, relationships, stress, and spirituality. Visits to medical doctors can mean long waits, much paperwork, impersonal interactions, embarrassing gowns, incomprehensible results, and huge costs. The focus can seem to be primarily on the body and what is wrong with *it*, not on the *person* whose body it is. To the extent that conventional medicine has overemphasized drugs, surgery, and technology as the answer to all health problems, it must take seriously the arguments for an alternative.

Alternative medicine's popularity is also influenced by the growing awareness of conventional medicine's limitations. Sickness confronts us with the reality of our mortality. Conventional medicine seemed poised to conquer illness, and maybe even death. It faltered with cancer, was frustrated by AIDS, and is now on the retreat from antibiotic-resistant bacteria. People's expectations in the all-powerful god of conventional medicine have been dashed. But many still want to believe they can be cured of any illness. They turn to alternatives when conventional medicine reaches its limits.

Alternative medicine is particularly attractive to Baby Boomers. Those who most commonly use alternative medicine in the U.S. are middle-class, middle-aged, and well educated.[13] Their bodies are starting

13. Eisenberg, p. 248.

to show wear and tear in spite of all their jogging, dieting, and refraining from smoking. They have made a cult of personal health, have never liked authority, and want to make all their own decisions.[14] The titles of Deepak Chopra's books offer what many want: *Perfect Health* and *Ageless Body, Timeless Mind.*[15] Hence, alternative medicine's self-care, self-healing, partnership model is very appealing. This generation is also attracted to two other factors important in understanding the popularity of alternative medicine: postmodernism and New Age spirituality.

Postmodernism

A type of thinking increasingly evidenced in popular society today has been called *postmodernism.* Proponents of alternative medicine frequently use arguments based on postmodern ideology. While postmodernism does not necessarily advocate alternative medicine, it has become the Trojan horse by which alternative therapies, with very little supporting evidence, have gained acceptance and credibility.[16] A brief overview of the main tenets of postmodernism is in order.

Postmodernism is a diverse group of perspectives most easily understood by describing what it reacts against and rejects. Postmodernism follows after, and seeks to supplant, modernity — the era of reason and science that received its greatest boost from the Enlightenment. Postmodernism dismisses the ideas of objective knowledge and absolute truth. Instead, each culture is said to "socially construct" its own meaning based on arbitrarily chosen methods and standards. There is not just one reality out there which we all try to understand. Instead, each creates his or her own reality based on experience and chosen meanings. If someone claims, "This is true," that does not mean it is true for anyone else except the speaker. Postmodernism denies the existence of absolute truth about anything (except, of course, the absolute truth that there is no absolute truth).

14. Claudia Wallis, "Why New Age Medicine Is Catching On," *Time,* 4 Nov. 1991, pp. 68-76.

15. Deepak Chopra, *Perfect Health: The Complete Mind/Body Guide* (New York: Harmony Books, 1990) and *Ageless Body, Timeless Mind: The Quantum Alternative to Growing Old* (New York: Harmony Books, 1993).

16. Dónal P. O'Mathúna, "Postmodern Impact: Health Care," in *The Death of Truth: What's Wrong with Multiculturalism, the Rejection of Reason, and the New Postmodern Diversity,* ed. Dennis McCallum (Minneapolis: Bethany House, 1996), pp. 58-84.

Much of alternative medicine literature uses these ideas. Near the opening of his book, W. Brugh Joy notes:

> It may strike your imagination, however, that large groups of people perceive reality very differently. . . . Many of these ideas contradict one another. . . . The shocker here is not that these people embody particular contradictions but the more basic fact that no belief systems actually represent reality; they are only structured ideas created out of a small part of the human mind's potential.[17]

Therapeutic touch, a popular nursing alternative therapy, was co-founded by Dolores Krieger, a nursing professor. She claims, "It is now recognized that the concept of multiple realities is valid. . . . Therapeutic Touch has benefited from being perceived in this more liberal perspective."[18] The idea of multiple realities brings immense power and control. Dr. Joy goes on to claim that we need to come to the "recognition that belief systems are only belief systems and not realities. *At this level of consciousness we can create anything we desire*"[19] (emphasis original).

This assertion resonates well in a society placing ultimate value on autonomy and control. If each of us creates our own reality, only the individual can decide what is best for him or her. To do otherwise would be paternalistic and repressive. Any group claiming to have found truth which applies to everyone is accused by postmodernists of marginalizing others. Hence, popular culture readily embraces many of postmodernism's implications, like ethical relativism and a lack of respect for standards of evidence.[20]

Scientists and physicians have been attacked for claiming to have found objective truth about one physical reality, and for seeking to impose those truths on others. Western, scientific worldviews, or paradigms, are labeled "male-dominated, exclusive, authoritarian, linear, and rigid."[21] These produce "reductionist medicine" which results in "continued dis-

---

17. W. Brugh Joy, *Joy's Way: A Map for the Transformational Journey: An Introduction to the Potentials for Healing with Body Energies* (New York: Jeremy P. Tarcher, 1979), pp. 18-19.

18. Krieger, *Accepting Your Power*, pp. 6-7.

19. Joy, p. 20.

20. For many examples, see Paul R. Gross and Norman Levitt, *Higher Superstition: The Academic Left and Its Quarrels with Science* (Baltimore: Johns Hopkins University Press, 1994); and Marcia Angell, *Science on Trial: The Clash of Medical Evidence and the Law in the Breast Implant Case* (New York: W. W. Norton, 1996).

21. Daniels, p. 186.

ease, dependence on 'management' with drugs and surgery (control over nature being a fundamental need of patriarchal science), poor quality of life, and tremendous cost to patient and community."[22] As such, scientific answers simply reflect male, white, European prejudices. "Such paradigms require (indeed on a subconscious level they beg) to be overthrown."[23]

Hence, under the influence of postmodernism, alternative medicine frequently calls, not for change, but for radical transformation. A naturopath trying to bring alternative medicine into managed care plans claims, "We need to change the way we look at reality."[24] Jean Watson, past-president of the National League for Nursing, in a talk entitled *Postmodern Nursing*, calls for a "radical rethinking" about health and healing that would "turn our ideas upside down."[25] Chopra calls for "a completely new worldview" that will give us "the makings of a new reality."[26]

Postmodernists claim that questions about the physical, biochemical world are no more reliably answered by science than by other ways of knowing, like intuition or mysticism. Thus, anecdotal evidence becomes just as important as double-blind, randomized trials. Narrative becomes more important than analysis since stories reflect people's experiences better than statistics. Thus, some managed care organizations are promoting alternative medicine even though they acknowledge there is little evidence to support its efficacy. What matters more is that the public perceives it as helpful and wants it.

If traditional standards for efficacy and evidence are not upheld, and claims for scientific validity not scrutinized, little credibility will be given to any study. When research does not support the efficacy of alternative therapies, the postmodern critique of science is used to discount those findings. For example, therapeutic touch practitioners claim to be able to manipulate human energy fields, which can bring about relaxation, pain relief, and healing. Proponents claim it is the best-researched of the nursing alternative therapies. Reviews of this research, however, have

22. Pauline McCabe, "Natural Therapies in Australia: A Nurse-Naturopath's View," *Nurse Practitioner Forum* 5 (June 1994), p. 116.

23. Daniels, p. 186.

24. Marcel Hernandez, "Integrating Alternative Medicine & Managed Care," Pre-Conference Symposium at the National Managed Health Care Conference (INFOCUS, 4 April 1997), audiocassette #320-S3B.

25. Jean Watson, "Postmodern Nursing," talk given at Mount Carmel College of Nursing, Columbus, Ohio, October 24, 1994.

26. Chopra, *Ageless*, pp. 5, 7.

consistently found very little empirical support.[27] The most recent review was rejected as male-dominated medical imperialism marginalizing female-dominated nursing.[28]

One influential nursing text rejected skepticism of therapeutic touch and dismissed the relevance of research. Rather than criticize the practice, nurses were asked to accept therapeutic touch as a way to "celebrate the diversity among us."[29] If therapeutic agents are to be selected on the basis of diversity, a wide variety of useless and harmful practices will be introduced.

While postmodernism makes some valid points (especially in its critique of materialism and scientism), Christians must reject its relativism and its blind emphasis on openness and diversity. The biblical worldview is not the same as either modernism or postmodernism. In the same way, alternative medicine should not be accepted and promoted just because it offers an alternative to the previous health care system that needs change. We can accept some aspects of alternative medicine, but there are others we must reject. We should not embrace anything just because it is part of a popular movement and claims to replace something we know has problems.

Christians must critically examine all the tenets of alternative medicine in light of God's word. The following section divides alternative medicine into five categories to help clarify our evaluations of some therapies. Admittedly, the lines between these categories are arbitrary and fuzzy. The same therapy is often practiced in different ways. Practitioners commonly intermix a number of therapies. Therapies will move from one category to another as more is understood about them and as their acceptance changes. But this categorization will help us better understand how to respond to the current interest in these very diverse therapies.

27. Barbara C. Walike et al., ". . . attempts to embellish a totally unscientific process with the aura of science . . ." in Letters, *American Journal of Nursing* 75 (Aug. 1975): 1275, 1278, 1282; Philip E. Clark and Mary Jo Clark, "Therapeutic Touch: Is There a Scientific Basis for the Practice?" *Nursing Research* 33 (1984): 37-40; H. N. Claman, *Report of the Chancellor's Committee on Therapeutic Touch* (Denver: University of Colorado Health Sciences Center, 1994).

28. Linda A. Rosa, "Therapeutic Touch: Skeptics in Hand to Hand Combat Over the Latest New Age Health Fad," *Skeptic* 3 (Fall 1994): 40-49.

29. Lynda J. Carpenito, *Nursing Diagnosis: Application to Clinical Practice,* 6th ed. (Philadelphia: Lippincott, 1995), p. 356.

Five Categories of Alternative Medicine

1. Complementary Therapies

Familiar practices such as good nutrition, exercise, stress reduction, marriage and parenting classes, support groups, massage, and spirituality are included in this category. Health care professionals and institutions have not necessarily viewed such practices as unimportant. Rather, they have not provided them primarily because they have not seen them as part of health care. Common sense and mounting evidence from studies show that these practices are important for healthy lifestyles and prevention of illness. However, traditional settings (family, school, church, community) provide these services less frequently and educate fewer people about them. Whether health care professionals and institutions should be the ones teaching these remains to be seen. However, third party payers want these types of services provided as part of their preventive care programs, often listing them as alternative therapies.

Christians should be leading the way in this area. The Hebrew term for healing, *rapa'*, was used to describe the repairing of a broken jar, the healing of a person, and the restoring of the nation of Israel. The fundamental meaning of the word, then, is to restore something to its original condition, or make it whole again.[30] God's activity as healer is not dichotomized into physical and spiritual realms, but refers to his work in every aspect of people's lives.

Thus, meeting people's relational, spiritual, and community needs is central to the mission of the Church. The Bible affirms that people are not just bags of chemicals, but are embodied spiritual, emotional, and relational beings (1 Thess. 5:23; Heb. 4:12). Any form of medicine that neglects patients' feelings, family dynamics, or lifestyles fails to care for the whole person. Good health involves one's mind and spirit. Proverbs 17:22 states: "A joyful heart is good medicine, but a broken spirit dries up the bones" (cf. 2 Sam. 13:2; Prov. 3:8). But Scripture, unlike modern or alternative medicine, also states that good health depends on having our moral guilt dealt with (Ps. 32:3-4; 1 Cor. 11:29-30). This starts with the forgiveness that is available only in Jesus Christ. Thus, he is the only true source of ultimate healing (John 6:35-40).

Christians should allow God's healing power to work in them and

---

30. Michael L. Brown, *Israel's Divine Healer* (Grand Rapids: Zondervan, 1995), pp. 28-31.

through them. The example of Jesus, the Great Physician, guides us as we interact with others. The belief that all people are created in the image of God should impact the care and compassion shown to all. If we exhibit "the fruit of the Spirit, which is love, joy, peace, patience, kindness, goodness, faithfulness, gentleness, and self-control" (Gal. 5:22-23), we will show a real alternative to the cold, impersonal ways patients are sometimes treated.

2. Quackery and Fraud

The second category is at the other extreme of the continuum of alternative medicine. Unfortunately, some people will intentionally deceive others about the efficacy of a therapy, especially to earn a profit. Quackery, however, includes ineffective therapies promoted by people with good intentions who believe they work. Good intentions are not enough in health care. Professionals should ensure that they have accurate information about what they provide and promote — especially about its potential risks — and that this information is based on trustworthy data.

While quackery and fraud is possible with any form of health care, alternative medicine is particularly prone to this problem. Those conditions most frequently leading people to pursue alternative medicine (such as cancer, AIDS, obesity, or chronic diseases) are the same conditions most susceptible to quackery.[31] Fraud and quackery thrive more easily in an environment where therapies are not expected to have clinical evidence to back up their claims, or where the medical research establishment is excessively mistrusted. When a therapy is promoted primarily by bashing physicians, or if it promises too much, people should be on the alert. Health care fraud remains a significant problem, estimated by a 1984 U.S. congressional committee to cost $25 billion annually.[32]

3. Scientifically Unproven Therapies

The third category covers empirically or scientifically unproven therapies that are based on established scientific principles. While anecdotal evi-

31. Robin Nishiwaki, Alice Morton, Carla Bouchard, James A. Peters, and William T. Jarvis, "Perceived Health Quackery Use Among Patients: A Physician Survey," *Western Journal of Medicine* 152 (Jan. 1990): 87-89.

32. William T. Jarvis, "Quackery: A National Scandal," *Clinical Chemistry* 38 (1992): 1574-86.

dence may exist for these, little or no clinical evidence backs up their claims. Much of herbal medicine would be included in this area. More than 1,400 herbs are sold commercially and promoted for various unproven medical benefits. Yet only nine of these have been judged by the U.S. Food and Drug Administration to be safe and effective. Even in Europe, where herbal remedies have been studied more, little is known about many products. For example, a German government panel has examined only 300 of the 1,400 herbal drugs available there.[33]

Chiropractic and acupuncture are other practices where scientific studies have revealed effectiveness for certain specific problems.[34] Uncertainty remains, however, about their use with other conditions, and there is debate over exactly how they work. It remains difficult to categorize these therapies because, while they are gaining in acceptance because of their empirical results, many resist them because they are unfamiliar. Such resistance is common when new therapies are first introduced. However, if they continue to show reproducible clinical results, acceptance of them will likely grow.

Regarding this group of therapies, uncertainty about their claims should be admitted. They should not be rejected outright, nor blindly promoted, without supporting evidence. They should be approached with the same caution given to any other unproven therapy. If there is little evidence of harm, and minimal burden and expense, it may be appropriate for patients to try them. However, particular caution should be exercised with herbal products. While many are marketed as food supplements, they are drugs and can be harmful. Most pharmaceutical drugs were originally developed from herbs. Just because something is natural and readily available does not eliminate potential harm. Tobacco demonstrates this dramatically. More research is needed to provide clearer recommendations for therapies in this category.

4. Scientifically Questionable Therapies

The fourth category of alternative therapies also have little or no scientific evidence to back up their claims, though they may have anecdotal support. These therapies differ, however, from the third group in being based on

33. Ellis Q. Youngkin and Debra S. Israel, "A Review and Critique of Common Herbal Alternative Therapies," *Nurse Practitioner* 21 (Oct. 1996): 39-60.
34. For a list of studies, see Gordon, pp. 2205-12.

principles or theories that contradict widely held scientific beliefs. One example here would be homeopathy, where dilution with shaking (even to the point of diluting out every molecule of the original "active" ingredient) is believed to increase the pharmacological potency of a solution. This goes against the common scientific finding that the greater a drug's concentration, the stronger its pharmacological action.

While proponents claim homeopathy is "the most effective curative system known to mankind,"[35] reviews of clinical studies on homeopathy show the findings are often weak, with many studies poorly structured.[36] In spite of the weak evidence, postmodern arguments are used to promote these therapies. For example, Dana Ullman, President of the Foundation for Homeopathic Education and Research, claims: "It is sad that in this land of freedom some people seek to 'protect' others from making their own decisions in health care. Hopefully as we approach the 21st century and as more and more countries experience 'glasnost' and 'perestroika,' America will re-commit itself to real freedom and real democracy."[37] Of course, Ullman means the freedom to do as one wants, not the freedom to do what is best.

Research-funding agencies must make decisions about which therapies to test. When a therapy is based on principles in direct conflict with widely supported scientific principles, it is difficult to justify using limited resources to study it. However, if carefully collected data shows that improvements occur with these therapies, some funding should be made available to test them further. Until then, it seems justified to remain skeptical of their claims.

5. Energy Medicine

The fifth category is a diverse collection of practices based on "life-energy" or "spiritual principles." The postmodern emphasis on diversity is used to promote acceptance of all forms of spirituality and religious beliefs. The only unacceptable view is one claiming to have truth that applies to

35. George Vithoulkas, *Homeopathy: Medicine of the New Man* (New York: Arco, 1979), p. 1.

36. Jos Kleijnen, Paul Knipschild, and Gerben ter Riet, "Clinical Trials of Homoeopathy," *BMJ* 302 (Feb. 1991): 316-23; C. Hill and F. Doyon, "Review of Randomized Trials of Homoeopathy," *Revue d'Epidemiologie et de Santé Publique* 308 (1990): 139-47.

37. Dana Ullman, *Discovering Homeopathy: Medicine for the 21st Century*, rev. ed. (Berkeley, Calif.: North Atlantic, 1991), p. xix.

everyone. Biblical Christianity is such a view. With the postmodern mindset has come an openness to spiritually-based healing practices.

Many of these practices are based on a nonphysical life-energy, or force, also called *prana, chi, ka,* or *orgone.* According to this outlook, the basic substance of human bodies is not matter, but energy and information. This life-energy is nonphysical and universal, animating and sustaining all living things. The energy of each person is a localization of infinite fields of energy, which pervade the universe. This energy enters the human body through channels called *chakras.* True health results from a balanced flow of this energy through the body and an unblocked exchange of this energy with one's environment. Imbalances or blockages in the flow lead to physical symptoms that we recognize as illness, aging, and death.[38]

Belief in this life-force is not just on the fringes of alternative medicine. It underlies the vast array of "energy medicine," and includes therapeutic touch, Reiki, reflexology, Deepak Chopra's ayurvedic medicine, Larry Dossey's healing words, and hundreds of other therapies. Some proponents even claim that, "No matter what therapies a traditional healer depends upon, he or she essentially is treating the life force itself."[39] Some claim that acupuncture, chiropractic, herbal medicine, and homeopathy also work by influencing this energy, but other practitioners use purely physical concepts to explain how these work.

Since this energy is nonphysical, no instruments can detect and measure it. Instead, humans must train themselves to become more sensitive to it. Meditation, or centering, is needed to enter a state of consciousness where one can detect this energy. Trained practitioners claim they not only sense the energy field, or aura, around a person, but see it in a variety of colors and shapes. Illness can be detected, and health restored, once imbalances or blockages in the field are detected because the fundamental essence of who we are is in our energy field, not our physical body. Many will recognize these beliefs as integral to Eastern mystical religions, or New Age, occult, and vitalistic belief systems. Yet they are growing in acceptance even among health care professionals and Christians.

Part of the reason for this acceptance is the use of postmodern rhetoric and wordplay. Postmodernism had its roots in literary theory,

---

38. Chopra, *Ageless;* Krieger, *Accepting Your Power;* Deborah Cowens, *A Gift for Healing: How to Use Therapeutic Touch* (New York: Crown Trade Paperbacks, 1996).
39. Cowens, p. 20.

becoming popular in reader-centered interpretation. Language is viewed as a field of play, where the meanings of words are stretched and strained to help make the author's point. At times this borders on deception. For example, one therapeutic touch book begins:

> Therapeutic touch is perhaps the first form of health care ever utilized. Every parent since Adam and Eve has used this practice instinctively when he or she has placed a loving hand on a child to reduce discomfort, help heal a wound, or alleviate a fever. Therapeutic touch is the most human of all forms of healing, using the hands to reach out in service to another person in a gesture of peace, balance, and love.[40]

Most would agree with these claims in reference to physical touch, but they are completely irrelevant to therapeutic touch because the latter involves *no physical contact*. What child would be comforted by a "hug" involving no physical contact? In therapeutic touch, contact is only needed between two people's auras (or energy fields). Practitioners sweep their hands over a client's body a few inches *above* the skin. Yet the above rhetorical wordplay connects therapeutic touch with commonly held beliefs about the value of touching, and distracts readers from the true nature of the therapy.

Chopra's book about aging provides another example. He claims that each person is an "ageless, timeless being" who can turn aging off and even reverse aging. He asserts: "If you don't want to grow old, you can choose not to."[41] Yet in a chapter entitled "Learning Not to Age" he states that aging is natural, inevitable, normal, universal, and fatal. The oldest we can expect to live is 115-130 years. What about choosing not to age? Actually, he is not going to help us stop aging, but will instead help us attain old age with the best possible quality of life. He has stretched the meanings of his words, intermingling metaphorical and factual statements. But people are drawn into his ideas by the attractiveness of his more extravagant assertions.

Alternative Medicine's Alternative Religion

People seeking advice on health are being drawn into a new worldview: a new religion. The turn to alternative medicine is as much a religious

---

40. Cowens, p. 1.
41. Chopra, *Ageless*, pp. 48, 82; cf. p. 31; for the following claims, see pp. 57-79.

issue as it is a medical one. Excessive rationalism and materialism have led to an overemphasis on the physical aspects of health and illness in modern medicine, and have also led to a rejection of spirituality and the supernatural in the modern church. But people's spiritual needs remain. They want to sense the reality of God in their lives. These healing techniques offer people a way to tap into divine energies and to use them in tangible ways. Unlike God, however, this energy field makes no moral claims on the person. What is promoted as alternative medicine is actually alternative religion.[42] As one advocate put it, "I got more from mind-body medicine than I bargained for: I got religion."[43]

Although this worldview is completely alien to Christianity, some Christians are attracted to these ideas on the assumption that the energy field is the power of God. Resistance to nonmedical approaches to healing is said to be based on the legacy of medieval church patriarchy and Enlightenment rationalism, not biblical principles.[44] Some Christians claim we should be open to alternative medicine since all healing comes from God.[45] Nothing could be further from the truth.

The Bible describes an intense conflict between legitimate and illegitimate approaches to healing. In the Old Testament, King Ahaziah was condemned for seeking out the god Baal when he was seriously injured (2 Kings 1:2-4). In contrast, King Hezekiah prayed to God when deathly ill and was healed (2 Kings 20; Isa. 38). Pursuing God as the source of healing was very important in ancient Israel since he alone was their healer (Exod. 15:26).

When King Asa developed a serious illness, he was condemned for seeking the aid of physicians instead of God (2 Chron. 16:12). This has led some commentators to conclude that the Bible advocates seeking only divine healing. However, the context is clear that the primary problem was Asa's refusal to turn to God for help. In fact, the physicians referred to here were most likely Gentiles who practiced pagan magical

42. Robert C. Fuller, "The Turn to Alternative Medicine," *Second Opinion* 18 (July 1992), pp. 11-31.

43. Marty Kaplan, "Ambushed by Spirituality," *Time*, 24 June 1996, p. 62.

44. Zach Thomas, *Healing Touch: The Church's Forgotten Language* (Louisville: Westminster/John Knox, 1994); Sara Wuthnow, Letters to the Editor, *Christianity Today*, 8 April 1996, p. 10; the same claim is made from a non-Christian perspective by Mary Chiarella, "The Magic of Nursing: From Witches and Warriors to Workers and Wonderers," *Australian Nursing Journal* 3 (Sept. 1995): 22-44.

45. Sara Wuthnow and Chris Jackson, cited in Joe Maxwell, "Nursing's New Age? Controversial Therapeutic Touch Methods Divide Christian Health-Care Community," *Christianity Today*, 5 Feb. 1996, pp. 96-99; Wuthnow, Letters, p. 10.

healing.[46] Ancient Israel was unusual in that a separate class of physicians did not exist. Neither did the priests practice medicine like people did in the surrounding cultures. One thorough study of healing in ancient Israel concludes, "However, it is likely that the battle for religious purity and monotheism militated against a thriving class of physicians in ancient Israel, given the idolatrous and magical nature of virtually all ancient Near Eastern medicine."[47]

However, Israel did not reject natural means of healing in favor of divine healing. A number of casual references in the Bible show that the Hebrews viewed certain medical practices as normal and religiously neutral, including cleansing, bandaging, and soothing with oil (Isa. 1:5-6) or balm (Jer. 8:22; 46:11; 51:8), and setting fractures (Jer. 6:14; Ezek. 30:21). Physicians were not viewed negatively (Jer. 8:22). If fact, Exodus 21:19 mandates the provision of medical treatment.

In the New Testament, the healing miracles of Jesus were obviously crucial to his authentication. Yet how did he heal? Did he tap into a healing energy field still available today to Christians? A number of authors have claimed that Jesus healed via magical practices very similar to these recent energy-based alternative therapies.[48]

Alternative energy-based therapies use the same principles as those generally believed to constitute magic. While difficult to define, magic is widely viewed as the attempt to manipulate supernatural powers by specified techniques to meet the immediate needs of individuals.[49] Energy medicine practitioners hypothesize the existence of a supernatural force they can manipulate by certain techniques to bring about healing in individuals. It is no wonder that sociologists of religion have long labeled this movement a "resacralizing of medicine," a turn to medical magic.[50]

46. Darrel W. Amundsen and Gary B. Ferngren, "Medicine and Religion: Pre-Christian Antiquity," in *Health/Medicine and the Faith Traditions: An Inquiry into Religion and Medicine*, ed. Martin E. Marty and Kenneth L. Vaux (Philadelphia: Fortress, 1982), pp. 53-92.

47. Brown, p. 53; cf. Amundsen, p. 65.

48. For an excellent review, with a complete bibliography for the claims made in the following two paragraphs, see David E. Aune, "Magic in Early Christianity," in *Aufstieg und Niedergang der römischen Welt*, ed. H. Temporini and W. Hasse (Berlin and New York: Walter De Gruyter, 1980), part 2, vol. 23.2, pp. 1507-57

49. Howard C. Kee, "Magic and Messiah," in *Religion, Science, and Magic: In Concert and In Conflict*, ed. Jacob Neusner, Ernest S. Frerichs, and Paul V. M. Flesher (New York: Oxford University Press, 1989), pp. 121-41.

50. Theodore E. Long, "Religion and Therapeutic Action: From Healing Power to Medical Magic," in *Religion and Religiosity in America: Studies in Honor of Joseph H. Fichter*, ed. Jeffrey K. Hadden and Theodore E. Long (New York: Crossroad, 1983), p. 145.

While the New Testament spends little time addressing magic explicitly (cf. Acts 19:18-19; Gal. 5:20; Rev. 22:15), a number of scholars have concluded that "the accusation that Jesus practised magic is a motif which permeates the gospel tradition" and "that an anti-magic apologetic permeates the gospels."[51] For example, when tempting Jesus, Satan asked him to perform feats common in magical folklore of the time (Matt. 4:1-11; Luke 4:1-13). Jesus' refusal to obey is a rejection of Satan's authority, but also implicitly condemns these magical practices. Also, Jesus was accused of being in league with Beelzebub, which was the equivalent of accusing him of practicing illegitimate magic (Mark 3:22-30). The words reported in the gospels as spoken by demons have many parallels in magical incantations. In effect, these incantations are presented both as illegitimate because of demonic association and as ineffective against the word of Jesus.

Leaders in the early church also frequently addressed illegitimate, magical means of healing. Responding to these issues was very important for the early church because of the existence of the cult of Asclepius, the Greek and Roman god of healing. This cult "was regarded by early Christians as the chief competitor of Christ because of his remarkable similarity in role and teachings to the Great Physician."[52] Few doubted that true healing occurred at his temples. Hence, for example, Augustine (354-430) frequently condemned magic, but distinguished between medicinal and magical purposes for using herbs. On the one hand he approved of Christians taking herbs for stomach pain, but disapproved of wearing them as charms for the same purpose.[53]

Early Christian leaders were accused of harming their disciples by preventing them from visiting physicians. Origen (ca. 184–ca. 253) responded: "But let it be conceded that we do keep away those whom we encourage to become our disciples from other philosopher-physicians."[54] He then condemns a number of physicians who use their position to teach philosophies that contradict Christianity, including physicians teaching reincarnation and the idea that all living beings have the same type of spirit. Clearly, the problem was the philosophy Christians were exposed to when they visited philosopher-physicians. The same remains true today.

---

51. Aune, pp. 1541-42.
52. Amundsen, p. 80.
53. Augustine, *On Christian Doctrine*, 2.45.
54. Origen, *Contra Celsum*, 3.75.

In contrast to magical or energy healing, the healing power of God is not an inanimate supernatural force. It is not an energy field people can use for their own purposes. Instead, we can humbly ask God to grant us healing if that is his will in this instance (James 5:14-16). Christians are not given the means to heal every illness. Jesus told those who questioned the lack of healing miracles that only one of the many hungry widows in ancient Israel was fed miraculously, and of all the lepers only Naaman the Syrian was cured (Luke 4:22-27). Miraculous healing is not an everyday event. But we are promised that God will remain with us and comfort us in our pain and suffering (Rom. 8:35-39). Frequently he does this through other Christians (2 Cor. 1:3-7).

When healing does not occur, we must have faith in the love of God. In these difficult times, we must turn to him and his provisions in this world, but not to spiritual healing from other sources. John Chrysostom (ca. 349-407) lauds a Christian woman for refusing to recite magical incantations and put magical amulets on her sick child.

> For what, even though those things are unavailing, and a mere cheat and mockery, still there were nevertheless those who persuaded her that they do avail: and she chose rather to see her child dead, than to put up with idolatry. . . . For these amulets, though they who make money by them are forever rationalizing about them, and saying, 'we call upon God, and do nothing extraordinary,' and the like; and 'the old woman is a Christian,' says he, 'and one of the faithful'; the thing is idolatry. . . . this is the device of Satan, this is that wiliness of the devil to cloak over the deceit, and to give the deleterious drug in honey. . . . How will not the Greeks laugh? how will they not gibe when we say unto them, 'Great is the virtue of the Cross'; how will they be won, when they see us having recourse to those things, which themselves laugh to scorn?[55]

Christians who use energy medicine should ask themselves this ancient question. Much of energy medicine has clear connections to the occult. For example, Dora Kunz was the President of the Theosophical Society in America when she co-founded therapeutic touch with Dolores Krieger. Theosophy is a syncretistic blend of ancient and occult religions and philosophies and remains an active promoter of therapeutic touch.[56] Earlier theosophical books, along with occult and witchcraft books, describe prac-

55. John Chrysostom, *Homily 8 on Colossians.*
56. Sharon Fish, "Therapeutic Touch: Healing Science or Metaphysical Fraud?" *Journal of Christian Nursing* 13 (Summer 1996): 4-13.

tices identical to therapeutic touch (usually in terms of pranic healing or auric healing).[57] Krieger admits there is a high occult factor in how therapeutic touch works.[58] She recommends divination to obtain insight for practicing it.[59] She has noticed that as her students learn therapeutic touch, "Sensitivity to others as well as personal psychic sensitivity deepens. . . . many who undergo these changes in awareness feel that they can also communicate with and understand other sentient beings, such as trees, birds, animals, as well as human beings."[60] She then describes how a very old maple tree once told her "in lucid terms" how to find a lost dog!

Other practitioners recommend the use of spirit guides.[61] Information about Reiki, an ancient Japanese therapy, is said to be available through channeling.[62] Shamanic medicine is being promoted in some hospitals. Shamans enter altered states of consciousness and "travel" to spiritual realms to gain healing knowledge.[63] One alternative medicine encyclopedia notes that life-force or *prana* "can be harnessed by the individual who sensitizes himself by certain occult practices," including meditation, deep breathing, chanting mantras, advanced visualization and "secret rituals which have been closely guarded secrets of the highest mystery schools on earth . . . and beyond"[64] (ellipsis original).

Such practices reflect the promotion of New Age philosophy in the guise of health care. Health care practitioners who promote these practices

57. Dónal P. O'Mathúna, "The Subtle Allure of Therapeutic Touch," *Journal of Christian Nursing* 15 (Winter 1998): 4-13. Some of the sources cited there are: Yogi Ramacharaka, *The Science of Psychic Healing* (Chicago: Yogi Publication Society, Masonic Temple, 1909); A. E. Powell, *The Etheric Double: The Health Aura of Man* (Wheaton, Ill.: Theosophical Publishing House, 1925); Janet Farrar and Stewart Farrar, *A Witches Bible Compleat* (New York: Magickal Childe Publishing, 1981); Raymond Buckland, *Buckland's Complete Book of Witchcraft* (St. Paul, Minn.: Llewellyn Publications, 1987).

58. Robert Calvert, "Dolores Krieger, Ph.D. and Her Therapeutic Touch," *Massage* 47 (Jan./Feb. 1994): 56-60.

59. Dolores Krieger, *The Therapeutic Touch: How to Use Your Hands to Help or Heal* (Englewood Cliffs, N.J.: Prentice-Hall, 1979), p. 80.

60. Dolores Krieger, *Living the Therapeutic Touch: Healing as a Lifestyle* (New York: Dodd, Mead & Company, 1987), p. 53.

61. Barbara Brennan, *Hands of Light: A Guide to Healing Through the Human Energy Field* (New York: Bantam Books, 1988); Jack Angelo, *Spiritual Healing: Energy Medicine for Today* (Shaftesbury, U.K., and Rockport, Mass.: Element, 1991).

62. Diane Stein, *Essential Reiki: A Complete Guide to an Ancient Healing Art* (Freedom, Calif.: Crossing Press, 1995).

63. Roger Walsh, "The Psychological Health of Shamans: A Reevaluation," *Journal of the American Academy of Religion* 65 (Spring 1997): 101-24.

64. Malcolm Hulke, ed., "Spiritual Healing," in *The Encyclopedia of Alternative Medicine and Self-Help* (New York: Schocken Books, 1979), p. 178.

have crossed the line of providing health care and become proselytizers. While Christians are called to share their faith, they should make it clear when they are sharing their faith as opposed to their health care expertise. New Age therapies not only hide their religious roots, they usually deny having any. However, people with discernment should see through this guise. After surveying the growing popularity of New Age nursing spirituality, Barbara Barnum asks some very pointed questions. "Is the practice of the New Age nurse deceptive? Do patients' weakened conditions simply make them targets of opportunity? If New Age nursing is care of the soul, is it also usurping the field of those perceived to be more prepared for that task, namely, religious priests, ministers, and rabbis? Or is the nurse a representative of a new religion?"[65]

The promotion of these New Age healing methods as part of alternative medicine points back to the problem of an overly broad definition. The field needs to be divided into categories, such as those suggested here. The difficulty with defining alternative medicine should caution us against quickly endorsing or rejecting the whole area. Rather, we must examine each therapy, and the general ideas and beliefs underlying it. As Christians we can welcome and affirm certain aspects of alternative medicine, but we must be cautious about others, and still others we must completely reject.

When rejecting therapies, though, we must be careful not to reject those involved with them. People are searching for spiritual reality. The church has been entrusted with the precious treasure of God's truth to provide them with answers (2 Tim. 2:1-2). Christians need to be people who reveal the reality of God. If we become the sweet aroma of Christ, people will be drawn towards his love, and will receive the healing they need (2 Cor. 2:16). If the church would be the true church, it would provide the true alternative that hurting people need.

The church has at times played this role, and dramatically changed the face of health care. As medical historian Henry Sigerist reminds us, the early church's impact on illness and health should give us a vision for what an authentic Christian church can accomplish.

It remained for Christianity to introduce the most revolutionary and decisive change in the attitude of society toward the sick. Christianity

---

65. Barbara S. Barnum, *Spirituality in Nursing: From Traditional to New Age* (New York: Springer, 1996), p. 81.

came into the world as the religion of healing, as the joyful Gospel of the Redeemer and of Redemption. It addressed itself to the disinherited, to the sick and afflicted and promised them healing, a restoration both spiritual and physical. . . . The social position of the sick man thus became fundamentally different from what it had been before. He assumed a preferential position which has been his ever since.[66]

66. Henry E. Sigerist, *Civilization and Disease* (Chicago: University of Chicago Press, 1943), pp. 69-70.

Conclusion: Change Health Care — A British Point of View

Stuart Horner, M.D., F.R.C.P.

George Bernard Shaw described England and America as two nations divided by a common language. Whatever the political incorrectness of such a quip, it aptly captures the international health care challenge today. As this book illustrates, the problems and concepts are common to the health care systems in the two countries; it is more the language and terminology which divide them. Indeed, most health care systems throughout the world must address exactly the same issues whatever their form of health care delivery. The exponential growth of medical technology in the last thirty-five years means that no country in the world can afford to give to all its patients all the potential benefits which medicine can offer. Some techniques are extremely expensive. We are now able to save, at enormous expense, the lives of premature babies who would have died only a few years ago. As people grow older, so their health problems increase. It is now possible to replace individual joints and transplant many organs. Should this technology be denied because a person has reached the biblical age of three score years and ten? Whilst we may applaud and support the use of such techniques to save the lives of individual elderly people and possibly to welcome a technique which may offer a further twenty years of good quality life, does our beneficence extend to a risky operation on a ninety-five year old, which might increase her quality of life (if she survives) for six further months before her inevitable death?

In the United States health care is bought and sold in a commercial market place, with buyers looking for the cheapest high quality option and vendors anxious to maximize income and profit. Because of the high cost of care, many Americans choose to insure themselves against the risk of medical and financial disaster. The Federal Government has taken tentative steps to ensure health care for certain groups. Medicare provides state help for medical care for the elderly, who can no longer work and are therefore not covered by employment insurance. Medicaid provides some support for some of the poorer categories in American society. Insurance companies are, however, in the business of making profits. Perceived political imperatives demand that expenditure from taxes be controlled. These so-called "third party payers" have come increasingly to dominate the American scene. Little wonder that many health care professionals think that the system is more interested in cost control than in patient care.

These problems are mirrored in the United Kingdom, where the 'third party payer' is the government. The National Health Service grew up in a period of communitarian idealism, which Richard Titmus described as *the gift relationship*.[1] We all give, according to our means, without any immediate expectation of reward. But we give in the expectation that, should disaster cross our path, society will come to our rescue. Titmus explored the specific example of blood transfusion. We voluntarily give blood, with no expectation of immediate reward. If, however, we need blood, we know it will be provided. We will not receive our own blood; that has been used for someone else's needs. We will receive that of some unknown donor, who also responded voluntarily to the needs of others. Significantly Titmus showed, in the case of blood, that "the gift relationship" provided the cheapest, safest, and administratively most efficient method of all. When the NHS began to buy blood products abroad on a commercial basis, disaster struck and many patients with hemophilia paid with their lives. Similarly in the provision of our own National Health Service (NHS) it is generally considered that, until the introduction of the 'internal market,' the NHS was the cheapest, safest and administratively most efficient of all health care systems.

This communitarian spirit broke down in the Thatcher years, as society became more selfish and individuals began to complain about the level of their taxes. In great secrecy, a group of political zealots tried to

1. R. M. Titmus, *The Gift Relationship*. Original edition with new chapters, ed. Ann Oakley and John Ashton (London: LSE Books, 1997).

introduce the commercial concepts of the American market into the British National Health Service. The result was a relentless drive not to maximize profit, but to reduce costs "whilst maintaining quality." Common sense tells us that such mutually opposing objectives must be to some degree contradictory, but the myth is widely believed because it is alleged to be achievable in private industry.[2] The result has been an explosion in administrative costs, a progressive devaluing of the staff, and a widespread perception that money is now more important than patients. As each new piece of research evidence becomes available, it shows that the hoped for beneficial gains have simply not emerged. The health care workers, whose tragedies Peter Bruggen so carefully documents,[3] would instantly recognize the ethical dilemmas faced by Barbara White (see her comments in the Introduction) and the nurses whose experience she records.

Rationing

Nowhere is the dilemma of language more apparent than in the central theme of this book, i.e. rationing. The very word has different meanings on either side of the Atlantic.[4] More right wing writers in the United States claim that a nationalized system of health care is, by definition, "rationing." The restriction of a free market, by the creation of a state-run monopoly, is for them a rationed system. They point to waiting lists, general practitioner "gatekeepers" and the capping of overall expenditure, as clear evidence that a rationing system is in operation. Although it has been alleged that rationing has existed in the National Health Service from the day of its inception, most people in this country believe that rationing is a recent phenomenon. As an editorial in *The Lancet* commented in 1995, "From now on the British public must learn to live without equity, comprehensiveness and universality of health care."[5] It was almost forty years before a secretary of state admitted that the National Health Service could not meet all the needs it was identifying.

2. J. S. Horner, "The Management Myth," *Journal of the Royal College of Physicians of London* 31 (1997), pp. 149-52.

3. P. Bruggen, *Who Cares? True Stories of the NHS Reforms* (Charlbury, Oxfordshire: Jon Carpenter Publishing, 1997).

4. J. M. Humber and R. F. Almeder, eds., "Allocating Health Care Resources," in *Biomedical Ethics Reviews 1994* (New Jersey: Humana Press, 1995).

5. Editorial, *The Lancet* 346 (1995), p. 651.

On the other hand, Europeans gaze on the American system incredulous that the American people do not recognize the rationing in their midst. How can a system, which excludes thirty-seven million Americans from any guaranteed health care provision, be described as anything else but a rationed system? Admittedly the rationing is by price, but rationing none the less. A free market which excludes individuals from participation within it is not only not genuinely free, but is rationing health care by excluding significant numbers of beneficiaries. As Titmus said in relation to blood transfusion, such a system cannot be described as efficient. It is also unjust. Onora O'Neill reminds us that "the core of justice is rejection of principles whose attempted universal adoption would foreseeably injure at least some."[6]

The groups most likely to be excluded from the health care system are the minority communities. The difficulties rehearsed by Frank and Barbara Staggers (pp. 202-13) have clear echoes in the United Kingdom. As the Staggers themselves point out, even where health care is provided free, disparities are still seen. In this country, for more than a decade, the link between social deprivation and ill health was denied. Even when the link could no longer be ignored, the political correctness of the time demanded that we should talk about "variations," rather than "inequalities" in health. Those who live in deprived communities may find it more difficult to access the highest quality of care. The most successful doctors and health care workers are likely to find practice in such areas less congenial than in the prosperous middle class suburbs. Despite praiseworthy exceptions, it should be a standing reproach to Christians that the best known doctor who committed his life to working in such a community[7] was motivated by his political rather than any religious convictions. Christians ought to be identified with such communities and be in the forefront of addressing their problems.

Arthur Dyck (pp. 74-88) defines rationing as the restriction of any procedures which are "medically appropriate, beneficial, and available." Yet surely each of these words is a debate in itself. In the United Kingdom where, as Dyck tells us, individuals over the age of sixty-five have been denied care from which many could benefit, we have begun painfully to disentangle each of these criteria in respect of individual procedures.

---

6. O. O'Neill, *Towards Justice and Virtue: A Constructive Account of Practical Reasoning* (Cambridge: Cambridge University Press, 1996), p. 64.

7. J. Tudor Hart, C. Thomas, B. Gibbons, C. Edwards, M. Hart, J. Jones, M. Jones, and P. Walton, "Twenty five years of case finding and audit in a socially deprived community," *British Medical Journal* 302 (1991), pp. 1509-13.

Abortion is available and may, in certain circumstances, be beneficial: but beneficial for whom — and is it also medically appropriate? Dyck also tells us that, "rationing refers only to the deliberate creation of scarcity." The confusion between American and European writers regarding when such rationing is occurring is evident, since Europeans would argue that in the United States rationing has long been a consequence of the particular approach to health care adopted.

Managed Care

The concept of "managed care" may not be as familiar to non-American readers as to American ones. This does not mean that it does not exist. In America insurance companies are increasingly deciding what is the most appropriate form of care for patients suffering from particular forms of illness. Hospitals, aware of the enormous cost of law suits in the United States, are increasingly demanding that all their staff pursue a particular program of care, so that it can be demonstrated that the appropriate investigations were carried out and the most appropriate treatment given. In other words, the care being provided for the patient is "managed." Although doctors may be involved, either as a group or as individual experts, in advising on the program of care, the final decisions will be made by non–health care staff, who will obviously factor considerations of cost and "risk assessment" into the equations. They may require all doctors to follow a particular program of care in, for example, the acute treatment of a coronary thrombosis.

Massive clinical trials have now been done which show that, on balance, some specific treatments are more effective than others. There is an increasing emphasis on such evidence-based medicine. There are a number of benefits. Investigatory television programs in the United Kingdom have drawn attention to the treatment lottery to which patients with early signs of cancer are exposed. Length of survival may be determined by one's general practitioner, the local specialist, and even the treatment offered at a specialist center. Managed care, which is being seen in the development of cancer services in the United Kingdom, is a response to this kind of unacceptable variability. Similarly, many hospitals now require doctors in training to follow particular protocols when confronted with an acute heart attack in the accident and emergency department. These protocols are based on the treatments which have been shown to be most effective.

There are two major problems with "managing care" on both sides of the Atlantic. The first is the increasing involvement of non-medical staff making decisions for other than strictly medical reasons. The commercialization of our own National Health Service has led to an increase in "risk assessment." This is a cold, objective, financial appraisal of the cheapest option. This may involve taking the risk because it is cheaper to pay compensation for the rare failure which may occur, than to pay for all patients to receive optimum care. Hospitals may decide not to defend a negligence case, since the cost of proving the doctor innocent may be more expensive than paying compensation to the patient. Yet by appearing to admit guilt (whatever legal words are used to avoid this implication), the doctor's reputation may be ruined.

The second problem with managed care is that medicine is still not an exact science. Individual patients sometimes do not benefit from treatment which has been shown to be ideal for a group. Other patients get better without it. For this reason, most doctors on both sides of the Atlantic believe that they must have the discretion to vary the protocol to meet the needs of particular patients. This tension between the needs of "third party payers" for cost control and of health professionals to provide the most appropriate care for the patient now receiving their undivided attention, is a source of many ethical dilemmas, which are well rehearsed in the contributions to this book.

The unusual terminology and the unfamiliar language should not blind the reader into believing that the dilemma is a peculiarly American one. Jeffrey Stout, whilst defending ethical diversity which results from the adoption by individuals of different ethical approaches to their problems, nevertheless concludes that the biggest threat to ethical values is the commercial market.[8] We must be constantly on our guard to ensure that its subtle demands do not erode our human values. The most important values in health care cannot be counted or measured. What is the financial value of feeding a frail, lonely old lady with a cup of water, compared with the cheaper financial cost of letting her do it for herself. What value should we place on the nurse sitting with a dying patient, gently squeezing her hand? What price should we attach to doctors spending time talking to their patients and ensuring that they fully understand what is being said, when the managed care protocol has factored in a shorter time for the medical consultation? Do health care

8. J. Stout, *Ethics After Babel: The Languages of Morals and Their Discontents* (Cambridge: James Clarke & Co. Ltd., 1988).

workers follow the system, or follow their ethical values? How can Christians reconcile their work within such a health care system with the injunction of the Master, *in as much as you have done it to one of the least of these my brethren, you have done it unto me.*[9] The dilemma is just as relevant in the United Kingdom as it is in the United States.

A major difficulty of managed care is the emphasis that it gives to economic appraisal and risk assessment. Faced with a patient who requires highly expensive long-term nursing and rehabilitative care, with no certainty that the ultimate outcome will not be death, a cold economic appraisal would suggest that it is in everyone's interests for the patient's life to be brought to a speedy end. Managed care carries within it the potential for managed death. Already there is evidence of ethical failure, with less access to required services for those on Medicaid and for the uninsured. The debate on both sides of the Atlantic about the active killing of patients has an important economic dimension. It also violates the principle of justice. There is convincing evidence that a disproportionate number of poor people are likely to be recipients of a premature death at the hands of their physicians, even though the debate itself is conducted by a vociferous minority of middle class enthusiasts concerned only about their own "rights." This concern is buttressed by indications that increasing reliance on managed care for the poor means more bed-days per year due to bad health for them as well as more serious symptoms and a greater risk of dying.[10]

Nurse Patricia Benner (pp. 119-35) adds the concern that managed care challenges the nursing tradition of caring for and meeting people in their suffering and vulnerability. Her wise words need little translation to the scene in the United Kingdom or elsewhere. She shows the way in which the move from hospital care to community care effectively insulates health care workers and their patients from one another and from the remote bureaucracy which finances care. Avoidance and neglect are very human temptations in the face of suffering. Her conclusion, that financial incentives in the health care system which seem to encourage that neglect must be resisted, is surely a sentiment to endorse. Compassionate strangers are needed to care for our vulnerability in situations where the support of close family and friends is not enough. When we read the New

---

9. Matthew 25:40 (A.V.).

10. J. E. J. Ware, R. H. Brook, W. H. Rogers, E. B. Keeler, A. R. Davies, C. D. Sherbourne, G. A. Goldberg, P. Camp, and J. P. Newhouse, "Comparison of health outcomes at a health maintenance organization with those of fee for service care," *The Lancet* 1 (1986), pp. 1017-22.

Testament parable, many of us identify with the Good Samaritan and hope he will be our example. Perhaps we should also identify with the vulnerable victim and reject a market model of health care which marginalizes the care ethic. In the present volume's Introduction, vulnerable patient Harold Brown gives a moving account of the attempts by a variety of doctors to limit the cost of his care within a health maintenance organization. The result was a failed diagnosis and near fatal outcome. There are, however, also British examples of patients who nearly died because they were overlooked on the waiting list. Indeed, it is now generally accepted that the market style NHS actually resulted in the deaths of some patients, whilst responsibility for their entitlement to care was being identified. As Patricia Benner concludes, this is deadly moralism. However, we must also always remember that no health care system can exclude the possibility of a missed diagnosis.

Radical Solutions

Arthur Dyck claims that "medical needs are not infinite" and that a rich country like America should be willing to invest more in health care. Although I doubt that any country can now afford to provide all available medical techniques for all its citizens, it is a valid comment to argue that any particular country should invest more in its health care system. The British Medical Association has consistently argued that greater investment is needed in our own National Health Service, irrespective of the problems resulting from a failure of the policies of the Conservative Government. At first sight, proposals to increase investment in the American health care system do not seem to be particularly radical. I would argue, however, that radical overhaul of that system is essential, before more money is invested in it. In America the health care system, like a number of other American institutions, simply does not work. Like the welfare state in the United Kingdom, more and more money is being spent for less and less return. For example, after 37 years of the most severe trade embargo in the world and with malnutrition of pregnant women documented by American physicians, Cuba still has an infant mortality half that of Washington, D.C.[11] Only radical changes in the American health care system and also in the British welfare state will justify a greater investment of resources. In this

11. C. Chelela, "Cuba shows health gains despite embargo," *British Medical Journal* 316 (1998), p. 497.

context, therefore, proposals to invest more resources are extremely radical and, of course, highly political. They involve increasing the overall burden of taxation and require hard choices between different programs of government expenditure.

James Hussey (pp. 227-34) describes a health maintenance organization which began in December 1994 and provides care based on biblical principles. It accepts those on Medicaid and some who are uninsured. In little more than two years, 150,000 patients have been recruited and all have access to treatment, regardless of their ability to pay. His four *Physicians Quality Care* principles constitute excellent advice to health care workers in the British National Health Service. His emphasis on building round the church, but nevertheless engaging the entire community, together with his emphasis on thorough preliminary planning, will hopefully prevent ill considered attempts to copy such a radical initiative.

Alieta Eck (pp. 235-44) is even more radical. She proposes that Christians should band together in their own financial gift relationship, each contributing on a regular basis according to their means, in the certain knowledge that, should the need arise, even the most expensive costs of necessary medical care will be met. The concept is less easily translated into the United Kingdom, but the proposal contains a most important message for Christians. The church in the West has often seemed impotent in the face of poverty, rampant global capitalism, and, in America, the crippling costs of health care which can reduce families to destitution. The Christian church has been in the forefront of many initiatives concerned with ameliorating the results of poverty and there have been initiatives in the Third World, such as Traidcraft, which are designed to help subsistence farmers and low cost producers to escape from the poverty trap into which global capitalism consigns them. Nevertheless, the Western church has been reluctant to face the causes of these problems head on and to adopt alternative, radical strategies to overcome them. Indeed we often seem resigned to their inevitability and apparently supportive of free choices and market forces. Many Christians have argued that we have no business being involved in political and social issues at all, but must instead concentrate exclusively on the proclamation of the Gospel. It is, however, difficult to reconcile such attitudes with the words of the Old Testament prophets and the teaching of Jesus.[12] Both gave overwhelming priority to the needs of the

---

12. U. Duchrow, *Alternatives to Global Capitalism: Drawn from Biblical History Designed for Political Action* (Utrecht, Holland: International Books with Kairos Europa 1995).

poor, ground down by the prevailing social system. Can we stand idly by, whilst the elderly die in poverty and the homeless roam our streets? Can American Christians stand idly by while the cost of health care and its burgeoning administrative costs and profits spirals steadily out of reach of increasing numbers of its citizens — like a child's balloon, inadvertently released from its moorings, because no one was sufficiently attentive to what was going on?

The Primary Care Physician

It has long been argued that the great strength of the British system is the general practitioner, who acts as a "gatekeeper" to specialist services. By their proficiency in limiting tests and referrals for specialist care, general practitioners are able to control health care costs. This restrictive gatekeeping lay behind the Conservative Government's concept of budget holding, which has subsequently been shown to have been an expensive failure, as well as unjust to patients. However, political imperatives have demanded that the new Labor Government retains a central role for 'gatekeeping' in controlling health care costs.[13] Gregory Rutecki (pp. 136-44) challenges this assumption. In America health maintenance organizations are growing rapidly. These provide health care very like that in the United Kingdom model. In particular, they enhance the role of a primary physician. Rutecki argues that in some situations at least, specialist care can be both cheaper and more effective. Reference has already been made to the lottery of cancer care in the United Kingdom. Protocols are being drawn up by specialists for general application amongst general practitioners for heart disease, lung disease, and a range of childhood cancers. Rutecki emphasizes that the Christian physician must take account of the needs of the wider community in developing a covenant relationship with individual patients. He also challenges Christian specialists to follow the practice of earlier generations of doctors, who reduced charges to poorer patients and accepted a responsibility to treat others free of charge.

Similarly, Sondra Wheeler (pp. 63-73) provides a timely warning about an overemphasis on the personal relationship between doctor and patient, which so many others stress as a healthy counterbalance to the insistent demands of "third party payers." Wheeler points out that the

13. Department of Health, *The New NHS*, Cm 3807 (London: HMSO, 1997).

Bible emphasizes the role of society, as well as stressing provision for the poor and needy. The Christian physician cannot ignore the needs of the whole of society by an overemphasis on the individual patient. Money spent on this patient cannot be spent on that patient, or upon the patient who has not yet reached the doctor's consulting room door. Christian justice means that every person has claims against attack, claims to fair treatment, and claims to an equitable share of resources. She argues that we must distinguish between strictly medical and non-medical criteria for treatment and for scarce resources.

Similarities at the Micro Level

It is not just in the broad sweep of health care economics that issues in contemporary U.S. health care resonate with the situation in the United Kingdom. Reference has already been made to Barbara White's excellent paper about the growing pressures on nursing ethics. Her problems of skill mix, unlicensed aides, restructuring and "down sizing," job security, and job stability will be familiar to any nurse manager in the United Kingdom. Indeed she gives a disturbing picture of likely trends in the National Health Service unless they are reversed. The relentless pursuit of so called "efficiency savings," which are little more than a disguised budgetary cut; the apparently never ending organizational restructuring, which destroys the organization's collective memory, as well as damaging staff morale; and the introduction of the private financing initiative, which is storing up truly horrendous problems for the next generation, are issues which must be addressed in the United Kingdom, just as much as in the United States. The traditional role of the nurse as the patient's advocate is slowly and relentlessly giving way to the new role of responsible steward of the resources allocated.

Judith Shelly (pp. 45-62) gives an insightful historical account of the development of the nursing profession, its secularization, and its progressive independence from medicine. Nurses are now being employed as case managers, with control over doctors' clinical decisions. Bedside nursing is being given by the least well educated and the least well trained nurses, whilst the most skilled nurses are being given ever more detailed managerial roles. Shelly believes that the standards are falling because of the emphasis on cost control, and that there is a need to awaken the church to a mission of healing. Although she is describing the American system, all of these concerns are equally reflected by nurses working within the

National Health Service. Her radical call back to true vocational nursing will surely be welcomed. Nevertheless, her suggestion that Christian nurses might work extra shifts and spend their own money on patients, whilst laudable, runs the risk of perpetuating the abuse of the goodwill of the staff on which the National Health Service has relied so much and which the internal market has wastefully frittered away over the last seven years.

Richard Olson's description of managed long-term care (pp. 192-201) seems initially difficult to translate into the United Kingdom scene. Yet we too have problems with long term care, to which short term solutions have been applied, with little thought for their more distant implications. The 1980s witnessed the privatization of old people's care in this country. Thousands of elderly people were decanted from our hospitals into nursing homes, initially funded by the National Health Service. As the hospital beds disappeared, new patients had no choice but to enter the nursing homes direct. It should surprise no one that, as in the United States, concerns are being expressed about the quality of care available to the residents. There is a vast difference between a nursing auxiliary working in a team of qualified nursing staff in a hospital setting, and a nursing aide working in a nursing home, with minimal supervision from a nursing qualified matron. Moreover, with the transfer of responsibility for long stay patients from the National Health Service to local authorities, the specter of the "means test" has reappeared, with elderly people required to spend their savings and sell the property they had so self-denyingly built up as an inheritance for their children.

It would be unfortunate if Christians were thought to be resisting change. The book's Introduction closes with William Atkinson providing a timely reminder of the need to adapt to change. Whilst the changes required in the health care system in the United Kingdom differ from those in the United States, the fact of change is no less dramatic. Atkinson urges Christians to be involved and to take a longer view. His emphasis on the need to put ethics first and economics second, will find resonance among the staff he manages. He also emphasizes the need for planning and integration, which have been so neglected in the National Health Service in the last few years and which are making a welcome reappearance under the new Government's proposals.[14] The essential message of a hospital chief executive, that Christians must actively influence the system, find alternatives to the prevailing ethos of health care manage-

14. Ibid.

ment, and resist hostile developments, has never been more needed. We have entered a vicious spiral in the West, where utilitarian philosophies, emphasizing the greatest good for the greatest number, are dominating our approach to health care. There are other ethical philosophies which are more distinctly Christian. The pursuit of virtue, an emphasis on justice, the pursuit of the patient's good, and the avoidance of anything that might harm, need to be woven across the inherent conflict between the rights of the individual (autonomy) and the requirements of a broader collective society.[15] Arthur Dyck brings out very clearly the dangers of utilitarianism with which health care systems on both sides of the Atlantic currently seem to be obsessed. His analogy between our current attitudes and those of ancient Greece prior to the advent of Hippocrates, is very apt. Even Hippocrates was critical of the medical market of his day.[16] The later Oath, which bears his name, almost certainly reflects a minority strand of Greek thought, opposed to the social mores of the day.[17]

While many Christians today are very wary about the shift toward managed care, several essays in the present volume show that a more collaborative posture is possible. William Atkinson emphasizes that change is essential in all organizations and within the health care system, inevitable. All will welcome his emphasis on the ethics of health care. Similarly, in the United Kingdom the Institute of Health Service Management produced a briefing paper in 1993 on *Values and the NHS*.[18] Even more recently, the *British Medical Journal* has argued for a single ethical code common to everybody in health care, commenting that "Statements of ethics that pit one stakeholder against another, as when doctors claim to protect patients against management's assaults, will deepen divisions and stall collaborative thinking."[19] The problem is how such noble ideals can be put into practice. Certainly this will not be done from the outside and Atkinson's plea for health care professionals to

15. J. S. Horner, "Ethics and the Public Health," in *Ethical Issues in Community Health Care*, ed. R. Chadwick and M. Levitt (London: Arnold, 1997).

16. Chadwick and Mann, *Hippocratic Writings*, ed. G. E. R. Lloyd, Penguin Classics (Harmondsworth: Penguin Books, Ltd, 1978).

17. P. Carrick, *Medical Ethics in Antiquity* (Dordrecht, Holland: D. Reidel Publishing Co., 1985); E. D. Pellegrino, "The Metamorphosis of Medical Ethics: A Thirty Year Perspective," *Journal of the American Medical Association* 269 (1993), pp. 1158-62.

18. A. Wall, *Future Health Care Options. Values and the NHS*. A Briefing Paper of the Institute of Health Service Management. University of Birmingham, Health Services Management Centre (1993).

19. D. Berwick, H. Hiatt, P. Janeway, and R. Smith, "An Ethical Code for Everybody in Health Care," *British Medical Journal* 315 (1997), pp. 1633-34.

become involved on the inside is very welcome. Similarly, no one could seriously disagree with Kenman Wong (pp. 145-61) that business ethics can help an organization to clarify its true objectives. He is right to point out that doctors have often placed self-interest before ethics. How else does one explain the astonishingly high surgical intervention rates in North America,[20] compared with western Europe? (Incidentally, American writers would argue that this further proves that rationing exists in western Europe.) Nevertheless, a somewhat different perspective is possible here, for expenditure on "good causes" espoused by the organization are not entirely altruistic. As the trend to so-called ethical investment in the United Kingdom shows, the pursuit of higher ethical ideals is also good business. Companies may well decide that even large expenditures can be justified by the improved customer loyalty achieved in the marketplace. Moreover, while few, if any, commercial mission statements include a wish to maximize profits, it is naive to assume that this is therefore relegated to a minor objective. Profit or, in the National Health Service, "return on investment," is essential to the survival of commercially run enterprises. Although business ethics must be inherently a good thing, the difficulty occurs when it conflicts with other objectives of the organization. More than ten years ago two Canadian academics pointed out that "today's health care managers find themselves drifting between idealism and pragmatism, outwardly committed to a human service ideal yet conditioned by a survival mentality to favor the bottom line of financial well-being."[21] As the British Government has found with its new ethical foreign policy, when objectives collide it is most unusual for the ethical imperative to prevail.

Between these two extreme positions (the radicals and the collaborators) are the pragmatists and the philosophers. Managed care was primarily conceived to address problems in the acute health care market. It translates less readily to care for the elderly and for the psychiatrically disturbed. Richard Olson's description of care for the elderly in America has its close parallels in the United Kingdom. Here, too, the decline in quality is palpable and the problems of "community care" in the United Kingdom need no further rehearsal. Stephen Greggo (pp. 177-91) describes twelve risks in the managed care programs for mental health problems.

20. J. C. D. Plant, I. Percy, T. Bates, J. Gastard, and Y. Hita de Nercy, "Incidence of Gallbladder Disease in Canada, England and France," *The Lancet* 2 (1973), pp. 249-51.

21. Levey and Hill, "Between Survival and Social Responsibility: In Search of an Ethical Balance," *Journal of Health Administration Education* (Spring 1986), pp. 225-31.

Although not precisely similar to those in the United Kingdom, the concerns about confidentiality, early discharge, use of standardized treatment plans, the emphasis on restoration to baseline functioning at the expense of addressing long term issues, and the general pressures of insufficient time, are all familiar to psychiatrists in this country. Indeed, our problem is that the particular managed care program imposed on psychiatry in the NHS has been shown unequivocally to have failed. Sadly there are no plans to change it.

Scott Daniels (pp. 91-102) believes that financial incentives are not necessarily bad: "There is no universal agreement among researchers or ethicists that financial incentives negatively impact the quality [of care]." In this country whilst general practitioner fundholding does not have direct benefit for the doctor, it does create indirect benefits which are intended to change practice behavior by reducing the drug budget, as well as investigation and referral rates. Moreover, at the outset of the new system there were persistent reports of patients with greater health needs being excluded from practice lists.

In the book's first chapter, meanwhile, Nigel Cameron worries that the medical profession is being turned into a consumerist-corporatist exercise in the delivery of saleable skills to the market. He urges Christians not to withdraw, but to become dissidents within the system, in the same way that Christians opposed the system in the former USSR. Health care professionals may have problems with this approach, especially in view of "gagging clauses," which restrict the ability of employees to speak out against unsafe practices. Such clauses have recently been outlawed in the United Kingdom.

Edmund Pellegrino (pp. 103-18) is equally critical of the ideology and ethos of the commercial model. As he points out, it "has no place for the vulnerable, the marginalized, the poor, the persons who have neglected their health, the uninformed, or the uneducated." The Good Samaritan did not withhold care in the belief that an even more deserving case might lie round the next bend in the road. Pellegrino specifically rejects "disenrolling patients and physicians who cost too much" and the redefinition of medical necessity. Both have occurred in the National Health Service. His comment that "physician administrators . . . are soon engulfed by the system itself" would resonate with the similar experience of medical directors working in hospital trusts in this country. In addition, Pellegrino, too, urges health care workers to resist and to protest. He points out that we cannot avoid complicity if we participate and, like many of the authors here, emphasizes the need for evidence-based medicine, the reduction of administrative costs, and perhaps even the need for increased insurance payments, i.e. higher taxes in the NHS context. Health care professionals need these timely reminders of the dangers of complicity with the system. As Jeremy Lee-Potter, former chairman of Council at the British Medical Association, writes in his book *A Damn Bad Business: The NHS Deformed:* "it may seem a far cry from the NHS trust surgeon instructed to operate on GP fundholders' patients first irrespective of clinical priority, to the Iraqi doctor ordered to amputate a hand under shariah law, or a psychiatrist in the old Soviet Union forced to certify and treat a dissident as mentally ill because of his political opposition. But the slope is a slippery one and any system which tolerates such faltering first steps must be rejected."[22]

Although medical litigation is a particularly United States phenomenon, non-American readers would do well to reflect on the analysis of Janet Michael, a lawyer (pp. 214-24). She shows that managed care is fraught with legal as well as ethical dangers. The piece also provides a timely warning of the trends likely to engulf the National Health Service. In this country we have already seen that the public is less ready to forgive the mistakes of privatized companies, even for events outside their control, such as the impact of adverse weather on water supplies, power supplies, and the late running of trains. It is therefore no surprise to learn that plaintiffs in the United States are less ready to give health maintenance organizations the benefit of the doubt. The evidence seems to suggest that this is already happening in the National Health Service.

Another sign of dissatisfaction with the medical care available in the National Health Service, and indeed with health care generally, is the growth of "alternative medicine." Dónal O'Mathúna (pp. 258-79) identifies a wide range of alternative methods of treatment in the United States. He sees it as part of a wider rejection of paternalistic style medicine in favor of partnership in the healing process, which tends to characterize these alternative therapies. There are dangers, however. Many alternative therapies derive their authority from postmodernism, which rejects absolute truth and stresses a variety of value systems. There are "multiple realities." Criticism of alternative therapy by conventional practitioners simply results in a "dialogue of the deaf" between those who distrust objective evidence while embracing ethical relativism and those who affirm the former and reject the latter. The author believes that many

---

22. J. Lee-Potter, *A Damn Bad Business: The NHS Deformed* (London: Victor Gollancz, 1997), p. 243.

alternative therapies border on the use of magic and are founded on New Age beliefs. The church should provide the true alternative medicine by revealing the reality of God and the implications of that reality for effective health care.

If the church cannot meet this challenge, the declining importance ascribed to human life observed by Robert Orr (pp. 162-73) may well continue. There has been much debate in this country about whether doctors should swear an ethical oath, and an attempt to find an all inclusive oath by the British Medical Association seems to have been finally abandoned. It is interesting therefore that oath taking in medical schools in the United States has increased almost fourfold in the last sixty-five years and is now virtually universal. However, only 14 percent of those oaths prohibit euthanasia; only 8 percent forswear abortion; and only 3 percent exclude sexual relationships with patients. This declining emphasis on the protection of human life and vulnerable patients is not peculiar to the United States.

Options for the Future

At many points, then, changes underway in the U.S. health care system are fundamentally similar to the changes which have occurred in the U.K.'s National Health Service during the current decade. In spite of the different language, the problems are much the same. Accordingly, some concluding reflections are in order as to the four types of response appropriate for people today, whatever their geographical location.

Active support. People must first do the difficult analysis required to determine if the newer approaches to health care today are truly harmful or if they represent a reasonable (though imperfect) response to other imperfect approaches that are even more harmful. If the latter is the case, people may actively support the newer forms. But the reasons for such support may be different. People may simply be narrowly viewing the current situation from a "medical ethics" rather than also from a "business ethics" perspective, or they may always consider it their duty to support whatever the government commends as the best approach. Both of these reasons for active support must be held up to critical scrutiny.

Passive support. Another possible response — but one not appropriate for Christians — is to "pass by on the other side."[23] Some health

23. Luke 10:31.

care professionals would argue that they have other priorities, either in mission or in teaching within their local church. Social involvement is somehow seen as non-Christian.

This attitude has very specifically been rejected in this volume. Author after author has urged Christians to become actively involved. This is not necessarily an appeal for overtly political involvement. Rather it is a call for Christians to understand and debate the issues. As Alastair Campbell, Professor in Medical Ethics at Bristol University, has pointed out, health care professionals can play a prophetic role within the society which authorizes them to practice.[24] There has been a considerable amount of mostly inconclusive debate about health rationing in the United States, the United Kingdom, and other countries of the world. Yet the Christian church has been significantly absent from these debates, as it has been largely silent about the priorities which should be adopted within the health care system. Christians have many important insights to contribute — the importance of caring for the poor and doing so in a way that enables rather than disables them is only one example.

Christian health care workers also need to become actively involved in resource allocation decision-making by accepting management responsibilities and experiencing for themselves the conflicting pressures that many of their colleagues already have to bear. Christian communities need to support them in prayer and in other practical ways such as stress counseling. Managed care organizations and various health authorities have tried to restrict the hospitals to which local general practitioners have access; to control high cost treatments; and to restrict or exclude treatment for particular conditions or particular groups of patients. Again, Christians need to seek positions with these bodies and in the governmental structures that oversee them, not out of a vague sense of being involved in charitable activities but to bring the Master where he belongs right in the center of the decision-making process.

Passive objection. Once people genuinely understand the system, they may discover that a less supportive type of response is necessary. Many caregivers are recognizing that some of the recent changes in health care represent not merely different approaches but an assault on important ethical commitments. In their care for patients, such caregivers may expend time and other resources of which the system disapproves. They may speak out at every opportunity, warning colleagues of the dangers

---

24. A. V. Campbell, *Moderated Love: A Theology of Professional Care* (London: SPCK, 1984).

that they perceive. They may use every democratic right offered to them to resist any proposals they find unacceptable. Nigel Cameron has described them here as "dissidents." As with Christians facing communist tyranny, their opposition may at times have to be conducted secretly. Like groups of Christians holding services in the east European forests, their discussions may take place with small groups of like-minded colleagues. Their opportunities for more open dissent may be extremely limited. Sometimes they are restricted by so-called "gagging clauses." Health care "elder statesmen" and "elder stateswomen" who have retired from active practice but not from active professional involvement can add their authority and prestige to criticism of the dangers inherent in the emerging system,[25] though their wisdom will remind them to critique the shortcomings of previous systems as well.

Active objection. Some people of all ages will be so ethically uncomfortable with the system that they are prepared to withdraw from it completely, as in the case of Alieta Eck and her family. Others who are deeply moved by the wrongs in the system will have the opportunity and courage to "blow the whistle" on those wrongs, often at the cost of their jobs or at an even greater cost. Relatively few are willing or able to walk this path, but those who do provide a great service whether or not they immediately right the wrongs. Martyrs in health care, as in life generally, are a tremendous encouragement to others who gain from them the inspiration to fight their own lesser battles.

People will differ in their responses to the changing face of health care, but respond we must. We cannot in good conscience "pass by on the other side." It is the fervent hope of this book's authors and editors that the writings found here will help motivate many to understand today's changes and will help equip them to reform the bad and affirm the good.

---

25. Sir Douglas Black, "A View on the NHS Reforms," *Journal of the Royal College of Physicians of London* 30 (1995), pp. 442-45.

Glossary

Managed Care
integrates the financing and delivery of medical care. Managed Care Organizations (MCOs):
- contract with physicians and hospitals
- negotiate utilization and quality controls
- offer financial incentives to use their facilities
- share financial risk and benefit with physicians

Accreditation
managed care organizations pay accreditors to assess and certify their quality, service, and facilities.

Adverse Selection
enrolling a higher percentage of high-risk members (i.e., high risk for high cost) than exist in the general community.

Any Willing Provider
AWP laws are hotly debated and usually require MCOs to accept any provider (physician, nurse practitioner, pharmacist, or chiropractor) who meets the plan's terms and conditions.

This glossary contains material adapted from *The McGraw-Hill Pocket Guide to Managed Care*, ed. John La Puma and David Schiedermayer (New York: McGraw-Hill Healthcare Management, 1996).

Basic Benefit Package
- primary care/ambulatory medicine services
- pregnancy care
- well child visits
- outpatient surgery
- limited inpatient medical or surgical treatment
- limited organ transplantation
- limited formulary medications
- limited mental health services

Capitation
a flat "fee per head per time."

Carve-outs
services excluded from capitation agreements, and not provided by the managed care plan.

Compensation
at least half of HMOs pay physicians using capitation, and most use withhold accounts, some placing the individual physician at risk. A smaller percentage of HMOs use discounted fee-for-service.

Concurrent Review
factors evaluated include:
- appropriateness of care
- anticipated length of stay
- discharge planning

Consumer Input
consumer complaints such as those voiced about the substitution of a less expensive drug (e.g., one antihypertensive for another) can result in:
- changes in the formulary (approved pharmacy list)
- changes in the information provided to consumers about the formulary
- particular physicians to be included on provider panels

Cost-containment
an approach to health care that seeks to reduce expenditures. Quality is generally assumed to be high but not optimal before costs are contained;

as the process of cost-containment proceeds, quality measures such as early re-admission and readiness for discharge are usually evaluated.

Cost-effectiveness

defined as a benefit to the patient divided by the cost; a minimal cost-benefit ratio in clinical cases, where benefit is defined beforehand.

Credentialling

utilization patterns, quality of care, service-orientation, and professional liability claims history are all part of the MCO credentialling process.

Credentialling, Economic

while generalized and explicit economic credentialling seems unlikely, as the concept is so unpopular among physicians, MCOs and hospitals often attempt to evaluate physician financial performance, and make it part of the feedback and planning process.

De-selection

managed care slang for being fired.

ERISA (Employee Retirement Income Security Act)

ERISA is federal law which is supposed to protect patients by pre-empting state laws that regulate or tax employee benefits provided by employers.

Fee-for-service Insurance

allows for payment based on cost per service rendered; it is the same as indemnity insurance. Many indemnity insurers (e.g., Blue Cross/Blue Shield) now use managed care techniques — pre-admission certification, concurrent review, and second surgical opinion.

HMO

An HMO (health maintenance organization) is an organized system of health care which provides a defined, comprehensive set of services to a defined population for a fixed, periodic per person fee.

Group Model HMO

a single multi-specialty group of physicians that contracts with the HMO. The HMO pays the group a set amount per patient to provide the services defined. Physicians own the group.

301

Staff Model HMO

a multi-specialty group practice owned by the HMO. Staff model HMOs often own their own pharmacies and hospitals. Physicians see only the HMO's patients.

Mixed Model HMO

has features of several different types of HMOs. No particular model form predominates in the mix. Fastest growing type of HMO.

Information Systems

information systems will attempt to create a lifetime record to which multiple caregivers can contribute. Real-time tracking and integrated care will be clinical goals; concurrent outcome analysis, cost-effectiveness analysis, and resource allocation tracking will be administrative goals.

Integrated Delivery Systems

vertical integration can provide care at several different levels: outpatient, inpatient, home, and long-term care.

Independent Practice Association (IPA)

an association of independent practices which have affiliated to negotiate with payers to provide medical services.

Medical Director

an executive, often with specialized training in administration or management, given responsibilities in the MCO for utilization management, quality improvement, coverage approval, and sometimes, physician recruitment and compensation.

Medically Necessary

payer's term for whether a test or treatment is or was truly needed (according to, for example, an expert panel review).

Milliman Guidelines

Milliman and Robertson is a consulting firm that writes and updates practice standards and guidelines. The guidelines focus on reducing "unnecessary" hospital admissions, services, and days.

Networks

exclusive networks restrict physicians' ability to contract independently with other plans, while nonexclusive networks do not restrict independent contracts.

Outcomes Assessment
outcomes can include survival, physical and emotional health, and patient satisfaction.

Patient Satisfaction
four factors explain most differences between physicians in patient satisfaction:
- personalness of care
- sensitivity to concerns
- promptness of follow up
- frequency of "on time" for appointments

Peer Review Program
the key elements of peer review:
- the review process is confidential
- the subject is practice matters (incidents, profiles, guidelines)
- the reviewers are physician peers
- physicians give permission for their evaluation
- permission is granted to contact third parties involved in the case
- there is a fair hearing and due process plan

reports of action are confidential; the goals of peer review are to:
- improve the quality of care
- maintain accountability
- decrease the incidence of malpractice suits
- minimize the external micromanagement

Physician Hospital Organization (PHO)
exclusive contracts between a hospital and a large medical group can circumvent economic credentialling, as only physicians who belong to the group can practice at that hospital. Many hospital-based groups, e.g., radiologists, anesthesiologists, and pathologists, have found this concept helpful.

Physician Profiling
aggregate data that describe particular clinical and financial characteristics of physician-practice patterns over time.

Point of Service Option

in exchange for a higher premium, enrollees can receive care from a provider outside the MCO.

Preferred Provider Organization (PPO)

a PPO is a network or panel of service providers, such as hospitals and physicians, that PPO members must use in order to have a certain level of services covered financially.

Primary Care Medical Services

features of primary care include general medical care, case synthesis, "whole person" medicine, accessibility, availability, and continuity, but these are not exclusive to primary care.

Report Cards

MCOs and other payers will grade and publicize physician performance, and compare it with that of other physicians in the service area and with nationwide standards. MCO report cards will be probably based on the HEDIS (Health Plan Employer Data and Information Set). Examples of HEDIS report card categories are rates of:
- vaccinations
- diabetic retinal exams
- mammograms
- pap smears
- C-sections
- hospitalizations for asthmatics and diabetics mortality

Risk Management

risk managers prevent or minimize potential loss and liability to the MCO. They also manage claims against the MCO.

Service Area

a service area is the population-based area for which a particular MCO is the direct provider.

Social Mission

providing ethical managed care entails social obligations:
- to assure competent medical care
- to make care accessible to people
- to make prudent use of resources available

Subspecialist Medical Services
subspecialists' cognitive expertise is needed in managed care, as are their technological skills. Subspecialists may have to promote themselves to payers by carefully and deliberately explaining their expertise, displaying patient success stories, and highlighting their efficiency in difficult cases.

Tax Status
MCOs and medical groups are either for-profit or not-for-profit.

Total Quality Management (TQM)
Synonym: continuous quality improvement (CQI). A management philosophy based on the concept that medical practice is an integrated system of processes, and that prospectively and continuously assessing processes and outcomes of care can improve them.

Withholds
MCOs withhold money from physicians as an incentive for efficient care. Withholds are to be paid back in part or in whole if the plan's utilization standards, such as length-of-stay targets, quality indicators, or per member costs are met.

Index